Shin Gi Tai

Shin Gi Tai

KARATE TRAINING FOR BODY, MIND, AND SPIRIT

MICHAEL CLARKE

YMAA Publication Center
Wolfeboro, N.H., USA

YMAA Publication Center
Main Office: PO Box 480
Wolfeboro, NH 03894
1-800-669-8892 • www.ymaa.com • info@ymaa.com

ISBN-13: 9781594392177 (print edition) • 9781594392450 (ebook edition)
ISBN-10:159439217x (print edition) • 1594392455 (ebook edition)

Cover design by Axie Breen
Edited by Dolores Sparrow

POD 1216

Publisher's Cataloging in Publication

Clarke, Michael, 1955-

    Shin gi tai : karate training for body, mind, and spirit / Michael
Clarke. -- Wolfeboro, N.H. : YMAA Publication Center, c2011.

      p. ; cm.

      ISBN: 978-1-59439-217-7 (print) ; 978-1-59439-245-0 (ebook)
      "Traditional karate's philosophy and fighting techniques
revealed"--Cover.
      Includes bibliographical references and index.

      1. Karate--Training. 2. Karate--Psychological aspects. 3. Martial
arts--Training. 4. Martial artists. I. Title.

GV1114.3 .C534 2011   2011934943
796.815/3--dc23   2011

Disclaimer: The author and publisher of this book will not be held responsible in any way for any injury of any nature whatsoever, which may occur to readers, or others, as a direct or indirect result of the information and instructions contained within this book. Anyone unfamiliar with the karate techniques or exercises shown should exercise great care. Traditional karate training is not recommended for people under the age of fourteen. If any doubts exist in regard to your health, consult a doctor before commencing. Always practice karate under the supervision of a qualified teacher.

Printed in USA.

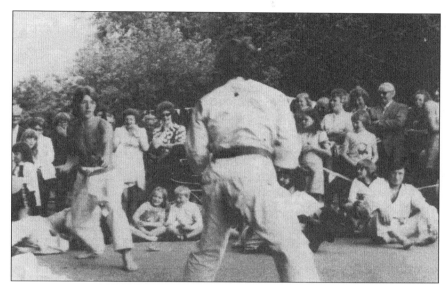

The author (right) and John Carey (1955–2010), ca. 1975.

Dedication

For John, who started it all by bringing me along to the dojo
one cold, wet night in January 1974. You changed my life.

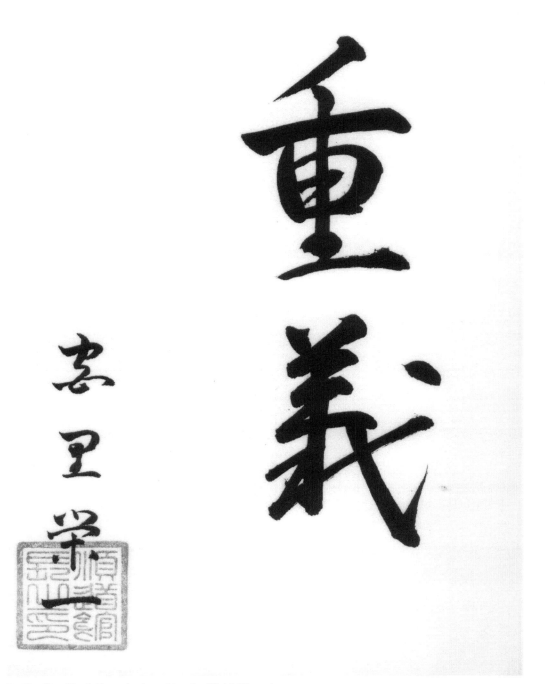

Ju Gi—Morality is Important, written by Eiichi Miyazato.

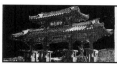

CONTENTS

4 Gi—Technique 93

5 Tai—Body 153

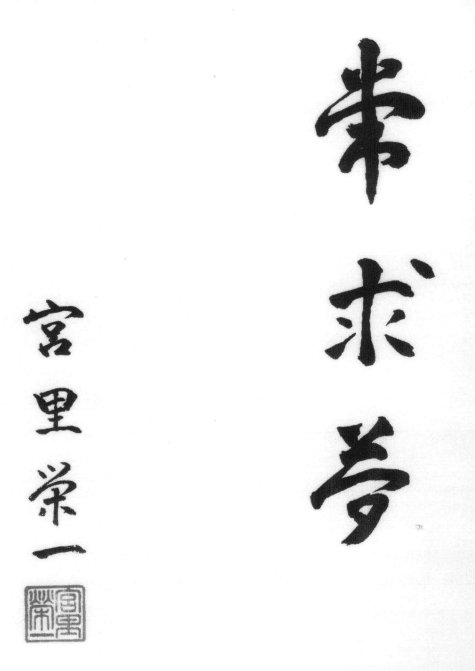

Jo Kyu Mu—Follow Your Dream, written by Eiichi Miyazato

Foreword

by Dr. Damon Young

Karate-do is no simple thing. To begin, it requires draining, painful, or dull physical labors—from hundred-pushup sessions to hours of precise *kata* and *bunkai* to vigorous *kumite*. To the novice, and perhaps to many naïve film-goers, this is karate: physical prowess, backed up by sweat and sometimes blood. And it's true: it is impossible to develop in karate without physical labor.

But for karate to be karate—rather than simply exercise, dance, or calisthenics—one must recognize its roots in Okinawa and Japan. Despite commonalities, these offer two very different experiences of lifestyle in general, and martial arts in particular. Where the latter stresses a more formal approach, the first is more informal—but no less austere or committed. What both traditions have in common is a long history of martial arts, known as 'te' in Okinawa, which must be understood if 'karate' is to have any meaning beyond kicks and punches. There are philosophies, scholarly and folk, which are bound up in the way of life, and the way of karate-do. One can be a fighter and ignore this, but not a karateka.

And yet sweat and study are not enough. Alongside physical and mental exertion, karate-do as *budo* asks something more: existential labor—in other words, a change in character and consciousness. This is neither a simple cognitive trick, nor a mystical epiphany. Instead, it is the transformation of one's psyche that comes with continual effort, challenge, and dedication. It involves the cultivation of virtues like sincerity, patience, restraint, and care. And it is characterized by a clearness of vision: a willingness to see things without delusion or confusion. The fight begins against others, but ends against one's own vices: one's vanity, ignorance, and laziness.

This is the journey of the karateka, and it is one I've taken only a few steps on. But even as a novice I recognize the importance of Michael Clarke's contribution with *Shin Gi Tai: Karate Training for Body, Mind, and Spirit*. It is many important things at once: an introduction to the culture, language, history, and rituals of Okinawa and Japan; a primer on karate's rites, techniques, and etiquette; a discussion of sport, fitness, and *budo* karate, and their value; and a very personal meditation on the 'inner life' of the dedicated karateka. It explores in detail the physical, scholarly, and existential dimensions of the martial arts and does so with an impressive balance of philosophical discussion and straightforwardness. Michael Clarke is erudite, meditative, without being pretentious or esoteric. If he refuses to name or describe something, he's not being mystical—the reader must experience the 'something' first hand.

If I may sum up the book in a single word, it would be 'gratitude'. Michael is certainly opinionated, confident, and sometimes blunt. He does not suffer fools, and in his youth many fools apparently suffered for this. This is not a book for those seeking glib happiness or easy answers. But the overriding mood of *Shin Gi Tai: Karate Training for Body, Mind, and Spirit* is thankfulness: to the masters, students, and teachers who keep karate-do alive; for the chance to train, learn, and live well; for the opportunity to literally change one's mind. This is the spirit of karate, and it is alive and well in *Shin Gi Tai*. And I am certainly thankful for the opportunity to read and re-read it.

Dr. Damon Young
Honorary Fellow in Philosophy, University of Melbourne, Australia.

Foreword

by Stan Schmidt, 8th dan Shotokan

Those who are truly keen and passionate about whatever art, sport, or devotion they have chosen will inevitably make a journey to the source. But sadly, some never take the risky path or have the guts to take that first step on a voyage of discovery in which their hidden potential is tested and brought into being.

Michael Clarke is an advocate of the traditional *way* of karate-do, which he explains throughout the pages of this book. To Michael this means immersing himself in daily training, as karate practiced in this manner doesn't build your character as much as it *reveals* your character. It means having to dig deep and uncover your true nature.

Michael is passionate about his chosen art of karate. This is evidenced by the four books he has penned already and by the hundreds of articles he has had published on the subject. But, first and foremost, he has 'put his money where his mouth is'.

In addition to interviewing many karate masters of all styles and descriptions, he has himself walked the walk—the long walk to Okinawa, the source and home of karate-do … a number of times … where he undertook the challenging rigors of Goju-ryu under a number of traditional masters, masters who had also been taught by masters.

Michael has earned the right to write about the deeper aspects of karate, as he does in this book, thus passing on valuable hidden treasures to other teachers and practitioners of the Art of the Empty Hand. The themes Michael writes about in *Shin Gi Tai: Karate Training for Body, Mind, and Spirit*—he has experienced first hand, and he knows well the actual culture surrounding karate training in Okinawa.

He has developed a good spirit, *Shin*, transforming his previously nasty temperament into a reasonable disposition; he has learned that by showing respect to a potential attacker he can often diffuse a threatening situation. He understands too, that cultivating a strong and pliant body, *Tai,* will help to keep him free from disease and other assaults upon his life; and finally, that such freedom comes at a price, the price being regular and ongoing hard work, while always seeking *Gi*—good technique.

Through my own experiences—by jumping in at the 'deep end'—that is, by training in Japan since the 1960s and having to face up to, fall down against, and rise above adversity, like Michael has, I have come to a similar conclusion to his with regard to Budo. In both life and *karate-do*, Spirit—*Shin* (good spirit)—is the platform from which *Gi* and *Tai* operate, thus giving the karateka self-knowledge and the ability to perform well when facing up to and dealing with life's numerous challenges.

Reading this book is a worthwhile start to a voyage of exploration for you through *Budo* training. Following the martial way with integrity, you will discover talents that lie within you, which are crying out to be released. Thus, if you want to know balance—be prepared to walk the tightrope. Aim high and train hard, go to the source of your karate, and seek its essence; by digesting the contents of this book, you will have made a good start!

Stan Schmidt
8th dan, Shotokan Karate-do
Melbourne, Australia

Foreword

by John Porta, 9th dan, Hanshi, Okinawan Goju-ryu

From its early beginnings in the Ryukyu Islands, the once obscure and little known civilian self-protection art of Okinawa known as karate has spread around the globe and has now become a world-wide household word. Today there are karate training halls in virtually every country, with multitudes of students. Over the past few decades, martial arts schools and teachers arose and various gyms, town recreation departments, and educational organizations all began offering martial arts and self-defense training courses under the heading of karate. However, much of the teachings lacked the physical training, philosophy, and internal workings of what was originally found in traditional karate.

For many years there has been a void in publications providing much insight to traditional karate in such a comprehensive way as presented in this book. Through a well-rounded presentation introducing the concept of Shin Gi Tai, the harmonious fusion of mind, body, and spirit, Michael Clarke re-introduces the traditional approach to karate training to the reader in a way that can be well understood.

As I proceeded through the contents, I was immediately impressed with the overall scope of the information provided and the many academic, historical, and philosophical references, including a vast number of pertinent photos and endnotes that enhance the information presented. The book surely captures the essence of traditional karate, and there are few persons qualified to write such a book. With Clarke's training experiences on Okinawa, continuing study and research, understanding of Okinawa culture, along with writing hundreds of articles and authoring four books, he has once again written an outstanding book relating to traditional karate training. I cannot think of a person more qualified to write such a book.

I have come to know Michael through the publication of his previous book *The Art of Hojo Undo: Power Training for Traditional Karate*. I was very impressed with the book's content and presentation of traditional power training, and I immediately knew it would be a success. Now, once again, Michael has written an outstanding book relating to traditional karate training. I highly recommend *Shin Gi Tai: Karate Training for Body, Mind, and Spirit* to teachers and students, regardless of karate style or affiliation. This book will contribute to a greater knowledge of traditional karate and will make an outstanding addition to everyone's martial arts library.

John Porta, Hanshi 9th dan
Okinawan Goju-Ryu Shobukan Karate-Do
New Jersey, USA

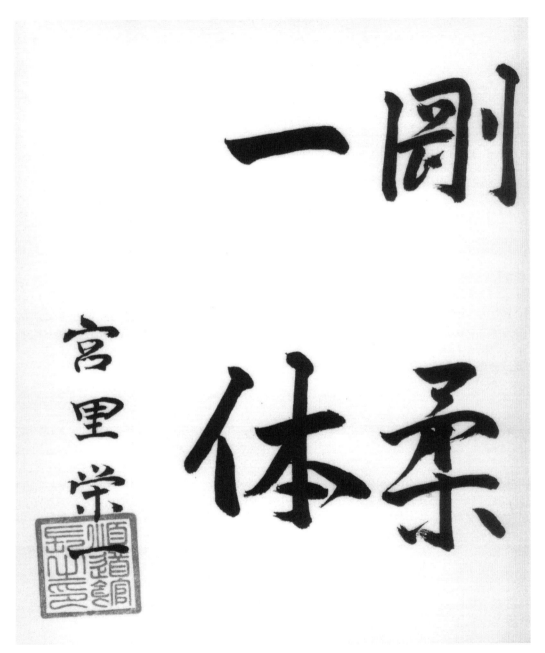

Go Ju Ichi Tai—Strength and Gentleness in One Body, written by Eiichi Miyazato.

Preface

Throughout this book, photographs and other images have been used to provide stimulus to what might otherwise prove to be a rather dry and dusty text: a picture paints a thousand words, isn't that how the saying goes? But this is not a karate book for children, nor has it been written to entertain; on the contrary, it has been written to question and challenge the established order of the day. To that end, readers will no doubt note a certain *tone* throughout the book: please don't mistake this for anything as facile as anger, animosity, or bitterness, for my thoughts toward others in the world reflect none of these things.

As I have endeavored to explain within the body of the book, I believe there is something "missing" in much of what passes for karate these days, and this book has been written to highlight this. I harbor no illusions of halting the decline in karate, but I hope this book will at least be the cause of some discussion: for from discussion and debate comes consensus and, sometimes, change. If just one person who reads this book begins to wonder about his involvement with karate, it will have been worth the writing.

I am no scholar, and this will become clear as you read on from here. What I know— or think I know—has come about through experience, and in this lies the source of my many limitations. I simply haven't experienced enough of life to know better! Any and all mistakes discovered within this book are mine and mine alone. I ask only that you view them in the context of my modest efforts to bring the world of budo karate once more before the public eye.

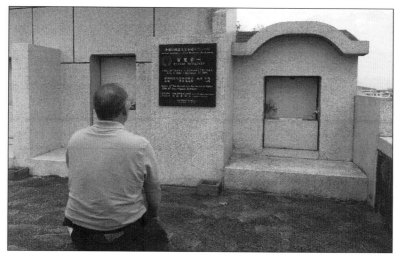

The author paying his respects at the grave of his teacher, Eiichi Miyazato.

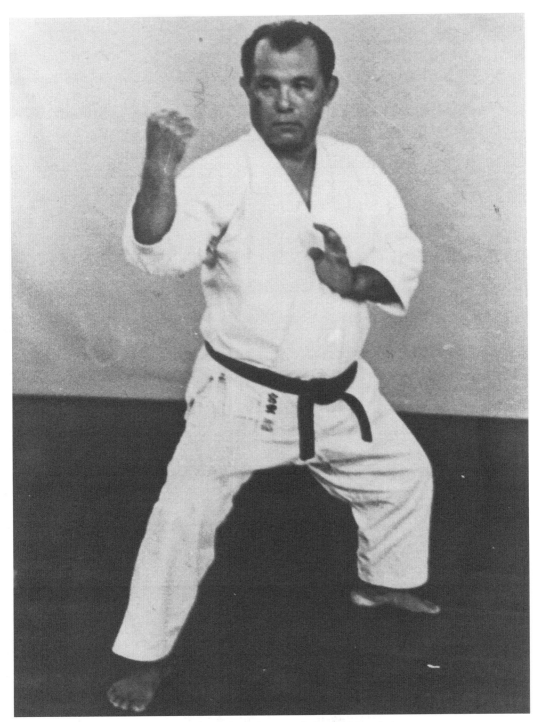

Eiichi Miyazato (1922–1999), Hanshi 10th dan Goju ryu, 8th dan Kodokan Judo.

Acknowledgements

The editor and I have taken the liberty to selectively italicize words of foreign origin in this text. This decision was taken to ease the flow of information. In most other matters of style, this book conforms to *The Chicago Manual of Style,* 16th edition. I have to admit that "conforming" to rules and regulations is not one of my strong points. There is a school of thought that believes rules—any rules—are put in place to be broken. I can't say I altogether disagree with that line of thinking. But I recognize that rules—sensible rules—serve a purpose; they give a sense of direction and provide boundaries we as human beings need. For make no mistake, life without boundaries leads irrevocably to psychological chaos. As sentient beings, we need boundaries if we are to remain intact spiritually and physically.

The discipline found in writing is similar in many ways to the discipline needed in the dojo; with both you have to apply yourself wholeheartedly to your endeavor and approach the task at hand with enthusiasm. Still, all the enthusiasm in the world won't make things right if you are doing something wrong, and this is where other people come in. We need other people in order to validate to ourselves who *we* are. Budo asks that we do this in a quiet way. Nevertheless, there comes a time when recognition is due, and when it is, it should be given with complete sincerity and clear humility. To this end, there are certain people whose contribution to this book cannot pass unnoticed.

I am most grateful for the use of extracts from Funakoshi sensei's autobiography and would like to extend my thanks to the publisher, Kodansha International. I am also grateful for the research done by Morio Higaonna, Tetsuhiro Hokama, and Masahiro Nakamoto, all of whom are important sensei living in Okinawa today, and to Kiyotaka Yamada of Japan, as well as Patrick McCarthy sensei of Australia, and Mario McKenna sensei of Canada. Without their scholarly efforts, many stories of Okinawa's past karate masters may not be known outside of Okinawa and Japan. To these teachers I extend my sincere gratitude and thanks.

I am indebted in no small way also to the skill and generosity of Dave Groves. As a professional photographer, but with no experience in studio photography, he accepted the challenge of capturing the sequential images found in the book. With a level of enthusiasm that characterizes his larger-than-life appearance as well as his approach to living, Dave took on the job and gave freely of his time and expertise with a camera. Without ever being in a dojo before, or throwing a punch or kick in his life, Dave's easy-going way exhibits many of the character traits found in those who understand the concept of budo, and it was an honor for me to have him involved with the making of this book.

Jesse Cottrell, John Mercer, and Mitch Turner are the three students pictured in the sequential photographs, and here too, I wish to express my sincere thanks and gratitude to them for giving so freely of their time over a number of days. It's not easy trying to capture the spirit of karate one click of the camera at a time. Without momentum, without intention, karate techniques lose their potency. Still, all three handled this task well, and the results of their efforts are to be found within the pages of this book.

It goes without saying, that you are reading this only because a publisher had sufficient faith in me as a writer to publish my thoughts and opinions. That publisher is David Ripianzi at YMAA Publication Center. Without his support and enthusiasm, this book may well not exist, for few publishers are willing to go into print with the subject matter found in these pages. For his vision and support, his advice, and sometimes challenging questions, I extend my thanks and appreciation once again, as I do to Tim Comrie and the rest of the team at YMAA Publication Center who work so hard to bring their writers' work before the public.

This is the second book of mine to be published by YMAA, and, as with all my books, the process of bringing these words to you has been long and at times arduous. A writer needs an editor, and on this project, that job fell to Dolores Sparrow, a woman of great depth and integrity. Over a number of months in 2010, she and I worked together to shape and form the words you are about to read. At times, our exchanges revealed strongly held opposing points of view on a number of matters, but with good communication and a shared desire to see this book come to publication, we remained on track to do just that. To put it simply, this book would not be the book it is without the skill, expertise, tenacity, and unflinching support of my editor, Dolores Sparrow.

When you reach the discussion on Japanese kanji toward the end of chapter two, take a look at the actual kanji embedded in the text. They are there because of Dolores and her unwillingness to let technicalities surrounding Japanese fonts and electronic compatibility stand in the way of their inclusion. It was her resolve to find them and establish a way by which they could be used that resulted in your eyes being able to fall upon them in this book … so ponder them awhile. My deep and sincere appreciation for her guidance and knowledge concerning the written word cannot be adequately expressed in a simple "Thank you!" but it is no less felt, for all that.

Photographic Credits

Most of the older images from Okinawa seen in this book have been in the public domain for many years, quite a few appear with kind permission, and a smaller number were taken by me. I have been unable to contact a small number of owners (the original photographers or others) of some of the images in the book. I apologize for this and request any unaccredited persons to contact me in writing. Upon proof of ownership they will be properly credited (or their photograph removed if they wish) in any future edition.

In particular, I want to offer a heartfelt thank you to the following people and institutions for the use of their wonderful photographs; without them, this book would not be able to deliver half as well the message I have tried to convey regarding the spirit of Okinawan karate: Blitz Enterprises, Shinzo Chinen, Donn Cuson, Derek English, Tetsuhiro Hokama, Daniel Lopez, Dennis Martin, Patrick McCarthy, Graham Noble, Okinawa Media Planning Co., Ltd., Terry O'Neill, John Porta, John Spence, Hiseo Sunagawa, Charlie Suriano, Stephen Turnbull, and the University of the Ryukyus.

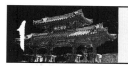 # INTRODUCTION

Standing in the doorway of the Kodokan in Kume, Okinawa, the silence of the empty dojo whispered to me. I could hear echoes of training from long ago when students of karate gave themselves fully to the learning of their martial art. And in the ecstasy of sweat they found a harmony of spirit, technique, and the intricate workings of their body. Those who devoted their lives to karate developed an internal ease and an economy of movement that belied the effort of their training. They found a sense of balance between mind, body, and spirit, so natural as to be rendered invisible to the casual observer. To others, karateka possessed almost mystical powers and were capable of superhuman strength. But nothing could be further from the truth, for karate training offers no such abilities. The potential to understand the essence of karate is innate in all of us. It lies dormant waiting to be discovered and is present in each individual who enters a dojo seeking instruction. The way we apply ourselves to the training reveals the reality of that potential. Long before karate became a pastime for children, a professional franchise, or a pathway to celebrity, it held a very different place in the hearts and minds of those who practiced it. In this book I want to explain what karate was intended to be, how the people of Okinawa learned the art, and how, having mastered its deadly techniques, also succeeded in cultivating a calm and peaceful mind.

Entrance to the Kodokan
dojo, Kume, Okinawa.

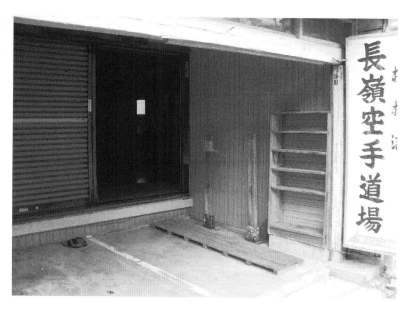

Karate did not originate on the battlefields of old Japan, as did some of the fighting systems that still exist today, albeit in diluted forms, such as *jujutsu, kendo, naginatado*, and more. As much as anyone has been able to ascertain, karate, as we know it today, is a development of the indigenous fighting ways of Okinawa, simply referred to as 'ti' (pronounced 'tee', meaning hand), combined with influences from countries with whom the Okinawans traded. Premier among these was of course China, but we should not forget Okinawa's other neighbors in the region, countries such as Siam (Burma), Indonesia, Thailand, and the Philippines, as well as others. All of which, even today, have strong fighting traditions that go back many centuries. It takes no great leap of faith to see how the flow of ideas from one location to another could have transpired. In the pirate infested waters of Southeast Asia, sailors who could not defend themselves were vulnerable to attack, and though I suspect the fighting styles of these men were somewhat less refined than we might imagine when thinking of skilled martial artists, I have no doubt they could handle themselves well and deliver a blow to be reckoned with.

Aside from the sailors and workingmen of the island, the landed gentry of Okinawa also pursued the martial arts. Shuri, the royal capital, has a long and illustrious history of residents who were highly skilled in the use of weapons and fighting with their bare hands. Almost always these men were connected to the royal household in some way for their employment, or held hereditary posts as village leaders. Within the culture of Okinawa, such men of rank[1] were revered in much the same way as the samurai were revered in Japan. They were referred to by the general population as *bushi*, a title bestowed upon those who excelled in both the fighting arts and the ways of scholarship. In truth, some who carried the title did not entirely live up to it by today's measure; be that as it may, such men were responsible for transmitting much of the fighting arts of Okinawa that exist today, and without them the gene pool of empty hand and weapon arts passed down to modern times would be much smaller. With successive generations of martial artists grew the notion that fighting should be used as a matter of last resort, although it is clear from the surviving literature that this idea was already well established in the Chinese martial arts. Throughout the 1800s, many individuals traveled from Okinawa to China with the specific goal of learning a martial art or improving upon the knowledge they already had. From these travelers, a fresh influx of fighting strategies and philosophical education began to filter into Okinawa's martial arts community; and as a result, the character building quality of training in 'ti' (today known as karate) and with weapons (today known as kobudo) began to make its presence felt even more strongly throughout the early decades of the twentieth century.

A glimpse of this evolution in thinking can be found in the March 1934 and January 1936 papers on Okinawan karate written by Chojun Miyagi, both entitled "An Outline of Karate-do" (*Karate-do Gaisetsu*).[2] In them he addressed the possible beginnings of karate in Okinawa and the state of the art at the time of writing. He touched on the subject of styles, the characteristics of karate, and the methods of training. Also, he hypothesized on the future of karate as it began its unsteady expansion outward from Okinawa to the rest of the world. In his book, *Tales of Okinawa's Great Masters,* Shoshin Nagamine[3] wrote: "When Higaonna, Miyagi's teacher, taught *'to te' jutsu,* he was always known to cite passages from the ancient book of Chinese martial arts called the *Wubeizhi,* a document perhaps better known by its Japanese pronunciation, *Bubishi.* Underscoring the eight principles of *chuan fa*[4] and the strategy of Sun-Tzu,[5] Kanryo Higaonna maintained that physical training without moral philosophy was not 'to te'." That Higaonna, an illiterate trader and sometimes drunkard,[6] was nevertheless stressing the importance of moral philosophy as far back as the early years of the twentieth century indicates that long before karate was known outside Okinawa, it had already obtained a mantle of character development, moving karate beyond the realms of mere physical self-protection. Indeed, over two centuries earlier, in 1683, the noted Okinawan fighting master 'Ti' Junsoku (1663–1734) offered the following advice regarding the underlying nature of training in the martial arts of Okinawa:

> "No matter how you may excel in the art of *ti* and in your scholastic endeavors, nothing is more important than your humanity as observed in daily life."

The behavior of men like Kanryo Higaonna may fall short of the bar by today's standards, but it would be wrong to take him out of his historical milieu and judge him by our present day understanding of what is and isn't considered decent behavior. If we today can live with a variety of political leaders around the world who have, on record, cheated on their wives and families, taken bribes, fixed elections, and smoked cannabis—without inhaling, of course—and still allow them to remain in office to decide the fate of humanity, then I see no reason why we should condemn those who lived less public lives in a time when their behavior was considered more acceptable.

Throughout this book, I have drawn primarily on my own experiences on Okinawa to show the value of practicing karate in the traditional Okinawan way. I have included accounts from Okinawan karate masters, both past and present, as well as stories and anecdotes from my time

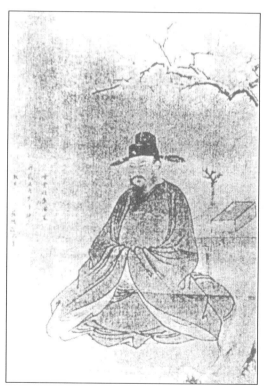

"Ti" Junsoku (1663–1734)

training in Japanese karate. In doing so, I tried to avoid accounts that, for me at least, have taken a few too many steps away from the reality that I am comfortable with. Such tales I will leave for others to tell. What I want to do here is remain as close to authenticity as possible. To that end, I have revisited the writings of Okinawa's great karate masters of the past and added my own observations on the present state of karate. It should be clearly understood from the outset that I am not suggesting parity in stature or importance between these teachers of the past and myself. I recognize my karate has been built upon the shoulders of the giants who came before me, people who in many cases had died before I was even born. Their thoughts, actions, and how they lived their lives have allowed me to gain access to training methods and ways of thinking that have long since fallen out of fashion, and these I want to share here. For without this education, I have no doubt my own understanding of karate would now stand upon much shallower foundations.

There has always been a sense of contradiction in traditional karate training: an obvious paradox. On the one hand, the schooling is extremely physical and sometimes even severe; on the other hand, those who persevere and endure such training for more than ten years develop a peaceful and cooperative nature. They appear gentle on the outside yet remain strong on the inside, but how does this happen? What is it about learning how to fight that opens the door to pacifism? In this book I will explore both the physical and the mental education that takes place in a traditional karate dojo, whether in Okinawa, Japan, or a dojo found in any other country. Such a place is where the "way" of karate takes precedence over profit and where the activities taking place should not be mistaken for the pastime being pursued in the commercial karate clubs found the world over. Both approaches to karate, traditional and commercial, are looked at in chapter two. While finding a commercial club these days is as simple as picking up the phone book, finding a traditional karate dojo is a little more difficult. Even when a dojo is discovered, access can prove to be easier said than done; you cannot simply walk in off the street and request instruction, for it has always been the prerogative of the teacher to pick the student, and in a traditional karate dojo this is still the case today. Karate was introduced to the West by the Japanese, and their language is now used around the world when discussing its techniques and even its philosophy. Because of this, where required, I have placed Japanese words in parenthesis to ease the flow of information; any errors are mine and mine alone. That said, the essence of the philosophical lessons you are about to encounter stems as much from Chinese and Okinawan thinking as Japanese. They have been mirrored in many different cultures throughout the ages. Therefore, it would be quite wrong to attribute too much credit for the underlying philosophy of karate to any one society alone.

I do not believe much progress can be made in karate without first developing a sense of balance, but the balance I speak of has less to do with standing upright and more to do with your overall approach to training and indeed, life. Karate insists you cultivate your body through your mind, and because of this you are obliged to fight your ego on two separate fronts, the cerebral and the physical. On the dojo floor, the mental and physical aspects of learning karate are regularly daunting and this alone causes many to stop training. Yet if you can endure the early years, the first decade, then there is an opportunity for real and lasting benefit. Once again, the term "balance" is pertinent here, for along with the physical doggedness needed to practice karate seriously over many years comes the mental tenacity necessary to open the mind to *tsu shin gen*: the piercing eye of insight. When the mind and body are healthy and in harmony, your true spirit emerges, and within this book you will find both physical training methods and psychological challenges. Karate is like everything else in life; the things you like, and those you don't, need to be reflected upon before you reach an understanding of them. It is essential not to offset the scales of reason with your own narrow-mindedness. Intolerance is not a character trait found in those who study karate seriously.

The expression *shin gi tai* has a literal translation: mind–technique–body. Additionally, the term has philosophical connotations that run much deeper and clearly point to a particular kind of concord in those who seek to gain an understanding of karate beyond the realms of mere kicking and punching. Although some may consider such an ambition to be fanciful, I would disagree; for regardless of how many people you learn to defeat in combat, the deeper aim of karate training since times long ago has always been to conquer your own ego, and by doing so, you increase the likelihood of avoiding conflict. When you can do that, you have an opportunity to establish a sense of balance in life, which is denied those who take as a measure of progress their increased ability to harm another. Such a benchmark may appeal to individuals who fear to face themselves in the dojo, but to a serious karateka, inflicting physical damage on others is always the last resort. Be that as it may, the use of force is an option that, if things should turn physical, allows a karateka to unleash an arsenal of techniques capable of producing severe injury, even death. As this is the reality of years spent training seriously in karate, it becomes clear why a person's mind (*Shin*) must be developed ahead of his technique (*Gi*) if he is to discover a sense of balance within his body (*Tai*). This is the essence, the spirit, of *Shin Gi Tai*. The way we learn karate is sometimes referred to as "do" (pronounced doe) meaning a path or road, and all those who choose to walk this path do so with the understanding that the way ahead will most certainly be a difficult one.

A word or two is also necessary to define the phrase "traditional karate" and what differentiates it from any other type of karate. While it is certainly true that karate as we see it today appeared relatively recently, the use of the word "traditional," for me at least, has always pointed to the role karate plays in my life, rather than the techniques learned or the kata practiced. The physical aspects of karate are the least of it; they provide only an opportunity to experience the essence of karate through training and, as Nagamine sensei put it, "the ecstasy of sweat." That so much is made these days of how things are done within a particular school of karate has taken the focus away from the individual striving to go deeply and, instead, placed it firmly upon the masses and their scramble to emulate their teacher. While the latter may provide the better business model, the former

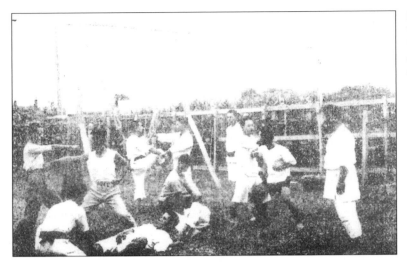

Kenkyukai kumite training, ca. 1928. The Kenkyukai dojo was an attempt to stop the spread of "styles" within karate.

still remains the only way to reach an understanding of yourself through the practice of karate. This to me is the tradition of karate, the way of karate, that I might discover through my own efforts strategies to live well and protect myself from adversity. It is, I believe, the same things others have striven for when they walked the earth and breathed the air, when they wiped the sweat from their face and took a deep breath, ready to go just one more time. Many years may have passed between them and me, but karate has endured. Long after you and I are gone, karate will live in individuals who have managed to avoid the distractions of their day and discovered what others found. This is the tradition I speak of when I use the word. The philosophy and the physical techniques of karate in this book do not represent the entire repertoire of either. There is much more to be found in the study of karatedo—the way of the empty hand—than any book can deliver. Indeed, even with daily training, I am not sure it is possible to master every karate technique or come to terms with every philosophical signpost we encounter; for as many a karate master will tell you, with karate one lifetime is not enough! That said, the information contained within this book should cause you to pause for a moment and consider your own situation. And in that reflection perhaps you will reaffirm, or possibly discover for the first time, your individual sense of direction within karate.

This book touches upon subjects many teachers of karate today are either unaware of or choose to avoid, but I am placing them back in the spotlight deliberately. Karate, as a martial art, is in danger of becoming homogenized, changed beyond recognition due to sporting and commercial concerns rendering it all but useless as a means of personal self-protection. Indeed, there are many voices within the martial arts community today only too willing to proclaim that karate's combat credentials have been lost already: but they are wrong! Karate techniques delivered correctly and with the appropriate mindset, continue to have the potency to maim or kill; what has changed over the past few decades is not karate, but the attitude of the majority who practice it. The original intention of karate has been hijacked by people who place form ahead of function. This book is not concerned with the 'look' of karate, or karate as a sporting or a business venture. What 'style' of karate you practice is irrelevant; the important thing to appreciate with karate is 'why' you practice; what do you expect the end result of all your efforts to be, and are those efforts being reflected in the quality of your life outside the dojo? The subject matter being presented here is for adults only and goes beyond the unchecked belligerence of the adolescent mind. In parts, you may feel offended by what you read, but hopefully not too much; I have not set out to offend anyone deliberately. As it has done for me and many others, traditional karate training has the capacity to change lives for the better, but only if you are prepared to move past the obvious. If you are prepared to swim in deeper waters than the shallows most people splash around in, you will discover more about yourself than you can imagine. Yet *budo* is a concept more often spoken of than put into practice, so you will need to gather all your courage and tenacity, and all your integrity, too, if you hope to walk the 'middle-path' of budo; for as difficult as it can be at times it is no less rewarding if you choose to accept the challenge. This book will provide an opportunity for you to consider why you practice karate, or why you are thinking of doing so. When you have read the book, don't get sidetracked by becoming a fan or a critic. I have no need of either. Only celebrities have fans and I am no celebrity; as for critics, this is what Theodore Roosevelt had to say about them:

> It is not the critic who counts: not the man who points out how the strong man stumbles, or where the doer of deeds could have done better. The credit belongs to the man who is actually in the arena, whose face is marred by dust and sweat and blood, who strives valiantly, who errs and comes up short again and again, because there is no effort without error and shortcomings, but who does actually strive to do the deed, who knows the great enthusiasms, the great devotions, who spends himself for a worthy cause; who, at the best, knows, in the end, the triumph of high achievement, and who, at the worst, if he fails, at least he fails while daring greatly, so that his place will never be with those timid souls who knew neither victory nor defeat.

Hopefully, you will take what you find of value in these pages and use it to spur you on to a deeper and more profound understanding of yourself, your karate, and the world in which you live. Whatever school of karate you study or whichever path you walk through life, endeavor to conduct yourself with humility and quiet confidence, make the most of your opportunities, and do the best you can with the resources available to you. Your life is yours, your karate is yours too, so accept ownership of both and reap the rewards.

Michael Clarke
Shinseidokan Karate Dojo
Tasmania, September 2010

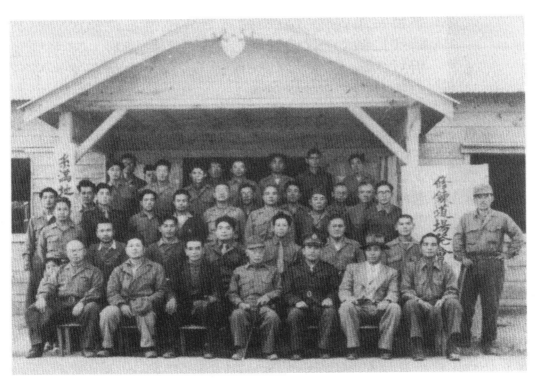

The new Shuren dojo, Itoman, Okinawa, opened just a few years after WWII.

2 THE DOJO

Borrowed from the Buddhist tradition, the word dojo means "place of the way." Originally used to describe a designated area or room in a temple complex where monks would go to receive instruction, it was borrowed by Japanese martial artists shortly after the fall of the Tokugawa Shogunate[7] and the end of the *bakufu*, or military government, in 1868. With the associated demise of the strict class system and the dissolution of the clans, many highly trained samurai found themselves without employment. Forced to earn a living, some turned their fighting skills to good use by teaching armed and unarmed combat.[8] Unknown at that time in mainland Japan, Okinawa's indigenous martial art, then known as ti (pronounced tee), was also undergoing its own inevitable revolution. Ti is the name Okinawans gave to their empty hand fighting art, but they were not the originators of the fighting strategies or techniques; for that, they depended heavily on China. Emerging from the shadows of secrecy in the later years of the nineteenth century, ti was now being taught openly for the first time. By 1901, karate had been established within the public school system on Okinawa and from that time on, sensei (teachers of ti) followed their martial art counterparts in Japan by opening up public dojo and began accepting paying students.

Although not as austere as the dojo found in Japan, Okinawan dojo have always been considered a special place by those who gathered to practice in them. On an island so bereft of space, setting aside a large room solely for the purpose of training in karate was rarely possible and so more often than not the early dojo of Okinawa meant training in the gardens and small courtyards that once surrounded the typical Okinawan home. Before this, ti, or as we call it today, karate, was a secret activity taught in graveyards

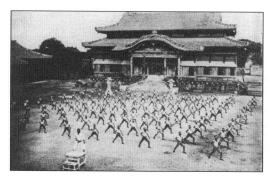

High school students demonstrate karate kata on the grounds of Shuri-jo.

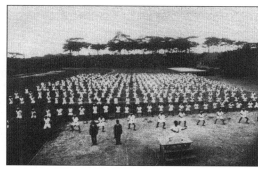

High school students taking part in a mass kata demonstration.

and in hidden groves late at night and in the early hours of the morning. It would take some time before the Okinawans followed the Japanese model and moved their training indoors, and for many years yet, it would remain an almost exclusively outdoor pursuit. There are still men alive today, many of them Americans, who began their karate training in Okinawa this way, in their sensei's backyard. But there can be no doubt that karate is an international activity now, no longer a solely Okinawan pursuit; therefore, the influences upon it come from many different cultural backgrounds. Be that as it may, the original karate of Okinawa still exists, and the once tiny island kingdom of Ryukyu that straddled the gap in the East China Sea between China and Japan remains karate's spiritual home. The very nature of karate training reveals in those who practice it much more than an ability to fight. Okinawans have always understood this and are acutely aware of the benefits of karate training to both the individual and the wider community. They knew, through folklore and legend, of the mental and physical severity students of karate endured and believed that because of this, their society was a better place to live, populated as it was by men skilled in the fighting arts and imbued with a sense of integrity. The best of these men were known in Okinawa as bushi, men who had mastered the concept of Bunbu ryo do: the way of scholarship and the martial arts. It was bushi who first established dojo in Okinawa and began teaching karate and kobudo (empty hand fighting and old style weapons) to the general public. These men were teachers without rank, as we understand it in the martial arts these days, but with real skill, abilities, stature, and reputations that often spread island-wide and beyond.

A dojo back then, as today, was never large, for the luxury of space was rarely available to those teaching. This, in turn, acted as a natural restriction to the number of people practicing at any one time, but with training going on each evening, some of the early dojo still attracted an impressive number of students. As indicated earlier, however, gaining entry to the dojo of a karate sensei (teacher) was not always so easy. Many of them took their lead for accepting new students from the Chinese tradition where prospective trainees often underwent long periods of character testing before being accepted as a novice. Personal introductions too played a significant role, and older family members with some connection to a sensei, perhaps as a neighbor or colleague at work, were often the way young men gained an introduction to their teachers. When a new student arrived at the dojo, it was his job to prepare and clean the training area, making it ready for the seniors when they arrived. Back then there were no changing rooms, as there was nothing to change into. The karate training uniform (*keikogi*) used today was almost unheard of in Okinawa at that time, and students often trained in nothing more than a loincloth or perhaps their trousers; afterward, they simply got dressed and returned home to clean up. No showers, no bathrooms, no member's lounge, and no cold drinks machines either. Unlike the "health club" atmosphere found in some commercial karate clubs at present, the only thing to be found in a dojo back then was karate! In Okinawa these days, it is still the same, with few traditional dojo offering much more than a place to train. If you are lucky, there may be a toilet available; if you are very lucky, there may even be a shower, but the confines of space on the island make even these luxuries the exception rather than the rule. I have met many disappointed visitors who arrived in Okinawa for the first time only to discover the *hombu* dojo (headquarters) of their association is no bigger than an average two-car garage. Used to training in buildings offering every amenity back home, they are unable to hide their disappointment at the relatively tiny dojo they find themselves training in on Okinawa: this saddens me. For in voicing their disappointment they not only show a lack of respect toward their teachers, but also a complete lack of understanding of what a dojo is.

Today there are different kinds of dojo in Okinawa. Some have an open-door policy and will accept anyone who is willing to pay the training fee, and, sad to say, there are some unscrupulous individuals who will offer—and issue—dan ranks and affiliations with the same ease as placing an order for large fries and a coke at McDonald's. From my point of view, these people and their establishments are to be avoided. The individuals involved in such enterprises have little if anything at all to offer, spiritually, mentally, or physically, all of which in my mind renders their tuition worthless. With the increased number of foreign visitors to Okinawa these days, it has become easier to fool those naïve enough to believe that all Okinawans are masters of karate. Let me state this fact quite clearly here: they are not! Even among those Okinawans who are teaching karate today, there are relatively few you might seriously consider a master of this indigenous martial art. Many are no better than their foreign counterparts, and quite a few I have met over the years are considerably less skillful. That said, Okinawa is still *the* place to go to discover for yourself the essence and original spirit of karate. For with careful investigation, patience, good manners, and with the appropriate introductions, it is still possible to find a teacher whose example is worth following.

A Map: Knowing Where You Stand in The Dojo

The size of an Okinawan karate dojo is likely to be smaller than its counterpart in America or Europe. It is also more likely to be attached to or form a part of the sensei's home. As already stated, space on the island is at a premium and few families can afford the luxury of leaving large sections of their home vacant and unused for most of the day. I have visited dojo where boxes full of stock from the family's shop, and even furniture, has had to be moved to one side first in order to allow enough space for training. I have to say that I never found this a problem; in fact, I always thought it added something to the experience of learning and somehow made the karate I was doing seem more natural and relevant to normal living. When a dojo is a place permanently set aside for karate or kobudo training, then in Okinawa it has a slightly different appearance from the dojo of Japan. As I follow the Okinawan way of karate training, so my dojo stands as a part of my home. When I established it I did so with my training needs in mind, and this in turn dictated the look and feel of my dojo. Like traditional dojo in Okinawa, you have to be invited inside; you cannot just walk in off the street and solicit instruction. Once inside there are some unspoken rules and a few invisible boundaries. These are borders

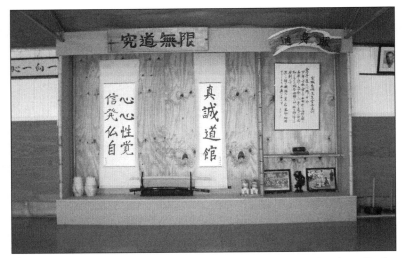

The shomen at the author's Shinseidokan dojo.

that you cross at your peril if you wish to remain in the dojo for longer than a single visit. What follows will give you enough information to find your way around a dojo without causing yourself unwanted problems due to a perceived lack of good manners.

In Okinawa the main wall, known as the wall of honor (*shomen*), will usually have some form of alcove (*tokunoma*) built into it in which are placed objects important to either the sensei or the type of karate or kobudo that is taught. It may also contain one or more hanging scrolls (*kakemono*). Along this wall, portraits of deceased teachers are placed high up, close to the ceiling, which is considered the most respectful position. Unlike the dojo of Japan, only a few Okinawan dojo I have been in had a small *Shinto* shrine (*kamiza*) on the shomen. Contrasting with the rather austere look of a Japanese dojo, the walls in an Okinawan dojo are usually cluttered with either weapons or the tools used in *hojo undo* and *kigu undo* training. Jars, barbells, and a collection of different weights and training devices can give an Okinawan dojo a full look. Nevertheless, the dojo in Okinawa are every bit as special to Okinawans as the Zen-like dojo found in Japan are to the Japanese. The training methods employed in each location, too, are often as different as the dojo. Whereas Japanese karate teachers are inclined to drill students in ordered lines up and down the dojo, in military fashion, in Okinawa the training is far less militaristic, and students often spend their time working individually or in small groups.

Perhaps it is the nature of all societies to arrange their activities in ways that reflect that society's underlying character. In a Japanese dojo, karate training has always been rather more formal than in Okinawa. Okinawan people live, by and large, in a very easy-going culture. Okinawan society, although hardworking, is built around a deep appreciation of its island home and tropical climate and bears only a passing resemblance to the big city lifestyle of Japanese salary men.[9] An American equivalent might be the difference between living in New York or Hawaii. Okinawans have a lifestyle that until recently saw an above-average number of them live well into their hundreds; and even with the relentless encroachment of modernity slowly eroding this statistic, island life is still lived at an unruffled pace seldom found on the Japanese mainland. In contrast to the more relaxed way of life in Okinawa, Japanese society has always been complicated; it may look simple from the outside but this is only how things appear on the surface. Ask anyone who has tried to conduct business in Japan and he will tell you tales of utter despair. The Japanese way of doing things, anything at all, is set firmly within the framework of how they believe a particular thing should be done. They have a word for this; it's called "kata." From how to meet and greet someone for the first time to how to go about serving or being served in a coffee shop, everything has a right way and countless wrong ways. I will return to this word "kata" again later in the book, but for now I want to look a little closer at the way the Japanese sense of conformity (kata) has shaped the place where karate is practiced: the dojo.

In Japan and in all dojo around the world where traditional Japanese martial arts are practiced, a similar blueprint, in accordance with the kata of a dojo, is used in the layout of the training facility. A large rectangular room or hall with sufficient space to accommodate several people training at the same time is divided into two halves, as well as four quarters. These demarcation lines are not obvious to the casual observer; that is to say, they are not visible. Rather, they divide the dojo in much the same way as the lines of latitude and longitude divide the globe. The entrance should be, ideally, located on the rear wall, the wall opposite the one being used as the shomen. Facing the shomen, senior students stand and train to the right-hand side, while the junior students use the left-hand side of the dojo. Each wall, and by extension the area closest to it, has a name; the wall and the area to the right of the shomen where the seniors train is called the upper seat (*joseki*), while the wall and area to the left is referred to as the lower seat (*shimoseki*). The wall at the back of the dojo and the place considered most appropriate for the entrance to the dojo is called the lower wall (*shimoza*). On the shomen in a Japanese dojo there would be a small Shinto shrine known as a shinzen or kamiza, or failing that perhaps a hanging scroll (*kakemono*) bearing some image or writing appropriate to that dojo or the martial art practiced there. You can also expect to see portraits of former sensei or perhaps the school's founder displayed on the shomen. If such portraits are present, they will inevitably appear in black frames as a symbol of respect to the dead. The side walls, joseki and shimoseki, are usually free of ornament, although this is often where you would find the weapons, if used, stored neatly in racks. The rear, or lower wall, the shimoza, is likely to have a number of items attached to it. These can include training aids, such as in the case of a karate dojo: *makiwara*, kick bags, and other equipment.

Immediately upon entering the dojo (in Japan or Okinawa), you enter an area known as the *genkan*. This is the place where shoes are removed before placing them neatly on a small shelf or tidily in rows along the floor. If shoes are in rows on the floor, time is taken to turn the shoes away from the shomen as a mark of politeness and also to facilitate an easy climb back into them at the end of training. You should not, however, remove your socks and leave them in your shoes; that would be a mistake. Instead, they should be

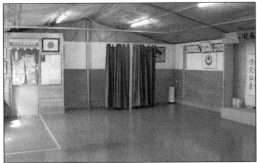

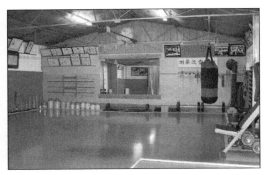

Shinseidokan shimoseki and genkan.

Shinseidokan joseki.

taken into the changing room and kept out of sight with the rest of your clothing until needed again when the training is over. A story I like from karate's past concerns the late master, Gichin Funakoshi. It was said that even well into the twentieth century, he observed many of the age-old taboos still governing people's behavior on Okinawa in the nineteenth century, and to this end, he would never use the words for certain everyday items. Things like toilet paper for example were unmentionable, and he would never speak openly about underclothes. Among these, socks were considered part of a person's *private* apparel and should not only go unspoken but for the most part unseen too. In his Foreword to Funakoshi's autobiography, *Karate-do: My Way of Life*, the president of the Japan Karate Do Shoto Kai, Genshin Hironishi, describes how Funakoshi's grandson tried to trick the old karate master into breaking this taboo and relates the story like this:

> To those of us who studied under him he was a great and revered master, but I fear that in the eyes of his young grandson Ichiro (now a colonel in the Air Self Defense Force) he was merely a very stubborn old man. I well recall an occasion when Funakoshi spied a pair of socks lying on the floor. With a gesture toward Ichiro, he said, "Put those away!"
>
> "But I don't understand," said Ichiro with a look of utter innocence. "What do you mean by 'those'?"
>
> "Yes," said Funakoshi, "those, those!"
>
> "Those, those!" Ichiro retorted. "Don't you know the word for 'those'?"
>
> "I said put those away immediately!" Funakoshi repeated, and Ichiro was forced to admit defeat. His little trap had failed. His grandfather still adamantly refused, as he had all his life, to utter the word for socks.

Today people do not adhere to such a rigid code of conduct; still, it is considered ill-mannered to leave your socks hanging out of your shoes in an untidy mess. If nothing else, it speaks to a person's laziness and lack of consideration for others, character traits that you don't want to put on display before you even step onto the dojo floor. There is also the question of odor and personal hygiene, neither of which should be taken lightly in the dojo. Being attentive to not only your surroundings but to how you interact with others is extremely important in the learning of karate, and neglecting such things is guaranteed to bring some harsh lessons your way.

> While Okinawan dojo share a similar layout to those found in Japan, I have observed that Okinawan students are often less restricted to which part of the dojo they train in than their Japanese counterparts. However, I have also noted that the lower-graded students tend to train toward the back of the dojo and always yield to a senior student who needs space.

What to Expect: Dojo Etiquette

Understanding your place in the dojo is vital if you are to avoid any misunderstandings, and so it may come as a surprise to some to learn that rank is not always the guiding force here. It is something many foreign visitors traveling to Japan or Okinawa for the first time can get confused by; seniority in a traditional dojo is as likely to be dictated by the length of time a person has been training as it is by the dan rank. As often as not, when people line up in a Japanese dojo, those who have been training the longest will line up closest to the joseki. This is also the area in the dojo where seniors spend the majority of their time training, moving to the lower end, the shimoseki, only to work with or assist a junior student. For their part, junior students should not loiter in the joseki area of the dojo and should go there only at the request of a senior or when cleaning the dojo (*soji*) at the conclusion of each training session. As time passes and progress is made students find themselves training in different parts of the dojo, and this acts as a reminder to them of the need to be attentive to their changing surroundings. When karateka begin to appreciate the dojo in this way, they begin to learn their place in the bigger scheme of things. They begin to understand that progress is marked not by the color of the belt they wear but by where they stand in the dojo. Even if someone who knew nothing of traditional martial arts were to stand in the doorway of a dojo and observe the training, he would realize that those farther to the right were more skilled than those to the left.

Etiquette in an Okinawan dojo is often less formal than that found in Japan, though it is considered no less important. Throughout karate's island homeland the etiquette being used can differ greatly from one martial art to another and even from dojo to dojo within the same martial art. Therefore, I do not intend to say categorically, "This is how things are done in Okinawa." For me, it is more important that etiquette is used at all in the dojo, rather than try to make a kata out of it. Still, we do well to often remind ourselves that etiquette is not merely considered important in the learning of a martial art: it is vital. My own teacher, the late Eiichi Miyazato sensei, was a stickler for punctuality. If he asked you to be at the dojo at a certain time, he expected you to be there, ready to go! An example of how he taught karate can be found in the following story:

A group of foreign karate students were visiting Miyazato sensei's dojo, the Jundokan, and like other visitors had spent a lot of money to be in Okinawa. Away from home, many foreigners like to play as well as train, and for some groups a kind of holiday atmosphere begins to prevail. At the end of training one evening this particular group had been asked by Miyazato sensei to return to the dojo at 10:00 A.M. the following morning. The next day they duly arrived at the dojo. They were no more than a minute late, two at most, but that was not good enough for my teacher, who met them at the door and asked them why they were late. They didn't think they were. Miyazato sensei then explained that he was ready to start at 10:00 A.M., not at 10:15 A.M., which is the time it would have been when they changed into their karate *gi*. He sent them back to their hotel and told them not to return for training until the following morning—at 10:00 A.M.! Some in the group took this badly, complaining to their friends that it had cost them a lot to be in Okinawa, and now they were going to miss out on a whole day's training. It seemed like a big price to pay for such a small indiscretion. Miyazato sensei however was not concerned about their hurt feelings; he had a lesson in good manners to deliver and so he delivered it. The next morning the group were in the dojo and ready to go when Miyazato sensei walked onto the dojo floor at 10:00 A.M. They were a day late, but they got their lesson. Whether they understood the importance of it, or confused the kicking and punching they did for the lesson my teacher was giving them, I'm not sure, but I hope they did.

When new students or visitors to my dojo, the Shinseidokan, walk through the door for the first time they often walk into a welcome they did not expect. The dojo forms a part of my home in the Okinawan tradition and so people cannot simply walk in off the street: they have to be invited. Sometimes, however, people arrive and fail to use any kind of etiquette at all on the way from their car to the door of the dojo, and so from my perspective the scene is now set for confrontation rather than harmony. It is a confrontation that is easily resolved once they are made aware of their ignorance; should their lack of etiquette stem from arrogance, then visitors are invited to leave. I realize this may sound harsh to some, but to me it would be unthinkable to arrive at someone's dojo, or their home, and behave as if visiting a football stadium. The importance of correct behavior cannot be overstated, and while I make allowances for different etiquette, I make no allowance at all for visitors who display none. To walk onto my property talking loudly, handling the makiwara or *ude kitae* that stands alongside the path leading to the dojo door, and then to walk through the dojo door itself without even pausing to stop talking has seen more than one group of visitors turned instantly around and escorted back to their cars. Bad manners and karate are like oil and water; they may sometimes exist in the same container, but you will never get them to blend. Etiquette (*reigi saho*) is yet one more aspect of traditional karate that seems to have been diluted or forgotten altogether by those who have prioritized their commercial interests ahead of everything else. Ironically, in some karate clubs and businesses these days, etiquette has become an instrument of control, or a means of shielding the instructor from the consequences of being lazy or out of shape. It is often overt and loud and takes on the feel of military discipline rather than quiet, good manners. All too often those involved in such practices have failed to understand the original meaning of the rituals they insist upon following. In his autobiography, *Karate–My Life*, Hirokazu Kanazawa, 10th *dan*, comments on this very subject:

> "'*Ouss!*' means never retreat from problems or hardships, but to stick with it, never giving up and achieving what you set out to achieve. Perseverance (*Nintai*), Effort (*Doryoku*), and Achievement (*Tassei*) are the underlying concepts of '*Ouss*'. I notice that there are many students nowadays who bandy the term around, endlessly saying '*Ouss! Ouss!*' They do so without actually paying any attention to what is happening around them or what the word actually signifies. In SKIF[10] [Kanazawa sensei's organization], we have stipulated clearly that '*Ouss*' means '*Nintai, Doryoku, Tassei*' and that this is the same for all members and countries."

Etiquette, or just plain old-fashioned good manners, allows the right frame of mind to be adopted in the dojo. It keeps the problems of the day outside where they belong and it allows us to immerse ourselves in the tradition we have come to the dojo to study. Often it can prove quite difficult to grasp the things being asked of us, and so learning to appreciate and apply the appropriate etiquette is often the key to unlocking the unfamiliar. Frequently students fail to make progress for no other reason than their erroneous attitude to etiquette. They may well develop wonderful techniques and yet still find advancement remains beyond their reach.

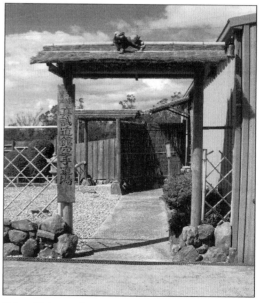

Shinseidokan entrance.

The legendary Okinawan karateka, Gichin Funakoshi sensei, famously proclaimed, "Karate begins with courtesy and ends with courtesy." Once we begin to appreciate that courtesy (*reigi*) is but an extension of the well-known attribute, awareness (*zanshin*), we can perhaps grasp the importance of the role etiquette plays in our overall karate education. Zanshin is a concept most karateka are familiar with, or at least have heard of, and from the beginning, karate students are encouraged to display zanshin at the beginning and end of each kata performance. The intensity of focus at the end of each kata is there to instill a strong sense of control that could, if left unchecked, see your newly acquired karate skills spill over into gratuitous violence. The media like nothing more than to flash headlines like "Martial Arts Maniac Murders Unarmed Intruder" or "Karate Killer Mangles Mugger With His Own Bare Hands." And even though the people involved have usually received very little in the way of serious training, such headlines point to the dangers of learning a type of karate that has been taken out of its historical context. Inherent in karate's techniques is the ability to maim or kill; therefore, a strong and overriding sense of self-discipline and humility must accompany the acquisition of the physical skills. To teach the latter without the former is akin to giving a child a loaded gun and hoping he won't do any harm.

Entering a dojo requires the adoption of a certain amount of reverence; you are not entering a temple, but it's not a gym either. To those who are serious about their education in karate, a dojo is a serious place to be; therefore, the space deserves its due respect. Stepping through the doorway should always solicit a bow toward the shomen. You should also check to see if there is a clear demarcation on the floor: where does the genkan stop? Where does the training area begin? Next, remove your shoes and place them accordingly. If you have to speak, do so calmly and quietly, but don't whisper. From the genkan proceed to the changing room; if this means stepping onto the training area, pause and bow toward the shomen once again. As a rule of thumb, it is best to bow whenever you leave or enter the training area unless told otherwise by the sensei. Returning from the changing room in your gi (karate uniform), move directly to the appropriate area on the dojo floor for your level and begin to warm up. Do not socialize on the dojo floor as this shows your mind is somewhere other than on the training you are about to undertake. Use the time before the training begins to get your mind on the task ahead and your body prepared to do what is about to be asked of it.

Although by no means the universal method for beginning a training session, the example I am about to give is fairly common across the karate world. With some minor adjustments here and there, most who already train in the traditional Okinawan or Japanese manner will recognize the routine. Often beginning with the sensei's call "*Shugo!*" that means "Line up!" the students take their place and prepare to begin formal training. As pointed out earlier, in traditional dojo, the students line up facing the shomen from the joseki, according to time served. However, this tradition has been superseded in many contemporary dojo by those with the highest rank lining up farthest to the right. Remember, though, it is not so important which etiquette is in place so much as etiquette is being used at all. The senior student present is the person calling the commands from here. "*Ki o tsuke!*" brings everyone to attention, before the call "*Seiza!*" directs the assembled students to sit (kneel) in the traditional Japanese fashion, with hands either resting on the thighs or cupped gently in front of the *tanden*, the spot about two inches below the navel. Then the command "*Mokuso!*" is given, and everyone sits still, with eyes closed. During this time students should regulate their breathing and, if they haven't done so already, should turn their minds to the training they are about to do. I have often heard it said that mokuso is meditation. Well, it might be for some, but it is not in any way similar to the kind of meditation found in Buddhist temples or other spiritual training. Mokuso is merely a time to prepare, a time to leave the events of the day behind for a while, and a time to turn your thoughts inward toward the polishing of your spirit (*sen ren shin*). After a few moments of quiet contemplation the senior student calls, *"Mokuso yame!"* (Stop mokuso!) at which point all those present open their eyes and prepare to stand. Before they do, however, the command, *"Shomen ni rei"* (Bow to show appreciation of your predecessors) is given. The sensei will then turn to face the students after which the call *"Sensei ni rei!"* (Bow in appreciation to your teacher!) is given. The students bow from their sitting position and the teacher bows in return. A small but important point to be careful of here is that the students' bows should always precede their teacher's and it should be deeper. They should also take care not to come back up ahead of their sensei. This can be tricky sometimes, but with a little thought and practice, it can be accomplished quite skillfully. *"Kiritsu!"* (Stand up!) is the call that brings everybody back to his feet, before training commences.

A similar observance is conducted at the end of the training; only this is followed in a Japanese dojo by the recital of the dojo *kun*, the ethics of the dojo. Although many Okinawan dojo have their kun displayed, I have never observed this custom of mass recital in Okinawa. Each dojo kun should be as individual as the dojo itself; however, in today's world of the karate conglomerate the dojo kun is sometimes used to enhance conformity within the group. Originally it was a set of precepts the sensei wanted their students to ponder, but the rise of the multinational karate organization has seen the dojo kun take on more of a "mission statement" rather than personal advice from a teacher to his students. Here are four examples of dojo kun; the first two are Japanese and are used by Shotokan and Kyokushin karateka respectively. The third comes from the Jundokan dojo in Asato, Okinawa, and was the dojo kun of my teacher, Eiichi Miyazato sensei. The final example is from my own dojo, the Shinseidokan. When written, each individual guideline is presented as the first. This is to stress that each piece of advice is of equal significance, and so, even though they may have been written in a particular order this should not be taken to be the order of importance. When kun are recited by the students in the dojo, each is preceded by *"Hitotsu!"* meaning "one" or "first." The chant, if done with spirit and determination, can be quite inspiring to younger students, especially when recited in Japanese.

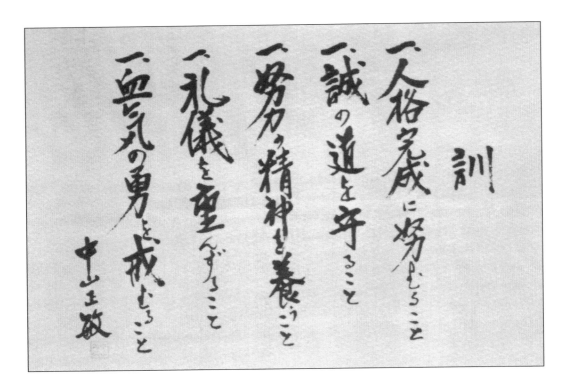

Shotokan Karate dojo kun

First	Work hard to perfect your character
Hitotsu	*Ginkaku kansei ni tsutomomeru koto*
First	Have fidelity in seeking a true way
Hitotsu	*Makato no michi o Mamoru koto*
First	Cultivate a spirit of endeavor and perseverance
Hitotsu	*Doryoku no Seishin o yashinau koto*
First	Always act with good manners
Hitotsu	*Reigi o omonjiro koto*
First	Refrain from violence and uncontrolled behavior
Hitotsu	*Kekki no yu o imashimeru koto*

一、吾々は身心を錬磨し
　確固不抜の心技を極めること

一、吾々は武の神髄を極め
　機に発し感に敏なること

一、吾々は質実剛健を以て
　克己の精神を涵養すること

一、吾々は礼節を重んじ長上を敬し
　粗暴の振舞ひを慎しむこと

一、吾々は神仏を尊び
　謙譲の美徳を忘れざること

一、吾々は智性と体力とを向上させ
　事に臨んで過たざること

一、吾々は生涯の修業を空手の道に通じ
　極真の道を全うすること

道場訓

Kyokushin Karate dojo kun

| First | We will train our hearts and bodies for a firm, unshaken spirit |
| *Hitotsu* | *Ware ware wa, shinshin o renmashi, kak-ko fubatsu no shingi o kiwameru koto* |

| First | We will pursue the true meaning of the martial way so that in time our senses may be alert |
| *Hitotsu* | *Ware ware wa, bu no shinzui o kiwame, ki ni hasshi, kan ni bin naru koto* |

| First | With true vigor, we will seek to cultivate a spirit of self-denial |
| *Hitotsu* | *Ware ware wa, shitsujitsu goken o mot te, jiko no seishin o kanyo suru koto* |

| First | We will observe the rules of courtesy, respect our superiors, and refrain from violence |
| *Hitotsu* | *Ware ware wa, reisetsu o monji, sobo na furumai o tsutsushimu koto* |

| First | We will follow our religious principles, and never forget the true virtue of Humility |
| *Hitotsu* | *Ware ware wa, shinbutsu o totobi, kenjo no bitoku o wasurezaru koto* |

| First | We will look upward to wisdom and strength, not seeking other desires |
| *Hitotsu* | *Ware ware wa, chisei to tairyoku to o kojo sase, koto ni nozonde aya-matazaru koto* |

| First | All our lives, through the discipline of karate, we will seek to fulfill the true meaning of the Kyokushin way |
| *Hitotsu* | *Ware ware wa, shogai no shugyo o karate no michi ni tsuji, kyokushin no michi o mattuo suru koto* |

道場訓

一、謙虚にして礼儀を
　重んぜよ。
一、体力に応じて適度
　に修行せよ。
一、真剣に工夫研究せよ。
一、沈着平静にして敏
　捷自在なれ。
一、摂生を重んぜよ。
一、質素な生活をせよ。
一、慢心せぬこと。
一、撓まず屈せず修行
　を永続せよ。

Jundokan dojo kun

First	Be humble and courteous
Hitotsu	*Kenkyo ni shite reigi o omon seyo*

First	Train yourself according to your physical stamina
Hitotsu	*Taiyoku ni oujite shugyo o omon seyo*

First	Practice earnestly and with creativity
Hitotsu	*Shinken ni kufu kenkyo seyo*

First	Be calm and yet quick to act
Hitotsu	*Heisei chinshaku ni shitei binsho jizai nare*

First	Take care of your hygiene
Hitotsu	*Sessei o omom zeyo*

First	Be conservative in life
Hitotsu	*Shisho wa seikatsu o seyo*

First	Do not be conceited
Hitotsu	*Manshin no senu koto*

First	Continue your training with perseverance
Hitotsu	*Shinamasu kusezu shugyo o eisoku seyo*

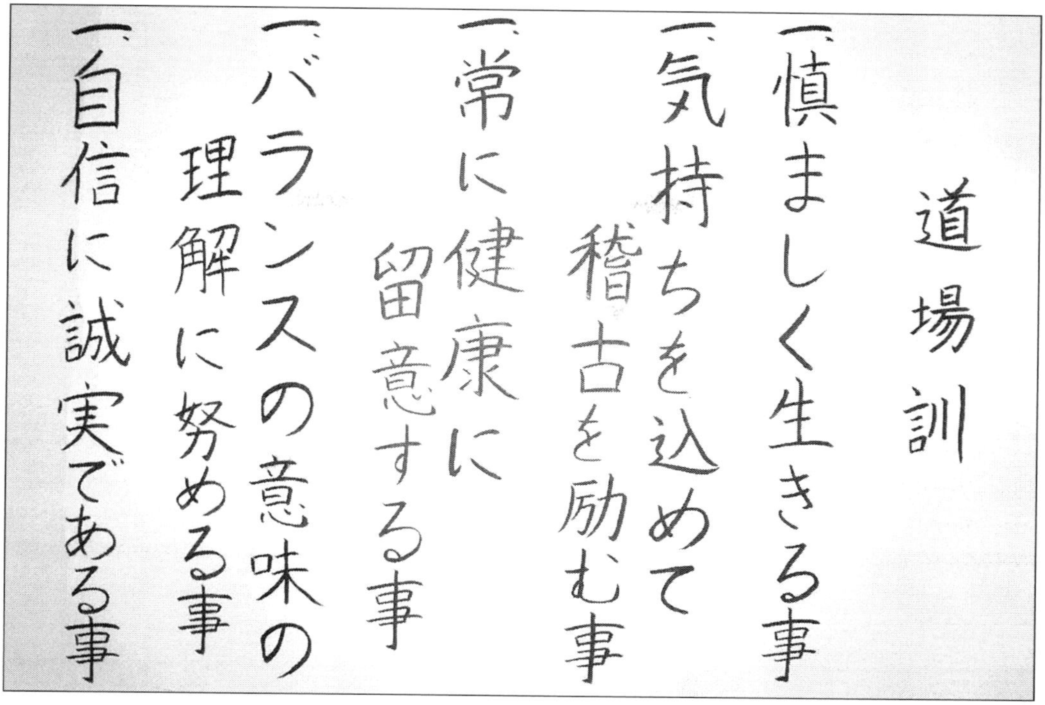

道場訓

一、慎ましく生きる事
一、気持ちを込めて稽古を励む事
一、常に健康に留意する事
一、バランスの意味の理解に努める事
一、自信に誠実である事

Shinseidokan dojo kun

First	Live within your means
Hitotsu	*Tsutsumashiki ikiru koto*
First	Practice often and with serious intent
Hitotsu	*Kimishi wo komete keiko hagamu koto*
First	Always consider your health
Hitotsu	*Tsune ni kenko ni ruisuru koto*
First	Learn to understand the meaning of balance
Hitotsu	*Baransu no imi no rikai ni tsutomeru koto*
First	Be honest with yourself
Hitotsu	*Jishin ni seijitsu de aru koto*

In my dojo, the Shinseidokan, the opening and closing etiquette is as follows: the commands are given in Japanese to familiarize the students with the language used internationally concerning karate. I call for the students to gather, "*Shugo!*" and the students line up facing the main wall (*shomen*) to begin formal training with a standing bow toward the shomen—where portraits of my late teacher and his teachers are located—and then toward me, their sensei. Once the students are lined up, the ritual flows as follows: the senior student calls "*Ki o tsuke!*" (Attention!) followed by, "*Shomen ni rei*" (Bow in appreciation of your predecessors) and then, "*Sensei ni rei*" (Bow in appreciation to your teacher). The second bow is accompanied by the students issuing the phrase, "*Onagaishimasu*" a polite adjunct used when making a request in Japanese.[11] We do not kneel in seiza, the traditional sitting posture found in Japan, as my sensei never did this in his dojo, nor did his sensei, Chojun Miyagi, sit this way in his dojo either. Those present follow the customary 'bowing in' ritual by forming a large circle facing inward toward the center, and from this position, the *junbi undo* exercises are performed together. At the conclusion of junbi undo the students engage in hojo undo training for a minimum of thirty minutes, before dispersing to work on their karate, either alone or with a partner, depending on what they are working on. My role in the dojo during this time is to offer advice and guidance, and where needed, an example. It is not my place to entertain with long demonstrations or to drill the students up and down the dojo. When formal training comes to an end, "*Shugo!*" is called once again, and the same procedure used to begin the training brings it to a close. Both the bows now, however, are accompanied by a second gesture of gratitude; as each student lowers his head and shoulders he issues the words, "*Domo Arigato Gozaimashita*," a polite way of saying "Thank you very much" in Japanese. Students then swing into action performing soji (cleaning), and the dojo is left fresh and ready for the following day. Although I have mentioned this point before, I want to stress again why the Japanese language is used in the Shinseidokan dojo instead of *Uchinaguchi*, the Okinawan language;[12] it is because Japanese is now the universal language of karate, and because of that, I do not wish the students at my dojo to be disadvantaged when they train elsewhere.

When you train in the traditional Okinawan way, you must bring your own enthusiasm to the dojo with you and in large measure too! To do otherwise is to risk your sensei losing interest in you. If this should happen, a student's presence in the dojo becomes untenable and before long he will be asked to leave—permanently. Although only rarely, I have witnessed my own sensei, Eiichi Miyazato, ask people to leave his dojo, and this has happened at the Shinseidokan too. Not so long ago there were two students, one with ten years of training and one with six years, who began to view the dojo as a place to go when it was convenient. Something on at the theater or a barbeque to go to, and my phone would ring with unsurprising regularity. On the other end of the line would be one or other of these students with his excuse for not coming to training that evening. Both were spoken to about the problem more than once over a period of a year, but neither managed to change his ways for more than a couple of months. So, as their sensei, I was left with little choice but to ask them to leave the dojo. There is a lesson to be had here for all those who see themselves as students of karatedo (the "way" of karate) and especially those of us who within that tradition also play the role of sensei to others. We must never shy away from making the difficult choices and taking the correct course of action. To do otherwise is to do karate, ourselves, and those who look to us for guidance, a huge disservice. Unless I am in Okinawa or sick and confined to my bed, I will not neglect my obligation to the students at the Shinseidokan. Over the years and with uncanny regularity, almost all the important dates in my life seem to fall on a student training day, even when the training days change. I have come to accept birthdays and anniversaries will *always* fall on a day I am meant to be in the dojo helping my students. Don't ask me how this happens, but I'm sure it's a phenomenon familiar to many. I am fortunate to have a very supportive wife who, as a nurse, understands only too well the meaning of commitment. And so, on those important personal days when I am scheduled to be in the dojo in the evening, celebrations are either brought forward or moved to another day entirely. On January 16, 2008, the same day my wife was diagnosed with Multiple Sclerosis, I took a phone call from my sister in England telling me my father had been diagnosed with Alzheimer's disease. To say I was sad that day would be a huge understatement; nevertheless, I was in the dojo that evening helping others and fulfilling my obligation to those who call me sensei. On March 30, 2009, at four o'clock in the afternoon, I took another call from my sister; this time it was to tell me my father had died. Two hours later I was in the dojo. Why? Because that is where I was obliged to be that evening. As difficult as it was for me to be there, the way I saw it I had no choice. I wasn't sick, although I was hurting very badly. In an interview some years ago, I was asked my opinion on the best way to teach karate. My answer was short and to the point: "By example!"

When we take it upon ourselves to display the correct etiquette for the situation we find ourselves in, we are cultivating our humility, and this in turn will act against the negative traits of vanity and arrogance. It is hard to be vain or smug when we are following sincerely the etiquette of karatedo. On a practical level, the display of good manners helps a dojo function properly, and so the tradition of karate is transmitted from one generation to the next without the ego of those who might see themselves as persons of stature or importance getting in the way. Students of karate who wake up to the significance of etiquette early on in their training often find themselves avoiding many potentially ill-fated situations; therefore, it is worth investing time in the observation of the dojo seniors. A word of caution is necessary here though; etiquette itself is only responsible for generating an atmosphere conducive to serious training and should never become an overwhelming presence. If this happens, it can be said with some confidence that the person imposing such etiquette has little understanding of its role or importance in the learning of karate. We should never become attached to the particular postures or gestures of the etiquette we use, but rather, quietly adhere to the principle of etiquette itself. That we use it at all is the important thing here. Although clearly visible, our actions should remain intangible; obviously present, our gestures should be subtle. Overt displays of etiquette are a fraud and contribute nothing to either the practice or transmission of traditional karate. It is therefore the responsibility of each of us to learn and use the correct etiquette required in the dojo we attend. For those trying to make some progress in life through the study of karatedo, ignorance is never bliss. Of course, if karate is merely a series of "kick-ass" moves perfected to make you look cool or live out some fantasy of being a martial arts master, then none of this applies. But for those who strive to go deep instead of high, the adoption of etiquette leads to the cultivation of character (spirit) and a sense of ongoing discovery about the kind of person you really are. Such personal development opens windows of opportunity in life that you often never thought possible.

When the training is over and in a Japanese dojo the dojo kun has been recited, it is time for soji (cleaning). This should be carried out with the minimum of conversation and with each student being systematic and thorough in the way he carries out his individual tasks. From a sensei's point of view, the way students approach soji is often a good indication of how they are doing in karate. Serious students will be precise in their approach to cleaning, less serious students, sloppy. Those who evade the challenges of training will also shun the challenges of soji; observing who takes his turn cleaning the toilet and who avoids it will tell the sensei what he needs to know about the student involved. Only when the dojo has been left clean and ready for the following day's training should the students change into their normal clothing and leave the dojo. Taking care to bow toward the shomen before stepping through the door and keeping their voices low if talking, they are now free to return to their normal life—slowly.

In 1992 when I was training at the Jundokan dojo in Okinawa for the first time, Eiichi Miyazato sensei devised a number of ways to reveal my character. He hardly knew me at the time and for all he knew, I could have been merely acting out the role of a conscientious student. Like other foreign visitors who have arrived in Okinawa for a few weeks training, my hard-working appearance in the dojo might have been just a performance. After all, it's easy to be a good student for three or four weeks; the challenge is to train with the same diligence and attitude when you return home. One afternoon, about two weeks into my training, he interrupted my lesson with Yasuda sensei and called me into the changing room, off which stands a large shower room. Measuring around eighteen square feet, and with a row of showerheads along one wall, it is a place of welcomed relief after a hard training session on a hot Okinawan night. But there I was at five-thirty in the afternoon. The afternoon influx of children had just left after their daily visit to the dojo on the way home from school, and like kids the world over they had left a bit of a mess. Miyazato sensei asked me if I would mind cleaning the shower room, pointing out it might be better if I removed my gi jacket first and rolled my trousers up before I did. He handed me a scrubbing brush and some cleaning liquid and said he would leave me to it, adding only a reminder to close the window when I was finished just in case robbers come and steal the soap. I loved that man's sense of humor.

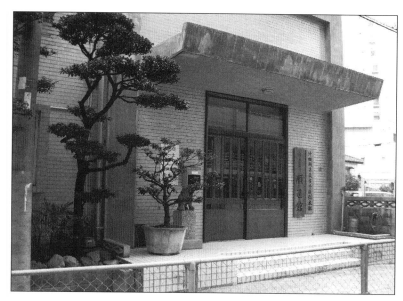

The Jundokan dojo, Azato, Okinawa.

The shower room was hardly dirty, just untidy, and didn't really need cleaning at all, but then, that was hardly the point. I was not being assessed on my cleaning skills but on my nature and what kind of character traits would emerge when faced with a challenge to my ego. Did I consider myself too important to help clean the dojo? Clearly not! So I scrubbed the walls and rinsed the cups next to the cold-water machine and took care to place them back in their proper place. I wiped down the showerheads and, finally, made sure the window was closed just in case somebody was, in fact, stupid enough to break into one of Okinawa's top dojo. I was back training with Yasuda sensei soon enough, and within a couple of hours found myself enjoying a nice hot shower in a lovely clean shower room.

This was the first of many little tests my sensei gave, over that and subsequent visits to his dojo. Now that he is no longer alive, my sense of gratitude for his lessons only grows deeper. If we fail to keep the practice of our karate wrapped in the etiquette of our tradition, we will lose the "art" of our martial art and be left with an activity that is in danger of becoming nothing more than testosterone-fueled brutality. The true value of karatedo lies not in its fighting strategies alone, but also in the way its training methods and discipline offer us a path we might take through life. Learning how to use karate to its greatest advantage takes place in the dojo. So we should treat the dojo with the respect it deserves by observing the etiquette our karate training demands.

What is the Difference Between a Karate Dojo and a Karate Club?

The problem with man is not that he aims too high, and misses;
but that he aims too low and hits.
                                                    —Michelangelo

From the public's point of view, the difference between a traditional karate dojo and a karate club may seem insignificant. The people who attend appear to be engaged in a similar pursuit, wear similar clothing, and on the face of it, behave in a way that looks just about identical, but this is where the similarities end. In much the same way as people might gather in the same place at the same time to take part in a similar activity, for example, having dinner at a restaurant, they may appear, on the surface, to be experiencing the same thing. But observe more closely and you will see this is not in fact the case at all. Staying with the restaurant analogy, we see that some tables are better situated within the restaurant than others; some chairs are better placed around individual tables to take advantage of the view through the window, while some chairs leave the diner facing the kitchen door. As well, the food each person eats differs in taste and texture, and the choice of drinks, too, alters the individual's experience of the evening. So what looked at first glance like a shared or similar experience is nothing of the sort. It is, instead, a group of people having individual experiences that just happen to be taking place in the same location at the same time. Training in a karate dojo is a little like this, and is why, should you find yourself among a large group of people marching up and down a "dojo" throwing the same punch or kick in unison for hours on end, it is a sure sign you are training in a karate "club." Imagine you are at a restaurant that served only one meal, the same way at the same time to everyone who came through the door; would you continue to eat there? I cannot envisage spending years of my life simply repeating the same limited movements over and over again. This is not my understanding of tradition, or karate. Yet I do, nevertheless, appreciate this kind of training is all some people are looking for and are more than happy to settle for the highly repetitive group experience. However, attaching yourself to the belief that by repeating someone else's idea of doing karate often enough will eventually lead to your own understanding of it is a questionable theory at best. At some point students must take responsibility for, and ownership of, their karate. In a dojo, this is encouraged from the outset; in a club, it is often not encouraged at all.

When you join a karate club, you become a member and are introduced to a syllabus. This is a road map of sorts and charts your course through each of the eight or nine *kyu* level ranks from beginner to black belt. The time between each promotion test (more commonly known as gradings) is laid out before you as are the minimum number of hours you are expected to spend in class. After each successful grading, you receive a different colored belt, but should the same color cover more than one rank, you get to wear a stripe on the belt to mark you out as being better than those without one. In clubs participating in commercial karate, it is not only important to make progress, but to be seen to make it too! When joining a karate club you may be asked to sign some form of contract, and you will almost certainly have to take out membership to at least one governing body or association. This organization will then "recognize" your future ranks in return for your annual membership fee. From here, you are all set to walk the well-worn path of commercial karate. The primary aim of commercial karate is not to preserve and promote karate; instead, it is to become commercially successful, and this consideration alone is enough to alter the fundamental nature of the training that takes place there. Karate clubs are the places to go if you harbor dreams of becoming a karate champion. Indeed, should such dreams be your motivation for training in karate, then a club, rather than a dojo, is the *only* place to go. In a dojo there is no place for sport or the state of mind the sporting approach to karate encourages in people. So what can you expect when you go to a dojo for the first time, and what marks a dojo as being distinctive from a club? Well, the differences have little to do with the architecture of the place or the way people dress for training; the distinction has everything to do with the nature of the struggle going on inside each individual.

When you enter a dojo, you are entering the world of budo. I will explain more about my understanding of what budo is toward the end of this chapter, but suffice it to say that budo training involves schooling both the body and the mind, and in doing so, engages the spirit. For without a spirited assault on your ego, the true value of karate will remain forever beyond your reach. The first thing that needs to be said here is this: finding a karate dojo these days is easier said than done. Dojo, as opposed to karate "clubs," are rare, and even when found, gaining access can be difficult. It requires patience and a display of good manners, and in some cases, even this may not be enough. Some traditional sensei just do not accept new students until they decide the time is right to bring someone new into the dojo. And even when they do accept a new student, they often use a variety of methods to test the student's character and filter out those who, in spite of pledges of dedication and commitment, are thought unlikely to have what it takes to train seriously and consistently. If all this is beginning to sound just a little bit elitist, then you are right. It is, but only in the sense that people who train in a dojo wish to avoid taking on the added burden of carrying someone who, having once gained access, looks to others to provide motivation. Budo karate is an individual activity, even when pursued in a group situation. If I may refer back to the analogy of the restaurant for a moment, students in a dojo may be training in the same place at the same time, but each person is having a different experience. There simply is no place in a dojo for those looking outside of themselves for the motivation that must come from within; insight cannot come from outside, even if the lesson does. And this is as true for those who pursue *kenko* and *kyogi* karate as it is for those involved in budo.

How do prospective students gain entry to my dojo, the Shinseidokan? Well, although the dojo is not advertised, it is well known due to my magazine work and books, so almost all initial enquiries begin as a phone call. A few come via email, but my response to them is almost always the same: "Here's my phone number. Please use it!" The exception to this is when the enquiry is coming from overseas or a long distance within Australia. When that happens, I will enter into a correspondence if the email seems genuine. Regardless of a person's gender, the procedure is the same. During the first phone conversation, I take note of a person's name, age, and where he lives. I ascertain what kind of work he does for a living and whether or not he is married, in a serious relationship, or single. I ask if he is still living with his parents or has his own home. I do all this to gather crucial information about the kind of person I am talking to. When people want something they can be very persuasive, but if, for example, a 27-year-old adult earning a good income is still living at home with his parents, I want to know why. He may have a perfectly good reason why he is not living an independent life at that age, but I want to hear it. Once I ask all my questions and talk a little about the dojo and what is expected of the students, I ask the caller if he has any questions of his own. Regardless of what the questions are, I draw the call to an end by asking him to visit the dojo blog. All my calls finish with the following advice: "When you have read the blog, if you feel you have found what you are looking for, please call me back." I am happy to say this strategy has worked well, accounting for around ninety percent of callers failing to get back in touch. When somebody does call back, I know he is at least looking in the same direction as I am. I ask a little more about his background and why he wants to practice karate. If all goes well he is invited to visit the dojo. However, only about half of those who call back receive an invitation, and this is due to their requests to customize their training in some way. This becomes apparent when they tell me they cannot always make training at the scheduled times, or they have a health condition prohibiting a particular exercise. And some people have said they felt unable to take part in certain practices, like bowing for example. Such requests are fine. Who am I to insist people do anything they are not comfortable with? But they always result in the caller being turned away. For good or bad, my karate is what it is, and my dojo operates in the way I think best. People are free to choose: accept what goes on in the dojo, or don't apply for membership. Of the few who do make it to the dojo each year, a month's assessment lies ahead of them, during which they are expected to be punctual and attend every formal training session, and above all, try their best.

The month's trial serves a dual purpose. It allows potential students to get over their nervousness of the first visit and to begin feeling at least a little more relaxed about their new surroundings and the students they are training with. They gain a small taste of the type of training that goes on at the Shinseidokan, and they come to some kind of consensus about me. This is no small consideration, for it is more important to find a good teacher than to waste time looking for the best "style" of martial art. If for whatever reason they dislike my approach to karate, or me, then it is far better for them to find someone they do like. For my part, the month gives me an opportunity to test the applicants and to gauge their reactions to the subtle challenges I give them. It is always interesting to witness a person's nature reveal itself once he relaxes enough to believe he has achieved what he wanted. For this reason, most of my "tests" are conducted toward the end of the month. When the trial is over, I sit with the applicants and discuss their time at the dojo. I listen to their version of events first before voicing my own thoughts. Seldom do the two accounts match, but for those that do, I issue an invitation to join the dojo there and then; for those that do not, I offer a list containing the phone numbers of the local martial arts clubs in the town where I live. I thank them for their efforts over the previous month, and I wish them every success for the future. Then I walk them to their car. On average, the number of students training at the Shinseidokan dojo grows by one new student per year. Each has his or her name written in Japanese *katakana*[13] on a small wooden peg called a *nafuda*, which is hung in the appropriate position on the *nafudakake,* a board found in all traditional dojo carrying the name and rank details of each student. At this point new students are required to wear a clean white gi when training and to familiarize themselves fully with the etiquette of the dojo. These days I seldom accept students who have not already achieved dan rank from a reputable teacher elsewhere. The rank does not have to be in karate; it can be any traditional fighting art, but I am more concerned with how long they have been training and with whom; this provides me with far more information than the rank they hold. The dojo blog has proven to be a highly effective way to filter out people who are looking for things I am unable to provide. My karate is exactly that, 'my' karate, and I will not pretend to make it all things to all people. Those who wish to train at the Shinseidokan these days have to use their initiative and approach with humility, not a list of requirements.

There are other obvious differences between a karate club and a traditional dojo, access being just one of them. When you join a karate club, it may appear as if you are joining a dojo, but you are not. With a karate club, you can simply walk in off the street, pay your money, and start training; but in a traditional dojo, the sensei decides who he will teach. Students don't get to choose what they do in the dojo either, but simply do what is asked of them. Now, although it may seem like the sensei is in control of the student's destiny this is not really the case at all, as all progress is made in direct relation to the amount of effort a student makes. Advancement comes about as a result of the student's improved understanding and abilities being observed by his sensei. When the student has reached a level where he is already displaying certain character traits and improved skills, then an invitation to test for advancement in rank is issued. In a traditional dojo, promotion tests are usually the sensei's way of affording the student one last chance to fail, to see if he has attached himself to the next rank, or perhaps to some self-imposed importance of the test itself. Should either of these things happen, the sensei will suggest he work on his karate a little longer. In a dojo, the level of trust between a student and his teacher is a powerful force. In rare cases it almost rivals love. Unlike love, however, the bond between a sensei and his student is never a relationship of equals. The sensei always leads the way, the students always follow, and in doing so, they create their own path based on their own experiences. A sensei will not hold on to students but, like a good parent when the time is right, will encourage them to step out on their own and make their own way in the world. This process of learning has been understood in Japan and

Okinawa by generations of martial artists and is known within karate as *shu ha ri*, to conserve, detach, and finally to transcend. Rather than the syllabus-based karate found in a club, where a long list of techniques and kata are used, in theory, as a kind of roadmap to progress, the concept of shu ha ri is used in a dojo to help explain why students may be feeling the way they are at particular times during their training. A syllabus looks ahead to where people might go. Shu ha ri, on the other hand, points to where people are now.

Perhaps more than most, the notion of shu ha ri (守破離) has been used to justify the incredible fragmentation over the past three decades within the various schools of karate. All too often martial artists wishing to establish their own "style" of combat or create a marketing opportunity, will quote shu ha ri as the rationale by which they are justified in doing so. A claim of training under a particular master or masters has, they say, led them to gain meaningful insight and thus produce their own "style" of karate, an innovative system of fighting the likes of which the world has never before seen. In truth, there are few things under the sun, let alone karate, which are truly *new* and even fewer that are unique. A personal discovery may feel new and unique to the discoverer, but more often than not, such things are nothing more than a re-discovery of something older and already known to others in the past. Only when someone begins to conduct his own research and starts to investigate the "way" of karate does he stumble upon ideas and methods that, once more, appear to be new. On the island of Okinawa, karate's birthplace, this "recycling" of ideas and methods has been well known and understood by many generations of karateka and is manifest most often in this proverb: "To know the future, look to the past." Over the past thirty-seven years since I began training in karate, I have found my own understanding was enhanced if I looked closer at the written word. Even a cursory glance at the meaning of a particular *kanji*, the Chinese characters adopted and adapted by the Japanese for writing, can often explain much and lead to a deeper level of appreciation. In the often heady rush to learn a martial art, people new to karate should avoid developing their external physical bodies at the expense of their most vital internal organ: the brain. Academic study of your martial art even at this basic level should not be neglected. In the long run the ideal is to develop a balanced character and become a person who can not only walk the walk, but also appreciate the talk. As everything you do physically begins in your brain, then clarity of thought is key to moving efficiently in the direction you wish to go.

Shu (守) has the essence of many different things: protect, obey, abide by, or conserve, and all of these are inherent in the feelings this kanji brings to mind when read. Conserving and protecting are, to an English speaker, perhaps the most informative meanings as shu is the realm of the beginner. Please remember also that in the pursuit of karatedo it is still possible to be a beginner even with years of training behind you. If you look at a person who is new to the martial arts and how he often perceives his training, you can see the principle of shu in action. He arrives at his first training session knowing nothing: a clean sheet. Even if his mind is full of ideas drawn from an over-exposure to movies, magazines, or books, the reality of traditional training will be an entirely new experience. What happens next is directly up to the sensei; new students have to remember only two things: do as they are asked and try their best. This is a time when physical fitness and a strong spirit are emphasized, a time when certain character traits are uncovered, and if found to be unhelpful, are whittled away until they present no more barriers to progress. It is also a time when attention to detail is stressed, and new students are asked to make every effort to follow the example of their teacher's movements, as well as his advice.

With an appetite that can sometimes surprise students and teacher, new students can become a little intoxicated at this stage. Their thirst for information and an opportunity to put that information to the test can often lead to problems. This is where the need for a sensei becomes apparent, and the skills of an instructor alone just will not do. Even the word sensei has hidden depths and layers associated with it, and people with only a few years of training behind them might do well to explore what they are. In karatedo, the kyu grade student can be compared to a child. Regardless of a person's physical age, in karate terms his grasp on the art is slight, and only the passage of time and regular hard work will make that connection stronger. As students approach the dan ranks they often take on similar attributes of the teenager who is approaching adulthood. Perhaps because they are too sure of themselves or a little too proud of their abilities, 1st kyu students often fail to make the step up to 1st dan rank for no other reason than their inability to behave like a sensible adult. A good teacher, like a good parent, will do what it takes to help his student's progress, and at times, this will cause friction between sensei and student. It must be understood that when this happens it is always the student who must yield; if he cannot accept his teacher's advice, then he should depart the dojo and seek assistance elsewhere.

With patience from the sensei and perseverance from the student, all obstacles can be overcome and progress can be achieved; thus, the tradition of karate is passed from one generation to the next. During this stage of learning, it is quite common for a student to see his training as being far more important than it really is. Students can become very patriotic and somewhat overly protective of "their art" or "their style" and develop the notion that somehow their training has more value than the training others are doing because their karate is faster, stronger, or more *traditional*. Such beliefs germinate from egos not yet disciplined enough to relinquish control of their thinking. It is the teacher's responsibility to draw these feelings from a student and demonstrate the flawed nature of such opinions. Before karateka move beyond this first stage of learning, certain aspects of their character and their physical ability become evident. These attributes are not like items on a shopping list that can be ticked off with the acquisition of each. Instead, students' physical prowess needs to be seen and felt by their teacher and seniors. These qualities, coupled with a character and personality that draws people close rather than pushing them away, are signs that a student has reached the borders of shu and is ready to progress to the middle kingdom of ha: a land where all things are possible, not least, the opportunity to become hopelessly lost.

Elements of tearing, breaking, and detaching point to the thoughts behind the kanji used to write ha (破). This is the stage of learning that sorts the chaff from the wheat, the mature from the immature, and the talkers from the doers. There is a kind of attraction to being at this level of learning. While in ha, a student's ability and knowledge, though in truth it amounts to little, stands him apart from the beginner, and yet, excuses him from the responsibility accepted by those who have progressed to the next level. Perhaps not unexpectedly, the majority of karateka when asked which stage of shu ha ri they have reached reply, "Ha!" No surprises here as most people, when asked, apparently choose to describe their social standing as "middle class" too. Regardless of the reasons people think this way, once within the boundaries of ha, students training under a traditional sensei will find themselves becoming explorers.

Though the idea of change has been present from day one of a student's education, nowhere is it more strongly felt than now, during this particular stage in his development. Armed with a body that can accomplish many of the demands his training makes upon it and equipped with a mind that can absorb information and convert it into knowledge, the karateka experiencing ha will inevitably start to make changes to the techniques he has previously been working so diligently to master and preserve. Such changes as do occur may not be visible to the casual observer, for many of them are nothing more than changes in the student's feeling for what he is doing. Any physical alterations may or may not be visible. During ha, a student's perception of what he is doing and his understanding of why he is doing it that way begins to gravitate inward toward his own character and personality. He does not invent new techniques but he does discover new and individual ways to do those he already knows. Remaining always within the scope of the tradition he is following, a student's technique nevertheless begins to take on a personal feel. In a cycle of exploration and personal discovery, karateka will slowly begin to comprehend the reality of their training and the true nature of its value to them.

The timeline for passing through each stage of development is not fixed. Different people spend different amounts of time at one stage or another. Some remarkable people manage to navigate all three stages of shu ha ri in a single lifetime spent training in karate, but the majority of those who enter a dojo never do. It may well be the sense of attachment many students retain, to this and other ideas found in the way of karate, which prevents them from progressing beyond a given point, a point, I might add, that is set by their own limitations and an inability to let go of certain character traits. But surely, the challenge of all budo is to continually meet such barricades and tear them down, to break through instead of backing away, to transcend the confines of the limitations you find yourself stranded in by "already knowing everything." If you know for sure, or even perhaps quietly suspect to yourself, that you have already reached ri, it is probably safe to say you got seriously lost somewhere back in ha.

Looked upon from a distance, the concept of ri (離) looks tantalizingly like ha, and for many that is close enough, but not for those interested in improving their understanding of life. The public might not be able to notice the difference, nor figure out where one concept ends and the other begins, but ask a serious *budoka* and he can spot the absurdity immediately, when an apprentice tries to pass himself off as a master. Often not tangible, but always noticeable, those who have achieved ri emit an energy and a presence that is impossible to imitate. Regardless of what rank or position a person achieves, it cannot be said he has progressed to ri if the characteristics of that concept cannot be clearly felt by those with whom he comes into contact. So, just what are these attributes? What is it that separates the few individuals who have been able to accomplish so much in a single lifetime? I'm not sure what to call it, for it defies description, but for want of a better word, I'll call it "oneness!"

In ri, no styles of karate exist, and while everything is possible not everything is achieved. A school of combat has been learned and absorbed and a tradition maintained, though not always passed on. The flow of energy and life is outward more than inward and this flow never stops. It is not part-time or temporary, but twenty-four hours a day, seven days a week, until death. It is apparent in people when they are in the company of others as much as when they are alone, for the essence of ri has become a part of them, and they a part of it. Ri is the closing off of one circle and the starting point of another. It is as profound and yet as complex as that. Those who reach this stage of development have done so by mastering not only a martial art, but also the art of living.

A secret, standing in plain view of us all that the majority often fail to see, shu ha ri, nonetheless, is real for all that: it exists. It cannot be bought or sold, nor can it be taken or given. It cannot be passed on from one to another either, although it can be pointed to. Each stage of shu ha ri grows within the karateka to a point where others begin to recognize it; therefore, no one can profess attainment of any stage, least of all ha, and yet, the level can be clearly observed in a person's behavior both on and off the dojo floor. If you are fortunate, you might know of someone who has progressed beyond shu and even beyond ha too; and if you do, you should take every opportunity to learn from him. But a word of caution here, such people are exceptional, so don't expect to meet them every time you meet someone dressed in a *do-gi*. If you cannot detect the level of progress a person has made for yourself, then it simply is not there, for there is nothing ordinary or widespread about shu ha ri. So be warned: if a person has to tell you his status, he is mistaken. In this respect, it is a little like being famous; if you have to tell people you are, you're not! To conserve, to detach, and to transcend are three vital steps for all who wish to walk the budo path and navigate the way of learning how to live well. To arrive in the place we started from and to know that place for the first time, due to the journey we have taken in order to return, this is the nature of shu ha ri.

Philosophical paradigms such as shu ha ri or shin gi tai that act as aids to students' education do not exist in karate "clubs" where the focus is elsewhere, on other things. In a dojo the attention is always squarely on the student and how best to assist him to make his own progress by means of personal discovery. Because of this, budo karate is a long and often emotionally difficult path to walk. Whereas a karate club offers a group activity, a dojo will often highlight the loneliness of the "way" of martial arts training.

In a karate club you learn to fight against others; in a dojo the fight is with the self, the ego; there are no others to do battle with, only your own sense of self. Even when you face another in the dojo, you are looking at your own behavior during such encounters. You are using the conflict with another to examine more closely the things going on in your own mind. For this reason, the struggle going on within the budoka never ends. It will at times have its less sombre moments, of course, times when the humor of our human frailties bubble to the surface, but the struggle never stops completely; at best it only ever eases for a while.

Who is Going to Teach Me: Your Teacher's Qualifications

"My sensei is a 5th dan," said one young man.

"Oh yeh, my sensei is 6th," said the other.

"My sensei has black belts in four different martial arts."

"Well, my sensei is a master of weapons!"

You might think this is the kind of conversation you could expect to overhear two six-year-old children having, but you would be wrong. I once stood within earshot of two young men in their twenties, both dressed in a *karategi*, and this exchange is a pretty good representation of their conversation. While on the face of it their discussion might seem facile, it is nevertheless symptomatic of the way rank in karate is viewed by many in the world these days. Given the long history of karate I am not sure if everyone appreciates that the issuing of rank is a fairly recent addition. The use of the black belt appeared around 1907 when the creator of judo, Jigoro Kano, replaced the use of a black sash with a belt similar to the one we see today. To people practicing their karate in a traditional manner, they mean very little. The founder of the Goju ryu tradition, Chojun Miyagi, like many of his Okinawan contemporaries, never felt the need to use belts to mark a student's progress, and therefore never issued one. In fact, his views on this matter were clearly explained to me one day by my sensei, Eiichi Miyazato, who was himself a senior student of Chojun Miyagi. He told me his teacher's views on the subject were clear: "If your karate is good enough you do not need a black belt to prove it, and if it is not, then you should not wear one." I have always felt this statement to be as true as it is straightforward, but as Miyagi sensei's views were not adopted by the mainstream of karate teachers at the time, the issuing of belts has now become a part of karate's tradition. It is worth mentioning, however, that although Miyagi had several very skilled students, he *never* awarded a black belt to any of them. Clearly, he meant what he said!

I think it is important to have a clear understanding of what belts are actually meant to represent. Many unsuspecting members of the public and even countless numbers of karateka believe a black belt symbolizes a level of mastery, when in reality nothing could be further from the truth. For example, there is no internationally recognized standard for the black belt ranks people are awarded in karate: it is all purely subjective. Unfortunately, although perhaps not surprisingly, given the reality of human nature, this has led to a kind of corruption of sorts. While harmless in many ways, due to the majority of

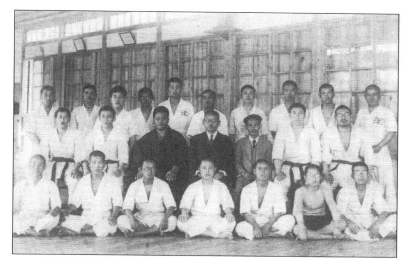

Chojun Miyagi at Naha Commercial High School karate club. Eiichi Miyazato is second from right, back row.

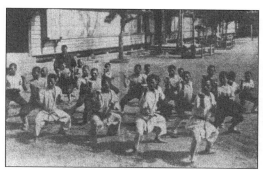

Chojun Miyagi sensei teaching saifa kata to students at Naha Commercial High School, ca. 1932.

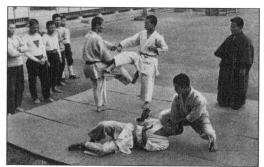

Chojun Miyagi's students demonstrate bunkai from saifa kata.

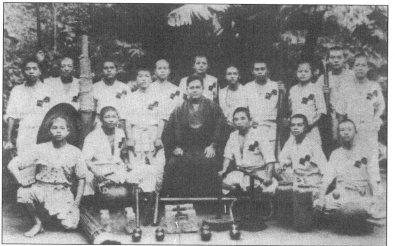

Chojun Miyagi with junior high school students in Naha, ca. 1942.

people in the world having no interest in karate, this corruption if I can call it that has in the past always led to problems for karateka, and I suspect will continue to do so in to the future. For those unwary individuals whose naiveté places them in the path of people out to make an easy buck, their experience with karate is often made far more difficult, and far more negative, than it needs to be. You would do well to remember when you go in search of a teacher to use ample amounts of common sense, and perhaps heed the age-old advice found in the expression *Caveat emptor!* Let the buyer beware.

In March 1971, the Federation of All Japan Karatedo Organizations, (FAJKO), tried to settle the matter of consistency by adopting a standard ranking system known as *dan-i;* they hoped all other countries would follow. But this never happened and each karate organization, to this day, continues to issue ranks as and when it sees fit and for all sorts of reasons, many of which have absolutely nothing at all to do with a person's skill or knowledge. Nevertheless, I am reproducing here the standards people were talking about forty years ago, and I'll leave it up to you to figure out where you would stand today if your present rank were judged by the benchmark people tried to set back then. I am presenting only the requirements for ranks from *shodan* to *godan*, as these are the levels most people today would think represent a serious student, 1st dan (*shodan*) through to master level, 5th dan (*godan*). Regardless of the rank a student may attain, the chances of fully mastering karate are slim. Even so, in much the same way as the joy of travel is in the journey and not the destination, the value of karate is found in the training, not the acquisition of rank. No kata names are given here as these standards were set for all schools of karate, regardless of which kata they practiced.

SHODAN (Black belt 1st *dan*): this level requires a mature level of ability. All techniques can be applied with force as well as applied in various combinations of technique.
Kihon (basic techniques): single techniques and combinations of techniques
Kata (fighting strategies preformed in thin air): intermediate
Kumite (sparring): from a freestyle position, can use basic techniques for defense and attack

NIDAN (2nd *dan*): applicants must have assimilated and be able to perform all basic body movements and techniques to such a degree that their karate reflects their own unique application of the techniques.
Kihon: combinations of all basic techniques
Kata: advanced kata
Kumite: free sparring, or self-defense from different directions against people with or without weapons

SANDAN (3rd *dan*): an applicant must be able to demonstrate, under a variety of circumstances and conditions, an understanding of all the underlying principles of basic body movements and techniques.

Kata: advanced kata

Kumite: sparring, or self-defense against multiple armed or unarmed attackers

YONDAN (4th *dan*): an individual applicant must be able to demonstrate exemplary knowledge of the principles of body movement and techniques, as well as the application of these techniques under different circumstances, and be able to demonstrate his ability to teach these theories.

Kata: advanced kata

Instruction: demonstration of his teaching ability

GODAN (5th *dan*): at this level a person has completed a research project into a particular area related to karate that looks at ways to make karate blend with the individual's physique.

Kata: advanced kata

Research: presentation taken from the applicant's written report on his research

As well as these requirements, time limits between each rank were also established, increasing in length between promotions, and ran as follows:

SHODAN: at least three years of training must have taken place

NIDAN: over one year after Shodan

SANDAN: over two years after Nidan

YONDAN: over three years after Sandan

GODAN: over four years after Yondan

From Rokudan (6th *dan*) and all the way up to Judan (10th *dan*) there were age limits imposed also; and given the plethora of karate "masters" we see in their twenties and thirties these days, I thought it might be interesting to include the age requirement details for these higher ranks as well.

ROKUDAN (6th *dan*): over five years after Godan and at least 35 years old

NANADAN (7th *dan*): over seven years after Rokudan and at least 42 years old

HACHIDAN (8th *dan*): over eight years after Nanadan and at least 50 years old

KYUDAN (9th *dan*): a minimum of ten years after Hachidan and at least 60 years old

JUDAN (10th *dan*): over ten years after Kyudan and at least 70 years old

As well as the dan-i ranks within karate, a separate layer of status known as *Shogo*, master titles, was also included with the following three titles: *Renshi*, *Kyoshi*, and *Hanshi*. Once again, these extra titles came with age and time requirements attached to them and were by no means bestowed automatically upon everyone who achieved a higher rank. Instead, these titles were meant to indicate the bearers' exemplary character or some exceptional achievement above and beyond the accomplishment of their rank. To be awarded the first of these titles, Renshi (skilled expert), you had to be at least 35 years old and had already held the rank of godan (5th *dan*) for at least two years. The second title, Kyoshi (teaching expert), required ten years to pass since the Renshi title had been given, and you had to be over 40 years old. Finally, the title of Hanshi (teacher by example) could be awarded only if you were 55 years old or over and had already held the title of Kyoshi for at least fifteen years. Besides these titles there are these days others, lesser titles that are used within some karate groups, with perhaps the most common being *Shihan*, which loosely translates as master teacher. This title is used widely in Japanese karate these days and is usually bestowed on people who reach 4th or 5th dan status. As well, one might come across the title, *Shidoin*. Where the title Shihan is used in conjunction with the higher dan ranks, Shidoin (instructor) is often attached to the lower ranks of shodan (1st *dan*) through to sandan (3rd *dan*). I never met an Okinawan who used either the Shihan or Shidoin titles, or its even lesser-known derivative, *Tasshi-shihan*, denoting exceptional master teacher.

As I have mentioned already, due to human nature being what it is and the lack of any commonly recognized and accepted levels of accountability, all karate ranks and titles these days need to be viewed with caution until verified. Quite simply, trying to standardize rank is like trying to catch fog with your bare hands. So a large amount of common sense is required when looking for a teacher. The standards put forward by FAJKO were never universally adopted, and even in Japan, individual associations and organizations have continued to issue ranks and titles to suit their own purposes. Now and then, the time between promotions from one rank to the next is surprisingly short, as can be seen in the case of the late Keinosuke Enoeda,[14] one of the finest karateka ever to emerge from Japan, and a lifelong member of the once prestigious Japan Karate Association. Known around the world as a master of Shotokan karate, no one who met him could ever doubt his ability and complete mastery of that particular school of Japanese karate, yet he spent a relatively short amount of time between promotions. According to Rod Butler in his book, *Keinosuke Enoeda, Tiger of Shotokan Karate,* (page 39), having gained shodan (1st *dan*) in November 1955, he was promoted to nidan (2nd *dan*) exactly one year afterward, in November 1956. Three and a half years later in June 1960 he was promoted to sandan (3rd *dan*), followed by yondan (4th *dan*) exactly two years after that in June 1962. Less than two years later, in March 1964, he was promoted to godan (5th *dan*). He held that rank for six years until April 1970, when he was promoted to rokudan (6th *dan*), and four years later to nanadan (7th *dan*) in April 1974. He remained at this rank until October 1985 when he was promoted to hachidan (8th *dan*). Enoeda sensei was awarded a posthumous rank of kyudan (9th *dan*) by the Japan Karate Association shortly after his untimely death in March 2003.

For me this example clearly illustrates why progress in karate cannot be homogeneous, or set out in a syllabus to suit people that like to have a step-by-step plan for everything. Enoeda sensei was an extraordinarily powerful man in every sense of the word. I would not like the inclusion of his grading record here to give an impression I doubted his knowledge or abilities in any way: nothing could be further from the truth. On the one and only time I met him, he was smiling and friendly, and generous with his time in the middle of a very busy day. He had an aura about him that was rare and unmistakable. Working freelance for martial arts publications around the world, as I have since 1984, I remain unable to explain fully what it is about the small number of sensei I have met who project this type of aura, marking them out as being special. Whatever it was, or is, I know that certain people possess a presence that is hard to define and yet I was always aware of it. I often wondered over the years if this might be something emanating from within me, a sense of awe, maybe. But I am not given to hero worship nor do I indulge in the immature foolishness of celebrity. I have no time for fame and even less for those who actively seek it. So meeting men, such as Keinosuke Enoeda, from time to time, and feeling the energy coming from them is always an interesting experience for me, to say the least.

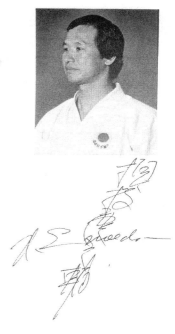

Keinosuke Enoeda (1935–2003)

Karate, like other martial arts, is just that, an art. It is not a science and therefore cannot be reproduced with any strict sense of uniformity in everyone who would practice it. Karate does not produce clones; it produces individuals who, at the deepest levels, share a common understanding. Consider for a moment the observation put forward by the English writer and playwright Francis Bacon (1561–1626) who wrote, "We rise to great heights by a winding staircase." With his comment, he points to success being achieved not by rote learning or linear progression from one stage to the next, but by the many twists and turns of your personal experience as you struggle to learn. A deep understanding of karate is not guaranteed merely by participation. The setting of ranking standards for karate failed in 1971, just as it continues to fail today within karate organizations that persist in this flawed method of recognizing an individual's level of improvement. Even though no two people reach an understanding in exactly the same way, nevertheless, education today is measured exclusively by exam results, endorsed by certificates and diplomas. This obsession with certification has now become the only acceptable benchmark, but is it accurate? People get lost in their own cleverness and ignore the value of personal experience. Budo, of which karate is but one expression, has never been merely a collection of techniques to be learned, memorized, and then regurgitated upon demand. It is instead an appreciation of certain combative principles and ways to live your life in harmony with your surroundings. This appreciation is born from the internal struggle endured over many years by the individual budoka, but should that endurance falter and the continuation of the training become too much, then progress also comes to an end.

Thus, trying to plan your progress in karate in this rigid way is, I believe, a mistake. Setting standards such as those proposed by FAJKO was never going to work;

its attraction to the Japanese was, I believe, its adherence to their notion of order. The Japanese wanted to devise a kata for making progress and this was their attempt at doing it on a global scale: thankfully, it failed. Still, the idea lingers. For it seems to be a driving force within human beings to arrange and control everything, from events to people themselves. Karate organizations, too, inevitably end up focusing more on the running of the organization and the control of its members than on the very thing they were set up to propagate: karate. Although verification of a person's status is simple enough these days and confirming that it came from a reputable source is no longer as difficult as it once was, thanks to the Internet, the best place to start is to simply ask the teacher directly. If doubt remains after this conversation, then invest some time confirming his qualifications. What type of karate a person is qualified to teach is, however, a different question altogether. Not all karate is the same, and this is a point of some importance when searching for a teacher. Let me explain. Within karate there are three distinct approaches to training: karate for sport (kyogi karate), karate for maintaining good health (kenko karate), and karate as a martial art (budo karate). It should be clearly understood that the physical and psychological requirements expected within each approach differ greatly.

Sport, Health, and Martial Art: Kyogi, Kenko, and Budo

For many people training in karate these days, there seems to be only one way to train … their way! Like other martial arts, karate has not escaped the glare of commercialism, and with that, the packaging and branding of each school, style, or association. But once you move beyond the marketing of different styles within karate and the different associations and organizations representing each style, you discover there are three distinct types of karateka. They are individuals who are involved in sporting competitions, those who are looking to stay healthy, and a relatively small group of people involved in karate as a form of budo. Wanting something is a start, but to be a tournament champion, live a healthy lifestyle, or to understand yourself more profoundly through the study of budo will take hard work and long hours of dedicated training. Regardless of which approach to karate you adopt, there are no shortcuts to success.

If you wish to get past the pedestrian level in anything you do in life and achieve something of value, then it *will* take hard work and it *will* take time. There simply are no fast-track methods and no easy options. The world of karate is large enough to accommodate all who want to visit, but it caters poorly to those who expect instant gratification. Some visitors will stay longer and explore more than others, but that's okay. What each person experiences is up to him. Metaphorically speaking, you can either hire a car or take a cab. But a word of warning here: while the distance between the driver's seat and the passenger's seat may seem small, the difference in the journey you experience, depending on the seat you choose, is massive. The road you travel may be the same and the view out the window may look similar, but the seat you occupy will dictate your personal experience, making your journey a totally altered one. In the passenger seat, you relax and let the driver make all the decisions about speed, direction, and even your personal safety. As much as it looks like you are having the same journey as the driver, you are not! But that's okay because you trust the driver … right? Wrong! If you wish to chart your own destiny in life, you must assume responsibility for it. In karate, you may well train under the guidance of your teacher, but you should never relinquish the responsibility for learning karate to anyone else; that remains yours—always. So, choose carefully which metaphorical seat you want to occupy before your journey begins because it's difficult to change once the journey gets started. Within traditional karate there are three distinct approaches to training: kyogi, kenko, and budo. Each approach has its benefits and each its drawbacks, and I will discuss them here. As I do, I will draw on my own experiences with the different approaches of training. Although my preference for the traditional Okinawan way of training is clear, it would be a mistake to assume I favor a similar approach to karate training for everyone. We must all make, and then walk, our own path.

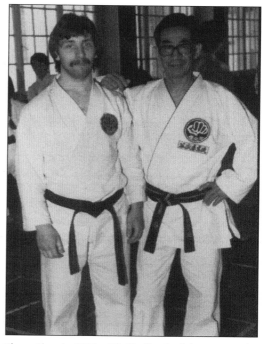

The author in 1980 with Chojiro Tani (1921–1998), the founder of Shukokai karate.

My own experience of kyogi karate—sport karate—stems from the time I spent as a representative of English Shukokai karate,[15] throughout 1976 and 1977. During that time I took part in competitions all over England and Europe, and even though I never placed higher as an individual than the quarterfinals, I was lucky enough to be on quite a few winning teams. Being a part of the Shukokai national squad within the Shukokai World Karate Union opened doors to European tournaments. I was never a great competition fighter, but I have certainly taken part in enough national squad training sessions and senior level competitions to have an insight into the mindset and physical training of those who pursue this type of karate. Kenko karate—karate training to maintain good health—has served me well on a number of occasions, most notably in 1982 when I was diagnosed with Legionnaires disease and was for a time very close to death, and again most recently in March 2009 when a lung infection developed into full-blown pneumonia. As your age advances and your body is no longer able to cope with the demands your once-youthful physique dealt with so easily, this approach to karate can have lasting benefits well into old age. As I have now reached my mid-fifties, kenko karate is beginning to appear larger upon my horizon. Soon it will be time for me to begin implementing a training regimen allowing me to continue my karate until I die. Budo karate—karate as a martial art—is perhaps the most difficult of the three approaches to explain clearly. I believe the unique demand it makes on an individual certainly makes it the most difficult of the three approaches to pursue. One could easily argue it was the rise in sporting competition that led to the proliferation of karate around the world; surely then, this has been a good thing … right? Well, not necessarily. I would say it all depends on what you are looking for from your involvement with karate. All karateka need to check that the kind of karate they *think* they are practicing is in reality the type of karate they *are* practicing. You need to take ownership for the choices you make and the people you become involved with. Many karate students in commercial clubs train for no more than an hour or so once or twice a week, and at that rate, it could take until Halley's Comet returns before they grasp anything of value from their training. Kyogi karate has many inherent weaknesses, but before I look at them, I want to highlight a few of its strengths. The most obvious positives include the high level of aerobic fitness and physical flexibility it brings to those who pursue it seriously. It encourages dedication to training and a high work rate over a prolonged period of time. All things being equal, it rewards hard work and effort, and in team events encourages comradeship. None of these things should be dismissed as unimportant. I would argue strongly that if handled correctly a young person's involvement in sport of any kind will have a very positive effect on his personal growth and future life. For those involved in kyogi karate these attributes, along with winning of course, form the backbone of their involvement and provide justification to keep training the way they do. Indeed, who could argue against the self-confidence gained from being able to walk in front of a large and often excited crowd and perform well in either kumite or kata. That such positive effects can come out of your involvement in sport (any sport) should never be in doubt, but what has any of this to do with karate? I would say very little, and here's why: because it is not just the physical mimicking of karate techniques that make karate what it is, but the mindset that underpins the movements we make, and why we make them. It is possible for a good dancer to look better than a competition kata performer if you put both of them in a gi and get them to move around. Tom Cruise looked great in the movie *The Last Samurai*, but hopefully no one would seriously argue he had grasped the use of the Japanese sword in the same way as a long-term devotee of kendo or *iaido* has. It's not the look of karate that gives it depth and therefore its value, but the way continual training over many years slowly reveals your true nature. In reality, what makes karate work is not the techniques but the mentality of the person using them. I walked away from kyogi karate in the early 1980s for a number of reasons, none of which had to do with getting older or no longer being a champion. I was only in my twenties when my dissatisfaction set in, and, as I was never a champion it wasn't as if I was in decline from some lofty place of success. My departure was due to a growing appreciation of the negativity surrounding this approach to karate, and the way the achievement of my personal success depended on the defeat of others. When I won, it was always at someone else's expense.

It fed my ego well, and perhaps this is sport karate's biggest draw card, but ultimately I found it shallow and pointless: pardon the pun.

The mindset (attitude) necessary to make karate work as a method of self-protection cannot be used in competition nor packaged into a sporting contest with all its rules and conditions, and in this basic understanding lies the limitations of kyogi karate. By their very nature, all sports have a single aim, to win! The Olympic ideal stating, "It is not the winning that is important, but one's participation" sounds wonderful. However, the vast amount of cheating exposed throughout the games' modern history, from the athletes themselves through to the judges and officials, clearly shows this particular Olympic ideal is in reality given scant consideration by many within the Olympic movement. For those athletes who work hard and make a great sacrifice over many years to represent their nation on the world stage, adhering to the rules and spirit of their sport, it must be disheartening, to say the least, to learn, once the games are over, that they were relegated to the list of 'also rans' by individuals who, intent on winning at all costs, cheated. You need look no further than Vyv Simson and Andrew Jennings' book *Dishonored Games: Corruption, Money & Greed at the Olympics* to discover the astonishing reality of 'The Games'; it makes for interesting but discouraging reading. Participation in any sport at an elite level has a limited shelf life and those who pursue it, a kind of built in sell-by date. Once a certain age is reached then you either stop altogether or continue with the same activity in a different, less intense way.

In karate, when your sporting days are over, you might, like many others, make the false assumption that you can simply move across to budo karate: if you do, you're making a big mistake! Actually, what happens is you move over to kenko karate, training to maintain an active body or lifestyle. Why so many make this error is unclear to me: people's egos perhaps? Nevertheless, the difference in training between kenko karate and budo karate is enormous. Perhaps budo karate has a marketing appeal not found in kenko karate, and this is why so much noise comes from commercial karate instructors about one type of training with almost nothing about the other approach. One might look no further than Tai Chi for an example of what happens to a martial art when successive generations focus on a single aspect of a multifaceted art. These days the "Grand Ultimate Fist" is considered by many karate instructors to be fit only for hippies and old people who are looking for an alternative cure for their arthritis. Clearly, they have no idea of Tai Chi's full potential and see only one particular characteristic of this martial art. It may be that karate instructors are keen to protect their macho image and so, regardless of the reality of what people are doing around the world, karate continues to be sold to an unsuspecting public as a deadly art of self-defense. On the other hand, commercial karate is advertised as safe for children! Another paradox, perhaps? I don't think so. I think when we hear more than one message coming from karate instructors, it is safe to say they have lost their sense of place in karate, as well as their sense of direction.

If your aim is to become a karate champion, then by all means pursue your goal with all you have. Find a coach with a proven record of success and a stable of people who win more than they lose. Go to the karate groups who advertise themselves as "The Home of Champions" and boast of their accomplishments in the contest arena. Look for the ex-champion who is now passing on his proven skills to others and sign up with him. For these are the people who are able to immerse you in the world of sport karate you are looking for. Whatever type of karate you wish to pursue you should first find a qualified teacher to guide you. In this regard, all three types of karate training share a commonality. Patience and common sense are needed at this important stage of karate training. The choices you make here are extremely important for they can have life-altering repercussions later on. Within the martial arts, and karate in particular, there are many self-proclaimed masters teaching improvised methods and systems that exist only to provide them with an income. In my opinion, once cash flow dictates a school's reason for existing, the person at the head of the class is no longer a reliable teacher. Kyogi karate offers its followers an exciting alternative to other sports. It provides a great way to gain and maintain high levels of fitness, and, like all good sports, works the brain as well as the body. With its potential for travel and personal achievement, it allows for individual success as well as team participation. It is possible to specialize in either sparring (fighting within a defined set of rules) or *seitei gata*, the solo gymnastic displays based on the traditional kata found in karate. Once you get too old to compete, you can remain involved by becoming a judge, a referee, or even a tournament promoter. If you have experienced a respectable level of individual success, then perhaps coaching the next generation of sports stars is also an option. Finding somewhere to learn this type of karate is easy. Almost every commercial karate club in the world is involved in kyogi karate. Phone books and Internet search engines provide easy access to people teaching karate as a sport. All you have to do is choose a decent coach and then give it all you've got.

> *"If you do karate you must always think about how to look after yourself, and if you don't look after yourself, one day you will have to stop. I am trying to be ready for training when I'm ninety!"*

This quotation comes from a conversation I shared with Hirokazu Kanazawa.[16] At the time, he was in his mid-sixties and looked like a man who was twenty years younger. In the dojo, he moved like a man forty years younger! Today, over two decades on from that conversation, and with his eightieth birthday already come and gone, Kanazawa sensei continues to live an impressively active life, traveling the world teaching karate. He once told me that anyone can train to run quickly over a short distance, but it takes more than muscles to run a marathon; it takes a certain type of spirit. He pointed out that those who excel in running the 100 meters have very dynamic but short-lived abilities and after a few years, it's all over, whereas those who run marathons can continue to run for most of their lives. He observed that the study of karate was like a marathon, not a sprint. If ever there was an example of kenko karate in later life, you need look no further than Hirokazu Kanazawa. There is a sense of harmony and balance about the man that

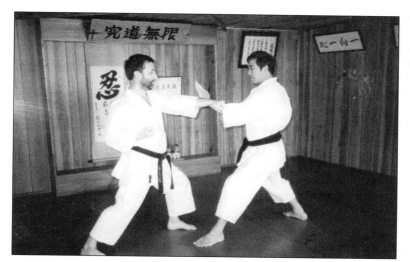

The author training with Hirokazu Kanazawa at the Shinseidokan dojo, ca. 1996.

should make all karateka stop and think for a moment, especially those people who in middle age insist on training as if they were teenagers. And while some might use their advancing years as an excuse for laziness, serious karateka appreciate the need to train smarter rather than harder, and above all, to remember the need to continue training and not spend all their time teaching.

When age or a change in your health begins to alter your ability to train as you used to, what should you do? How can you go on training seriously enough to continually develop your body and your mind as you move forward toward old age? Exactly what kind of training should you be doing? If your reason for training in karate is aimed at maintaining good health, you need never worry about fighting or gaining an ability to defend yourself. In fact, you never have to consider anything that will take you out of your comfort zone at all. All you have to do is turn up once or twice a week and have a bit of a workout kicking and punching, mostly in thin air. Every now and then, you can go berserk against a bag or a partner holding a pad and in that way reaffirm in your mind that the "skills" you are learning are somehow "real." You can train in a warm, safe, family-friendly environment, and at regular intervals throughout the year, you can pass your next grading test. You could do all of these things, but if you did, it would add nothing to your health or sense of wellbeing. For kenko karate, like kyogi and budo karate, requires a sense of honesty and sincerity that will test all who pursue it. If you want to maintain mental, physical, and spiritual good health, you are going to have to work for it. You are going to have to earn the benefits you are looking for in your advancing years. I know of no traditional approach to karate training that offers an easy option. Modern commercial karate might. But I don't consider the commercial activities certain people and organizations engage in today as karate. It's just business wrapped up in a black belt.

Those who enter a dojo for the purpose of maintaining good health engage in a training routine that may look similar to those engaged in budo karate, but this similarity exists only on the surface. The physical movements may look the same to the casual observer, but in the mind of those training in kenko karate there is a sense of recreation, enjoyment even, that is absent from the mind of a budoka. Kenko karate does not require its participants to understand the meaning of the kata they practice. There is no necessity to make the techniques work at all. Neither is there a sense of having to deal with someone else … in kenko karate there are no unfriendly adversaries. The kata in kenko karate have no *bunkai*. They are the same kata we find in budo karate, of course, but not the same as those found in kyogi (sport) karate. Kata training in kenko karate is done in order to help the body maintain a sense of balance and flexibility, and the constant repetition of the kata engages the mind too! Try repeating the same kata twenty times and see how often the mind wanders from the task at hand; you might be surprised at how often it will, and how difficult it can be to remain on target and complete the challenge. Over time, the practice of kenko karate keeps the mind sharp, develops healthy breathing patterns and physical flexibility in those over sixty. However, as beneficial as kenko karate may be, it is of little use if you fail to take a similar approach to your life outside the dojo. Smoking, overeating, or the excessive consumption of alcohol will undo any positive characteristics of training and may perhaps negate them altogether.

When you hear the terms "karatedo" or "the way of karate" being applied to your training, you need to think of the bigger picture. You should take your thoughts out of the dojo and into your life as a whole. If you do not, then maybe you don't understand what karate is. Of course, your karate is what *you* understand it to be, so if you perceive it as merely a different method of fighting to that used by others, then in my book at least, your training has limited value. Like the sprinter Kanazawa sensei spoke of, your karate has a short-lived shelf life and a "sell-by date" that is never far away. If your karate produces a way of thinking grounded in negativity and conflict, or a sense of suspicion toward others, then you can say your karate is creating conflict in your life instead of harmony. If karate is your way of maintaining good physical, mental, and spiritual health, you need to remember that none of this is achievable while you're living a life filled with discord. While your body may be kept healthy through physical exercise, you should not neglect the mind or the spirit. If you identify your karate as budo karate, a martial art, then you need to cultivate not a warrior's mind but a calm and well-balanced mind: for budo is all about balance.

Kenko karate is not concerned with fighting nor effective self-defense techniques, but it is nonetheless a difficult and demanding pursuit. Finding a person teaching kenko karate should not be too difficult. As previously stated, all commercial clubs are practicing either kyogi and kenko karate, or a mixture of both. They may not advertise it; indeed, the local instructor may not even be aware of it. He may be under the misapprehension he is training in and passing on some form of budo karate; however, the differences are fairly easy to spot if you take the time to look. While those involved with kyogi and kenko karate look to external markers as a sign of progress, a budoka understands the importance of the internal journey being made. The signs of progress by budoka are less obvious to those walking the path and are, rather ironically, usually observed first by others. Kenko karate is good for young and old, male and female, able and disabled. It has real value and adds to the overall quality of your life. It is a way of expressing yourself and can act as a tremendous release mechanism against the pressures of everyday life. It affords an opportunity to escape into another culture and in doing so adds to the understanding of your own. By training the body, mind, and spirit, kenko karate offers the world a uniquely balanced approach to healthy living. The main requirement is honesty between teacher and student, and a willingness to make a commitment. Oh yes … and a desire to live a healthy, happy, and contented life.

I read an article written by a teacher about what he referred to as a *reality*-based martial art. I wondered for a moment what this was saying about karate. In a world where cage fighting, in all its manifestations, has reduced the image of martial arts to entertainment similar to that found in ancient Greece and Rome, it would appear karate is no longer considered real enough to be effective in a *real* fight. Reading the article, my initial indignation soon eased as I realized it was not based in any reality I ever came across when fighting on the streets, but instead was geared toward the writer promoting himself as the answer to every frightened citizen's fears. If his article was to be believed, you are in danger of being attacked by a knife-wielding thug every time you leave the safety of your home. I began to wonder what kind of a world this guy lived in … and if it had anything in common with my own. I had to admit, his assertion that traditional karate just doesn't work seemed to have credibility, at least on the surface. But in reality, I think this claim has more to do with the abysmally low personal standards of many who teach karate to the public these days, not karate itself. Making easy money, pampering your ego, or seeking celebrity are all poor reasons to teach karate. When "traditional karate" is spoken of, people are almost always thinking about budo karate, a type of training that produces well-balanced individuals who are able to defend themselves against unwarranted violence. These people have learned how to do this by facing the challenges presented to them by their sensei in the dojo, individuals who have learned to look inward at themselves, and in doing so, found what it takes to be outwardly modest and unpretentious from a position of inner strength. In this simple statement, you can observe the essence of budo. A strong and determined mind coupled with a strong and healthy body are the results of budo training. The humility required to keep that strength under control is the hallmark of a budoka. For if you do not aspire to strength and gentleness in equal measure, if you develop one at the expense of the other, then you are not expressing the balance necessary in budo karate.

There are a number of errors people make when training in budo karate. To begin with, budo will not bring wealth, celebrity, or pamper the ego. Nor will the training produce a fearsome fighter, as believed by the more immature members of the karate community. Budo will not connect you to the mindset of the samurai warriors of old Japan, but it will demand you do the right thing for no other reason than it is the right thing to do. Budo will often make you appear to be less successful when compared to other (commercially successful?) karate people. And finally, budo will continually ask of you the following question: are you the person you think you are? Within karate today, there is an obvious problem, and this is it: the majority of those who put on a plain white gi believe they are training in budo karate, when actually they are engaged in something else. Now, although it might not be budo, the activity can still be a positive force in life if you remain true to yourself. The trick is to match your dreams with your reality, something I would suggest many karateka never really manage to achieve. When people gather in groups, there is a pecking order to establish. This may be done overtly if those involved are crude and uneducated, or more covertly if people put a little more thought into it. Either way, if you find yourself thinking there is a need to establish yourself, then you don't understand budo at all. You see, with budo no one needs to establish anything; it's always obvious. When people wear badges that say "teacher" or "sensei," to let everyone know just how important they are, then budo is the last thing they are involved in. Budo addresses the self and does battle with the self: it cultivates a person from the inside out, while other forms of karate training tend to set different goals and use different benchmarks for progress.

Budo karate is slow to understand and difficult to learn, for within the study of it you must face both physical and psychological hardships and discover for yourself how to overcome them. You meet your true self when your physical self steps aside, when you have pushed your body close to its limit, and when you can no longer hide who you truly are behind the disguise of your physical fitness and stamina. When you exhaust yourself, only then do you catch a glimpse of your real self. You can remain in your comfort zone if you prefer, but I guarantee you this: if you do, you will never meet your true self.[17] Budo karate is all about such meetings and what you do as a result of them; rather than being a soft option when it comes to learning, it is instead the most difficult of all forms of karate training. It asks the weak to become stronger and the powerful to calm down, the lazy to be less idle and the forceful to learn how to yield. It asks the ignorant to educate themselves and those who are already educated to be humble in their dealings with others. For everyone who would pursue it, budo karate demands you find a sense of balance. Because it does not indulge your ego and because it cannot be bought and sold, budo karate has always been unpopular among the majority of karateka; and yet it is exactly this kind of karate training most people dream of when they first decide to seek instruction.

Chojun Miyagi, the founder of the Goju ryu tradition, advised his students to become strong and from a position of strength, to be gentle in their dealings with other people. From my conversations with several of his direct students, I have learned this idea formed part of Chojun Miyagi's thinking when he was asked to put a name to his karate, and why he named it the strong (*go*) and gentle (*ju*) school (*ryu*). Although it is well documented that the name was taken from the line "*Ho wa goju wo tondo su*" contained in a poem found in the *Bubishi*,[18] it would be erroneous to assume that Chojun Miyagi was thinking only of the breathing methods employed in his karate. It is clear to me, having spoken with a number of his students, that he also appreciated why the acquisition of physical strength came easier to people than understanding the powerful potential of gentleness: hence, the order in which the kanji are written. You come to appreciate the potential of "ju" only through the acquisition of "go." So as budo karate toughens the body and mind through years of physically demanding training, it leads to a calmer nature in those who continue to train themselves daily with a budo mind. It is perhaps the simplicity of the message found in budo karate that deters many from training this way. All it has ever asked is that you train regularly and be honest with yourself.

So what good is budo on the street? Well, if nothing else, budo karate will teach you to see life differently. It teaches how to look past the obvious and observe what is really happening. This clarity in turn allows you to gauge other people's intentions and potentially dangerous situations that may be developing around you. When this happens, you can make a controlled withdrawal from either the individual or the situation, hopefully before physical solutions have to be employed. However, if the

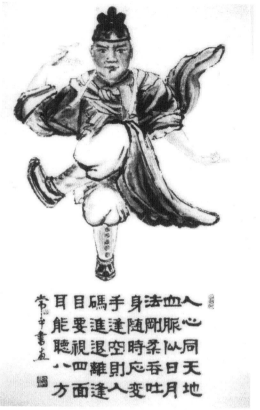

The deity Busaganashi above the Kenpo Haku, which is also known as the Eight Principles of Chuan fa.

situation turns physical, then the years of strong bodily training will improve your odds of dominating, controlling, and bringing the altercation to a successful conclusion. And by this I mean the budoka has eliminated the threat, stopped the violence, and closed the situation down permanently. In this way, budo karate is as potent a fighting system now as it ever was. No fighting method on earth will make you invincible, but many will, and do, improve the odds in your favor. Within the three approaches to traditional karate training, only budo karate provides a balance between the martial elements and the artistry of karate. Kyogi (sport karate) and kenko (karate for maintaining good health) both offer a chance to excel in the 'art' of karate, albeit in different ways. Kyogi is best suited to the younger person, while kenko is better for those who have no wish to compete against others or who may be past their physical prime. Both have value and both will require a commitment to regular and diligent training. Neither, however, should be confused with budo karate. When you face yourself in the mirror, you see only the outer shell, the face that others see. When you face yourself in the dojo, you get to see your true face. Neither kyogi nor kenko training are concerned with looking so deeply at controlling the self: but budo demands it. For inherent in the way of budo is the fundamental principle that you can never expect to control another until you can first control yourself. Once this is understood and the challenge of self-control is accepted, then you can say you practice budo karate. When your vanity overrules your sense of reality, you lose your grasp on budo karate. So regardless of which way you train, kyogi, kenko, or budo, the most important thing is to remember that the value of your training derives from your ability to be honest with yourself and with others, and then learn to become an outstanding example of the kind of karate you practice.

Interpreting The Kanji

Studying an Asian martial art can be a daunting task for a non-Asian student. Not only do you have to learn the physical postures and how to move from one to the other, you also strive to master the seemingly endless number of techniques. As well, the cultural milieu in which the martial art developed is often confusing. Many times the task you undertake is compared to climbing a mountain, and for good reason. Like those who aspire to ascend geographical peaks, martial artists must equip themselves with the right tools, and perhaps more importantly, with the correct attitude; setting out on either journey without these is a guarantee of failure. In karate you sometimes hear people talk of the Budo Mountain, and you learn that the path to its summit is a long and difficult one. You also learn that for each of us the way to the top is an individual and unique experience. If you want to arrive at the summit, you will have reached it by your own path. Once there, you will soon realize the view is the same for everybody who makes it to the top of the Budo Mountain. In reality, the study of karatedo is an internal journey, not a race to any external summit. In one of the many apparent contradictions found in the study of all martial arts, the higher you go on the symbolic climb of your personal Budo Mountain, the deeper into yourself the journey takes you. Now, when I say this, I am not trying to be mysterious or esoteric; I am merely highlighting the shifting sands of reasoning Western students have to navigate when coming to terms with the philosophical ties binding the physical training together. Implicit from the outset is the belief that the way of karate (karatedo) is not just a physical pursuit. This concept alone often requires a change in thinking for many Westerners, as does the level of openness and acceptance to an alternative set of values from those you may have grown up with. While you should always guard against abandoning an inquisitive and enquiring mind, there are many concepts in karatedo that appear at first to be contradictory. Remember, karate is a child of Okinawan culture. With its genesis in Asia and its birth in Okinawa, developing at least a modicum of insight into the history and traditions of this part of the world will assist your own passage. If you wish to make progress, to climb higher on your Budo Mountain while at the same time to go deeper into yourself, you will have to learn to reconcile the apparent inconsistencies you meet along the way. Failure to do so will result in a failure to perceive karate as anything other than punching and kicking.

When I began my karate training as a teenager, I sometimes wondered if practicing karate in England was really so different from training in Japan. I can remember being told that kneeling in seiza (the traditional Japanese sitting posture) in the dojo was easy for Japanese people because this is how they normally sat at home. It was not until years later, after I made friends with Japanese people, I learned that seiza was just as difficult at first for them as it had been for me. I also discovered that karate was no easier for them to learn either. My Japanese and, later, Okinawan friends did have one advantage over me, however; they already understood the way karatedo was transmitted from one generation to the next. They understood this because karatedo, indeed all Japanese and Okinawan martial arts, follow the same pattern as every other learning situation in the two societies: shu ha ri. I was yet to discover such ideas and so for my fellow students and me, it was a matter of trying to remember as much as possible so when promotion tests came around, we could repeat what we had committed to memory. Learning that things were done differently in Japan came as a surprise to me. In fact, many things I took for granted growing up were done differently by the Japanese. Doors opened outward in Japan; they open inward in England. Handsaws cut on the backward stroke in Japan; they cut on the forward stroke in England. Where an English sword cut by way of slashing or stabbing forward, the Japanese sword was designed to slice on a backward stroke. Even the bells in Japanese temples and those found in English churches not only look different, but are also used differently to make sound. In England, bells have an edge or lip that points outward like a trumpet, and it is struck from the inside producing a sound that soon fades to silence. In Japan, the larger temple bells have no lip and are struck on the outside, their deeper tones hanging in the air longer. The smaller bells in Japan are even more dissimilar to those found in the West, as they look more like a bowl and stand on a cushion with the opening facing upward. These bells curve inward at the lip and are often not struck at all; instead, a wooden baton moving gently around the rim brings forth the sound. It is a pulsating resonance that has the ability to penetrate the body and has to be experienced to be believed.

> It is interesting to note that the Western handbell produces its sound as a result of collision (conflict) between the bell and the striker. The smaller Eastern bell, on the other hand, finds its voice by harmonizing with the baton. To maintain the sound with a Western bell, after the initial strike, it must be struck again. The Eastern bell will sing for as long as the baton caresses it.

I eventually came to appreciate how the key to understanding karate, and everything else, could not be found by trying to remember everything I was taught ... actually it's closer to the opposite. Instead, it had to do with my being open to learning this martial art in the way it had always been taught. Many years after my small epiphany, I came across a quote by Professor B. F. Skinner (1904–1990), the noted American psychologist, which seemed to capture the essence of the contradiction I was facing. It read: "Education is what survives when what has been learned has been forgotten." When I read this for the first time, I knew I was no longer lost. I still did not have a clear vision of my destination. I needed more education, but I now understood that my education in karate would not depend on remembering a syllabus or on the attainment of a particular rank. All I had to do was take each day at a time and be attentive to the bigger picture instead of looking only a few months ahead to my next promotion test; as a young man who was eager to make progress, this was easier said than done. When it came to grasping the meaning of the ideas I was struggling with, I found one way extremely helpful, which was to look closer at the kanji, the Chinese characters used when writing the Japanese language, and in this way I would try to gain at least some insight into the meanings behind the words.

Budo

The word budo is made up of two characters *bu* (武) and *do* (道). Each of them is further made up of symbols that carry their own meaning. According to Hadamitzky and Spahn in their excellent reference book, *Kanji & Kana*, these symbols are known as "radicals" in English. Among Western linguists there is some dispute as to the exact meaning of radicals when put together to make up an individual kanji, or character; and they counsel against trying to deconstruct what amounts to modern kanji in order to find deeper meanings from long ago. They cite changes in both the written form and the evidence that the Japanese language has undergone a number of changes since the era that many martial artists look back to for inspiration. Linguists point to this orthographic shift within many kanji to explain the difficulty in obtaining a definitive interpretation and why an accurate reading is now perhaps beyond the casual researcher looking to find meaning in the written word. With this in mind I want to offer here only the most informal of explanations as to the meanings inherent in the kanji in the hope that even this briefest analysis might bring forth some advance in knowledge to those who have never before explored this particular avenue. "Bu" (武) is translated these days as meaning "military" and is made up of two radicals, the first meaning spear or lance (戈), and the second meaning to stop (止). Hence, the kanji is said to represent the idea of "stopping the spear." This in turn has been taken to mean "stopping violence." However, I believe this is a fairly modern interpretation, as my own research leads me to believe the original meaning was more like "advancing the spear," that is to say, advancing with the spear and subduing, stopping, one's enemies. A second explanation for the idea of stopping (someone or something) comes from the use of the radical (止), which itself is derived from an older pictograph representing a foot (in a shoe), or perhaps more specifically a mark left by a foot: a footprint. This suggested a feeling of standing still, at least long enough to leave a mark on the ground, and from that the idea came the idea of stopping or coming to a halt.

Do (the kanji can also be read as *michi,* 道) is somewhat easier to explain; it simply means a road or a path. Secondary to this however is the suggestion of a path through life or a road toward something, a goal of some kind. The Japanese, who had no written language of their own, adopted the written form of their giant neighbor, China; consequently, while the sound of a word differed, the meaning contained in the written character often remained the same. In Chinese, the character read as "Tao" is the same in its written form as "Do" in Japanese; and both carry the same meaning. When training in the martial arts ceased to be exclusively for use on the battlefield, or in the case of karate, a matter of individual self-protection, then "do" was added as a suffix to the majority of martial arts. The radical representing "movement" (辶) placed beside the symbol for "head" (首) completes the kanji. Chinese Confucianists used this character to convey the "ethical way" people should live, while the Taoist believed it expressed the "way of nature." To the Japanese, the use of this kanji indicated the rationale behind their training had now changed, shifting their focus away from unadulterated combat and survival skills, and turning instead toward a physical and psychological path to personal development. Thus, karate-jutsu became karatedo, ju-jutsu became judo, ken-jutsu became kendo, and aiki-jutsu became aikido. Still, this did not mean the training became effortless or undemanding; what it meant was this: the focal point of training was no longer one of killing or maiming an external opponent but was turned inward instead, toward the subjugation of the extremes existing within our own nature. As an alternative to simply learning techniques to deal with an assailant, budo sought to use the training itself to bring about a refinement of character in the individual, and by extension, the world. Budo therefore offers a great deal to those individuals who pursue it in any of its many forms and to a wider community that benefits from the positive character traits such individuals carry within them.

Budo—Bushido

The concept of budo (武道) as it is commonly understood today is a comparatively new idea and did not come into widespread use until a long time after the Tokugawa Shogunate established peace and stability throughout Japan. Some would argue it was unheard of until as recently as the early years of the twentieth century, and this may indeed be so; however, I am more concerned with finding value in budo as a concept, now, today, rather than pinpointing when it was first used as a word. Before the year 1600 and the decisive battle of Sekigahara,[19] in which Ieyasu Tokugawa defeated the combined armies of his main rivals and consolidated his grip on power over all of Japan, samurai warriors concerned themselves only with the making of war. Because of this, they needed to find a psychological counterpoint. When human beings engage in war, there is a need to make sense of the madness; the samurai found their answer in a code of ethics that we today know as *bushido* (武士道). But the samurai way of looking at life was something altogether different from that of the average person, Japanese or otherwise; and the two concepts of budo and bushido should never be confused for two ways of describing the same outlook on life. With the exception of the siege of Osaka Castle in 1614–1615[20] and an unsuccessful Christian-inspired uprising in 1637–1638,[21] there were few serious conflicts to occupy the samurai after the rise of the Tokugawa, and so came a time of peace and subsequent growth in the arts and philosophy. So when Tsunetomo Yamamoto, the attributed author of *Hagakure,* retired to his hermitage close to Saga Castle on the island of Kyushu in the year 1700, the term "budo" had yet to emerge as a way to describe a more philosophical approach to living now being sought by members of the samurai class. Although Yamamoto had been in the service of his lord, Mitsushigi Nabeshima, the *daimyo* of Saga, since he was a boy, he never fought in a battle nor, as far as I am aware, ever drew either of his swords in anger. To me at least, this casts a shadow over Yamamoto's credibility when giving advice on combat strategies, although he must have impressed the young Tashiro Tsuramoto,[22] the actual author of the book, for he continued to visit the hermit for ten years. Over seven of those years, Tsuramoto took notes of their conversations and later arranged over thirteen hundred of them into the book we now know as *Hagakure,* meaning *Hidden by the Leaves.* But as interesting as many of his thoughts are, they are also contradictory in places too. Yamamoto's lack of personal experience in dealing with the realities of living a normal everyday life or of engaging in deadly combat has always lessened their importance for me. I believe experience to be our greatest teacher. Opinions expressed without experience are, as far as I can tell, usually aired for the benefit of the person expressing them.

A later book, *Bushido: The Soul of Japan* by Inazo Nitobe was first published in 1907 and became standard reading for all those martial artists wishing to gain some insight into the mentality of their Japanese instructors. *Bushido: The Soul of Japan* is considered by many the best book to capture the essence of what it meant to be a samurai, but as with *Hagakure* I have little confidence in the value of this tome as a document to help present-day students of Japanese or Okinawan martial arts, for a number of reasons. Prominent among them is the time the book was written and Dr. Nitobe's own religious leanings: he was a Christian. Although his book may address concepts and behaviors that share a certain amount of crossover with ideas found in budo, such as developing a sense of justice, personal courage, politeness, truth, sincerity, and self-control, I think, in reality, his writing was more an attempt on his behalf to cast a softer light on his nation's past practices and make them more palatable to a Western (Christian) world into which Japan was at that time still emerging. That the book is still available may bear testimony to a certain level of success in this regard. Even today, the Japanese as a nation have yet to address their attitude toward the reality of their past; the massacre of many thousands of defenseless Chinese following the siege of Nanking[23] in December 1937 is one example, an event which took place a mere thirty years after the publication of Nitobe's book. Even the way of thinking within successive Japanese governments that keep such reality out of the school history books used by Japanese children is reminiscent, at least to me, of Dr. Nitobe's attempts to gloss over the darker side of the Japanese psyche in an attempt to give the nation's past a history it never had.

Karate—Karatedo

Originally written and referred to in Okinawa as *toudi* (唐手), meaning China hand to reflect the fighting arts of Chinese origin, the name karate meaning "empty hand" appears to have come into general use as late as the third decade of the twentieth century. However, the noted Okinawan karateka Chomo Hanashiro (1869–1945)[24] admitted to using the kanji for "empty hand" (空手) when compiling his personal research notes, as early as 1905. Popular history has recorded that the change in name for Okinawa's empty hand fighting art, like the change in the names of many of its ancient kata, rests squarely on the shoulders of Gichin Funakoshi (1868–1957) alone, but, as is so often the case, history is written by those who write it, which is seldom the same as those who actually made it. Although we can look to Gichin Funakoshi to discover who *Japan-ized* many of the kata names, identifying a single person as being responsible for renaming the entire art is not so clear. As already mentioned, Chomo Hanashiro was using the "empty" kanji (空) in his written notes almost thirty years before Gichin Funakoshi is said to have made the change. In his book, *Karate-do: My Way of Life*, published in 1975 under the heading "Chinese Hand to Empty Hand," (pages 33, 34), Funakoshi wrote the following passage:

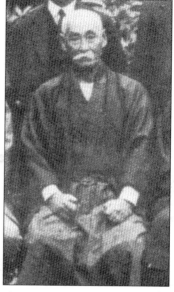

Chomo Hanashiro (1869–1945)

The Japanese language is not an easy one to master, nor is it quite so explicit as it might be: different characters might have exactly the same pronunciation, depending upon the use. The expression *karate* is an excellent example. *Te* is easy enough; it means "hand(s)." But there are two quite different characters that are both pronounced *kara*: one means "empty," and the other is the Chinese character referring to the Tang dynasty[25] and may be translated [in a broader sense to mean] "Chinese."

So should our martial art be written with the character that means "empty hand(s)" or with those that mean "Chinese hand(s)"? Here again we are in the shadowy realms of conjecture, but I believe I am safe in saying that before I came to Tokyo from Okinawa in the early 1920s, it was customary to use the character for "Chinese" rather than that for "empty" to write karate, but this certainly does not mean that the use of the "Chinese" *kara* was correct. True, in Okinawa we used the word *karate,* but more often we called the art merely *te* or *bushi no te,* "warrior's hand(s)." Thus, we might speak of a man as having studied *te,* or as having had experience in bushi no te. As to when *te* first became karate in Okinawan usage, I must refrain from offering even a conjecture, since there is no written material in existence that would provide us with the vaguest hint, much less tell us whether the character was that for "Chinese" or that for "empty." Most probably because Okinawa had long been under Chinese influence and because whatever was imported from China was considered to be both excellent and fashionable, it was the "Chinese" *kara* rather than the "empty" *kara,* but this, as I say, can only be the merest guesswork.

For many years the man considered to be the Western world's foremost authority on Japanese martial culture, the late Donn F. Draeger,[26] recorded the name change as the sole work of Gichin Funakoshi. Draeger did this first in his influential publication, *The Martial Arts and Ways of Japan,* vol. 3, *Modern Bujutsu and Budo* (1974) and later, repeated his hypothesis in his book *Comprehensive Asian Fighting Arts* (1980). In chapter seven, "Karate-do," in *Modern Bujutsu and Budo,* he had this to say about the renaming of karate: "In 1933 Funakoshi changed the concept of 'kara' which was originally written with an ideogram meaning 'China'. By substituting another ideogram, also pronounced 'kara,' Funakoshi changed the meaning to 'void' or 'empty'. Thus, Funakoshi's new karate-jutsu meant 'empty hand art'. Two years later Funakoshi discarded the word 'jutsu' in favor of 'do'. Thus 'karate-do' was born in Japan, and the literal meaning is 'empty hand way'. In Okinawa, Funakoshi's changes angered many exponents, who considered them to be gross insults to tradition. But by 1938 almost all Okinawan exponents were calling their systems either karate-jutsu or karate-do."

In 1936, the same year Gichin Funakoshi opened his Shotokan dojo[27] in Tokyo to propagate his own particular brand of karate, a meeting of prominent karate teachers took place in Naha, the capital of Okinawa. On Sunday, October twenty-fifth at 4:00 P.M., in the Showa Kaikan hall, the *Ryukyu Shinposha* newspaper hosted a gathering of many of the island's leading teachers of karate. Present at the meeting were Chomo Hanashiro, Chotoku Kyan, Choki Motobu, Chojun Miyagi, Juhatsu Kyoda, Choshin Chibana, Shinpan Gusukuma, Chotei Oroku, and Genwa Nakasone.

The following guests were also present: Koichi Sato (head of the Educational Affairs Office), Zenpatsu Shimabukuro (Okinawan prefecture's chief librarian), Kitsuma Fukushima (vice commander of the regional military headquarters), Eizo Kita (a high-ranking police officer), Chosho Goeku (a section chief from the Prefectural Department of Peace), Gizaburo Furukawa (a director of the Prefectural Physical Education Board), Sei Ando (author), Choshiki Ota (president of the *Ryukyu Shinposha* newspaper), Kowa Matayoshi (editor-in-chief of the *Ryukyu Shinposha*), Zensoku Yamaguchi (a director of the *Ryukyu Shinposha*), and a Mr. Tamashiro (a leading journalist from the same newspaper). All of the guests joined the veritable "who's who" of Okinawan karate

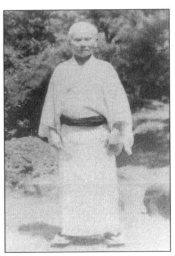

Gichin Funakoshi (1868–1957)

teachers at the meeting. What follows is a part of the communal conversation that took place that day. It was recorded as an appendix in Kanken Toyama's[28] book, *Karatedo Dai Hokan*, (1960), and this account is based on that record as translated into English by Kiyotaka Yamada. For a more detailed examination of this meeting, you can do no better than consult the work of Patrick McCarthy, the renowned karate historian, writer, and teacher, who published a complete record of the meeting, a translation from the original minutes, in October 1994. Copies of this important document can still be obtained directly from the International Ryukyu Karate Research Society, Brisbane, Australia.

GENWA NAKASONE: When karate was first introduced in Tokyo, the capital of Japan, "karate" was written in kanji as "Chinese Hand" (唐手). This name sounded exotic, and gradually became accepted among people in Tokyo. However, some people thought this kanji reading "Chinese Hand" was not appropriate in schools. In order to avoid the use of this kanji, some karate dojo wrote "karate" in *hiragana* instead of kanji. This is an example of a temporary use of the word. In Tokyo, most dojo use the kanji "Empty Hand Way" (空手道) for "Karate-do," although there are still a few dojo using the kanji "Chinese Hand" (唐手). In order to develop Japanese martial arts, I think the kanji for "karate" should be "Empty Hand" (空手) instead of "Chinese Hand," and "Karate-do" should be the standard name; what do you think?

CHOMO HANASHIRO: In the old days, we Okinawan people used to call it *toudi* or *tode*, not karate. We also called it just "ti" or "te." It means fighting with hands and fists.

CHOSHIKI OTA: We too called it "toudi" or "tode."

ZENPATSU SHIMABUKURO: Mr. Nakasone, I hear nowadays people say "karate-do" for karate. Does this mean people added the word "do" (道) to the name "karate" to emphasize the importance of spiritual training like with "ju-do" and "ken-do"?

GENWA NAKASONE: They use the word "karate-do" to mean the cultivation of the mind.

CHOSHIKI OTA: Mr. Miyagi, do you use the words "Chinese Hand" for karate?

CHOJUN MIYAGI: Yes, I use the kanji "Chinese Hand" (唐手) as most people do so. It is not so important. Those who want to learn karate from me come to my home and say, "Please teach me "ti" or "te."" So I think people used to call karate "ti" or "te." I think the meaning of the word "karate" is good. As Mr. Shimabukuro said, the name ju-jutsu was changed to ju-do. In China, years ago, people used the words "Haku-da" or "Bai-da" for Chinese *kempo* or *chuan fa*. Like these examples, names change according to the times. I think the name "karate-do" is better than just "karate." However, I will reserve judgment on this matter, as I think we should hear other people's opinions. We had a similar debate on this matter at a meeting of the Okinawan branch of the Dai Nippon Butokukai.[29] We shelved this controversial problem. In the meantime, we members of the Okinawan branch use the name karate-do written in the kanji that says "The Way of the Chinese Hand" (唐手道). A *shinkokai*[30] will be formed soon, so we would like to have a good name.

CHOTEI OROKU: Mr. Miyagi, didn't you go all the way to China to study karate?

CHOJUN MIYAGI: At first I had no plan to practice *kung fu* in China, but I found the *kung fu* was excellent, so I began to learn it.

CHOTEI OROKU: Has there been our own "te" here in Okinawa for many years?

CHOJUN MIYAGI: There has been "te" in Okinawa, and it has been improved and developed, like ju-do, ken-do, and boxing.

JUHATSU KYODA: I agree with Mr. Nakasone's opinion. However, I am opposed to making a formal decision here at this meeting. Most Okinawan people still use the word "China Hand" for karate, so we should listen to karate practitioners and karate researchers in Okinawa. Also, we should think about this question thoroughly at our study group before making a decision.

CHOJUN MIYAGI: We are not at this meeting to make a decision immediately.

KOWA MATAYOSHI: Please express your opinions honestly.

CHOMO HANASHIRO: In my old notebooks, I found I was using the kanji "Empty Hand" for karate (空手). I have been using "Empty Hand" to write karate this way, such as in "karate kumite"[3] (空手 組手) since August 1905.

CHOSHO GOEKU: I would like to make a comment, as I have a connection with the Okinawan branch of the Dai Nippon Butokukai. Karate was recognized as a fighting art by them in 1933. At that time Chojun Miyagi sensei wrote "karate" as "Chinese Hand." We should change his writing of "Chinese Hand" into "Empty Hand" at the Okinawan branch if we change it to "Empty Hand" here. We would like to approve this change immediately and follow the correct procedure, as we need to have the approval of the Dai Nippon Butokukai hombu [headquarters].

CHOSHIKI OTA: Mr. Chomo Hanashiro was the first person to use the kanji "Empty Hand" for "karate," in 1905. If something becomes popular in Tokyo, it will automatically become popular and common in other parts of Japan. Maybe Okinawan people do not like the idea of changing the kanji used to write "karate." But we would be marginalized if the word "Chinese Hand" were regarded as a local expression, while the rest of Japan regarded "Empty Hand" as the name for a Japanese fighting art. Therefore, we had better use the word "Empty Hand" for "karate."

GENWA NAKASONE: So far the speakers have been those who have been living in Okinawa for a long time. Now I would like to hear from Mr. Sato, the director of the Schools Affairs office, and who has come to Okinawa only recently.

KOICHI SATO: I have almost no knowledge about karate, but I think the word "Empty Hand" is good, as the word "Chinese Hand" is groundless according to those who have researched the matter.

GIZABURO FURAKAWA: The kanji written as "Empty Hand" is attractive for us who come from outside Okinawa, and we regard it as an aggressive fighting art. I was disappointed when I saw the kanji "Chinese Hand" being used for "karate."

GENWA NAKASONE: At this time I would like to have a comment from Mr. Fukushima, the lieutenant of the regional military headquarters.

KITSUMA FUKUSHIMA: The kanji "Empty Hand" for "karate" is appropriate. The kanji "Chinese Hand" for "karate" is difficult to understand for those of us who do not know karate.

CHOSHIKI OTA: It would appear there is no one who does not like the word "Empty Hand" for "karate," but there are people who do not like the word "Chinese Hand" for "karate."

CHOJUN MIYAGI: Well, when I visited Hawaii,[32] the people there seemed to have a friendly feeling toward the word "Chinese Hand" for "karate."

ZENPATSU SHIMABUKURO: Here in Okinawa we used to say "ti" or "te" for "karate." To differentiate the techniques from China and those of Okinawa, we would use "toudi" or "tode" for the karate that was brought from China.

GENWA NAKASONE: I think we have almost settled on the name for karate, so now I would like to discuss ways of promoting karate.

At that point the meeting moved on to discuss other topics, but it is clear from these records that the changes to the way karate was written and even which spoken word would now describe the fighting art from Okinawa were not altered at the sole discretion of Gichin Funakoshi. That he used the Japanese preferred kanji is not in doubt, but he was clearly not alone in doing so. (Author's note: It is interesting to see the way the conversation regarding the name of karate ended, steered to a rather abrupt close, I thought, by Nakasone. Sato's comment that the reference to China is "groundless" is curious, to say the least, although not altogether surprising. Fukashima, a military man, and Furakawa, a director of the prefectural physical education board, both make their feelings clear to the Okinawan sensei: stop using language that refers to China! The final comments by Miyagi and Shimabukuro seem to have been largely ignored.)

As far as I know, no specific date was settled upon to sever the link to China through the abandonment of the older kanji, and it would appear, as with most changes in society, a gradual transformation from the old to the new drifted over the karate world. No doubt the militarization of Japan at that time quickened the pace of change on the mainland, but on the far away island of Okinawa it was an altogether slower process. Still, as Chojun Miyagi said: "Names change according to the times." Therefore, I think it would be a mistake to focus on the trappings of the art if it diverts your attention away from its essence. Whatever name is given to the training people do, karate's worth should not be measured by its name or practical fighting applications alone, but by the value it brings to the individuals who practice it, as well as to the community at large. For the sincere study of budo karate has helped transform many aggressive individuals into well-balanced members of society.

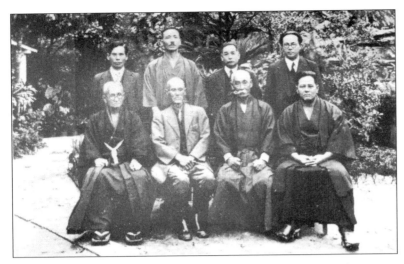

The 1937 meeting of prominent karate sensei on Okinawa.

In the photograph shown here taken a year later, in the Spring of 1937, many of the karate masters present at the 1936 meeting, and others, gathered again. They are, from left to right:

Back Row—Shinpan Gusukuma, Tsuyoshi Chitose, Choshin Chibana, Genwa Nakasone
Front Row—Chotoku Kyan, Kensu Yabu, Chomo Hanashiro, Chojun Miyagi

With over three and a half decades of training in karate, almost every day, I am aware there are no specific lessons I can give or receive that will produce a guaranteed level of ability or understanding. The way each person arrives at a point of appreciation—a lesser peak on the way to the summit of the Budo Mountain—is as individual as the number of paths to the top. All I can say with some confidence is this: the answers you seek cannot be found in the actions or thoughts of another. They are found in your own observations and the actions you then take as a result. Thoughts do little but identify a course of action; when you fail to act, you stop discovering new ways to think. The belt you wear, the rank you attain, and the title you may have bestowed on you by your seniors are nothing more than outward signs of progress being made in the internal struggle that is budo. To focus on any of the paraphernalia of karate is a bit like a mountain climber believing he cannot fall because he has all the right equipment. The external paraphernalia of either karate or mountaineering is a poor substitute for skill. Having the best equipment in the world will not keep a mountaineer from falling if he doesn't know how to climb. Similarly, wrapping a belt around your waist and calling yourself a master will do nothing for the karateka who may hold a particular rank, but has no skill. Therefore, each time you enter the dojo, it is perhaps no bad thing to remind yourself of why you are there, what you hope to achieve, and to provide yourself by the early adoption of correct etiquette with the means to receive the lesson your teacher has to offer. To do otherwise, it seems to me, is an opportunity lost.

3 SHIN—MIND, SPIRIT

The Circle of Budo

Concerning the concept of seishin tanren—the forging of your spirit ...

In Budo, it takes one thousand days to learn a technique,
ten thousand days to polish it; the difference between
victory and defeat is measured in a fraction of a second.

—Japanese martial proverb

The typically sober piece of advice above reflects a cultural outlook that is not altogether shared by many of the Okinawan masters of karate I have met and trained with over the past quarter of a century and more. Although no less serious in their endeavors than their Japanese counterparts, Okinawans also possess a certain sagacity when it comes to the significance of living a balanced life. The secret of Okinawan karate, if I can use such a phrase, lies not in the mastery of the technique but in the challenge of practicing karate every day. As Ralph Waldo Emerson (1803–1882), the great nineteenth-century essayist, philosopher, and poet wrote, "What lies behind us and what lies before us are tiny matters compared to what lies within us." I strongly doubt Emerson was aware of karate or even Okinawa, for that matter, and yet in this one short statement he managed to point to the very heart of budo and to capture with great elegance the direction in which all budoka should focus their attention. Possibly the most common error people make when they begin training in karate is trying to learn and remember everything. I did it, and I am sure most people reading this book did it, too; be that as it may, progress in karate is not measured by an ability to remember every technique and repeat each of them on demand. For those of us striving to master Okinawa's way of the empty hand, it is the unrelenting pursuit of physical movement free from conscious thought that lies at the heart of what we do. We aspire to move lightly and yet hit hard, blend instinctively with the incoming energy of a determined attack, and remain calm when all around is in turmoil. Is it any wonder then that reaching such a state of physical and mental balance takes, at the very least, a lifetime.

I traveled to Okinawa for the first time in February 1984. Back then, the airport was called Naha Field, and it had neither modern, sophisticated buildings nor the monorail link it has today. International flights were limited to Taiwan and Hong Kong. My journey from England took thirty-two hours and I passed through four countries as my flights hopped from London to Amsterdam, Dubai, Bangkok, Taipei, and finally into Okinawa. It was an isolated place back then and very few karateka from England had made the trip before me. With the notable exception of Mark Bishop,[33] karateka from Britain who had reached Okinawa before my arrival had mainly been students of Uechi ryu.[34] When I arrived in early 1984 I began to search for the dojo of Morio Higaonna,[35] who at that time had yet to acquire the kind of status he holds these days. He had become well known among British karateka due to a television series produced by the BBC, called *The Way of the Warrior*. At the time, it was a revolutionary six-part look at the martial arts of Asia, and even though it was made so long ago, few subsequent productions have, in my opinion, managed to repeat its intelligent and insightful approach to the subject matter. The episode featuring karate, entitled "Karate, the Way of the Empty Hand," featured Morio Higaonna in his dojo; he was forty-eight years old at the time and in his prime. I had been training in karate for ten years when I sat wide-eyed in front of my TV and watched a display of karate that left me questioning all I had been doing up to that point. Then, I held the rank of nidan (2nd *dan*) in Shito ryu karate,[36] had represented England in both kata and kumite competitions, and was teaching karate to others, but the importance of all that began to evaporate as I watched and listened to Morio Higaonna. It was as if a fog was lifting and I was catching a glimpse of how karate should be. It was not the first time I had seen Morio Higaonna; I had trained with him already, during a tour he made of Europe in late1982. However, I was in a huge sports hall with perhaps three hundred others, and even my place on the front line did not provide me with much personal contact. There is an old Zen proverb that says, "When the student is ready, the teacher will appear." I was ready, and there he was; the time was right for me to travel to Okinawa, and by a fortunate set of circumstances, I had the time and the finances to do it. All I needed was a contact. But as I mentioned earlier, few people in Britain had been to Okinawa back then, and of those who had, I knew exactly none! So I booked the flight anyway and trusted in karma[37] to see me through. My girlfriend, Kathy,[38] came with me and together we left a cold and wintry London on February 2, 1984, bound for exotic Okinawa. This part of my life has been well-documented already

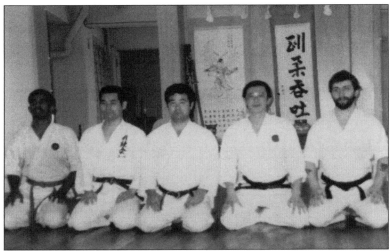

Before morning training at the Higaonna dojo, Makishi, Okinawa.

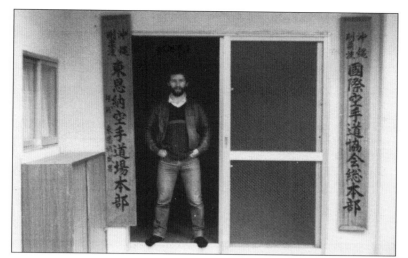

With training over, the author is about to leave the Higaonna dojo.

in my first book, *Roaring Silence,* so I do not intend to go too deeply into my experiences of that time again here; the book is still readily available for those who wish to read it, and details can be found in the "Recommended Reading" section at the back of this book. I do, however, want to explain how the quantum shift in my understanding of the tradition of karate came about and how this first visit to Okinawa changed the course of my karate and my life; but to do this, I need to take you back to a time before I first entered a dojo.

Even before my Shito ryu sensei, Keiji Tomiyama,[39] returned to Japan unexpectedly in the summer of 1982, I began to feel my involvement in Japanese karate was coming to an end. My training had begun almost ten years earlier, within a month of my release from prison in December 1973. As a teenager, I had been steadily falling deeper and deeper into a cycle of violent altercations, and often even more violent retribution, which was a common enough path for teenage boys on the streets where I grew up.[40] A trail of arrests over a number of years led to my eventual incarceration, just three days before my eighteenth birthday, on charges of causing grievous bodily harm to one guy, actual bodily harm to another, and the wounding of a third. All three had been members of a gang who had regularly terrorized a retarded brother of a school friend. For me it was a simple matter of introducing these gang members to the same fear and humiliation they liked to visit upon others. While I looked upon the events of that night, and still do, as natural justice, the judge saw it somewhat differently. Sentencing me to two years in a maximum-security young offender facility, he said he hoped the time would give me an opportunity to reflect on the direction my life was taking. Well, it certainly did that. I make the point of discussing this part of my life again here only to illustrate my attitude at that time toward aggression and violence; I had dished out plenty and been on the receiving end of much as well, including being stabbed, so when it came to fighting for real, I already held rank. Even within the walls of my prison, the choice to fight or walk away was not always taken wisely, and within ten days of my arrival I found myself residing in the punishment block for ten days due to an altercation that left a fellow inmate battered and bloodied, and with sizable bald patches where I had, literally, pulled his hair out. Long before I entered a dojo for the first time, or even heard the word karate, I knew what fighting was and how to do it well. What I saw in karate initially was a better way to fight, but the more I trained the more I began to feel the karate I was learning was lacking something. I fell in love with the discipline of training and the reality that my progress was not dependent on others, as it is in team activities. But, frankly, within a few years of training I began to doubt its effectiveness on the street, and I came to believe that my contemporaries and I were merely becoming better at training in karate in a dojo environment rather than being able to use karate as it was intended. This is no reflection on my first teacher, or on Keiji Tomiyama as an individual. It is, if anything, a comment on the way karate was being practiced, through the lens of Japanese rationality, and how it had been spread around the world bound up in technical detail and a rigid belief of right and wrong. Whatever the instructor was teaching was right. Everything else was wrong!

In Okinawa I realized for the first time that karate was about more than self-protection; it was an integral part of life for many. I began to realize where the real fight in karate was taking place, and it was in the last place I had thought to look: inside myself. Some years later I came across a passage from a poem that seemed to capture what unfolded for me on that first visit to Okinawa. Entitled "Where is God?" it read as follows:

> I tried to find him on the Christian cross but he was not there.
> I went to the temples of the Hindu and to the old Pagodas but I could not find a trace of him anywhere.
> I searched on the mountains and in the valleys but neither in the heights nor the depths was I able to find him.
> I went to the Caaba in Mecca but he was not there either.
> I questioned the philosophers and the scholars but he was beyond their understanding.
> Then I looked into my heart and it was there that he dwelt that I saw him; he was nowhere else to be found.

This poetry was written over eight hundred years ago by Jelaluddin Rumi, a mystic who was born in 1207 in present day Afghanistan; I came across this passage, in of all places, on the sleeve of a CD. For me it was a very welcome bonus to the music, music I still enjoy listening to.[41] Within the poet's words, I saw the truth clearly, that we need to look inside ourselves for the answers we seek in life. Our connection to reality can at times be tenuous, disrupted by illness, shock, or even self-delusion. I am not a psychologist, nor do I possess wisdom not already well known to others, yet in this verse, I had stumbled across a centuries-old confirmation that my progress in karate and my contentment in life lay not in the hands of others, but rested squarely upon my own shoulders.

You need no endorsement from others to look inside yourself to see who you really are, to penetrate the outer image and connect with the person behind the mask. You need no endorsement, but you do need integrity and courage, qualities that for all the talk are rare. I wasn't sure I had what it takes to stand in the blinding glare of self-criticism and remain honest, but I was about to find out.

More than just a part of the Ryukyu cultural tradition, karate seemed to give those who practiced it a sense of perspective on the world that offered clarity and a well-defined sense of balance. It offered a way to live without conflict and yet furnished the tools to deal with it should it arise. It schooled its followers in the ways of fighting; it also taught them to reject violence and to resolve problems by peaceful means if possible, resorting to aggressive tactics only when all others had failed. Above all, I saw in Morio Higaonna a man who seemed to have achieved this sense of balance in life, a man who was humble from a position of strength. So I immersed myself in the training and over the length of my stay learned as much from him outside his dojo as I did in it. Back then, his students trained twice a day, morning and evening, on alternate days. This, in theory, gave days of rest in between the days that were given over to karate practice. The only problem was Higaonna sensei often announced extra training on the days when the dojo was supposedly closed. This usually took the form of early morning training that lasted until around midday, followed by a trip to either a traditional Japanese bathhouse (*sento*)[42] or perhaps lunch at a local family restaurant (*izakaya*).[43] During such outings I had many conversations with my first Goju ryu teacher about the purpose (*hosshin*) of karate. I listened intently to his words and saw in them certain truths I felt were missing in my karate education leading up to that time. In Okinawa I learned for the first time about the concept of shin gi tai, the blending of body—and mind—with the techniques of karate, through the development of one's spirit. I came to understand that when karate training failed to take into account this 'development of the spirit', i.e., character, it became something else; it was no longer budo karate. I was introduced to the concept of sen ren shin, cleansing or polishing of the spirit, and through such concepts came to realize that on its own, physically tough training without the development of a strong spirit was not enough. Karate had to become a part of who I was if I were ever going to appreciate it in the same way as those who had gone before me had appreciated it. For some odd reason, a passage from the Bible came to mind at the time and seemed to encapsulate the nature of karate training across an entire lifetime. Without wanting to sound cliché here, by quoting chapter and verse, I do so only to further illustrate my point. In the King James Version of the Bible, Ecclesiastes 3:1 reads, "To everything there is a season, and a time to every purpose under heaven; a time to live and a time to die." For me this put in a nutshell the way karate training might be best approached as we move through the different stages of our lives. Each age—youth, middle, old—has its strengths and weaknesses, and knowing how to train according to them seemed to me to be the smart thing to do.

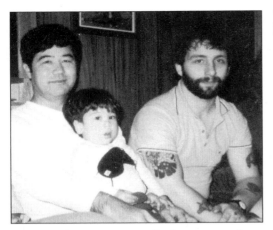

The author relaxing with Higaonna sensei at his home in Okinawa, 1984.

In Okinawa, I was finding examples every day of people who had learned this lesson well and were reaping the rewards of doing so. The island is world famous for the longevity of its inhabitants.[44] Even though I was only twenty-eight years old when I was training at the Higaonna dojo, I already felt my 'youthful' karate needed to change if karate was going to retain any relevance when I entered my thirty-something years. By the time I was in Okinawa, I had left behind the violent and irascible young man I had once been and had abandoned the idea of trying to resolve all my personal problems through violent confrontation. To obtain a lasting sense of contentment in life, I would have to adopt ways of coping within the rules of society. It was at this time I began to understand that karate, like all forms of budo, was in fact a life art and as such would take a lifetime to understand. My youth was over, although I did not consider myself old; but just as my body had begun to lose something of its youthful vitality, my mind was opening up to thoughts, ideas, and concepts I would have rejected out of hand only a few years earlier. Something was happening for sure, something inside; I just wasn't sure what it was. Still, it became clear to me that I would have to alter my idea of what karate was and chart a new course through life, or risk faltering when a tired body and an indecisive mind became too weak to manage, bringing my training to a halt altogether.

Shinjin: Awakening

My character did not change overnight, nor did that first journey to Okinawa transform me from the still rather 'rough-house' type of karateka, familiar in dojo throughout Britain in those days, into some all-knowing sage who was at one with the universe. Instead, my time training at the Higaonna dojo had opened a doorway, just a little, into something entirely different and totally unexpected. I instinctively knew I had to step through; for it was clear to me I would inevitably abandon karate altogether if I did not. This was not going to be easy. My character did not lend itself well to the esoteric, the cryptic, or the obscure. I was raised, and remain still, a very down-to-earth person who sees no value at all in blind faith. I believe strongly that intelligent people who follow without question are not followers at all; they're just lazy!

On my return to England, I began to read as much as I could about the history of karate and those who had preserved and promoted it over the years. Unfortunately, finding reliable sources of information on the history of Okinawan karate in the mid-nineteen eighties was almost impossible. People like Patrick McCarthy, Joe Swift,[45] and others had yet to begin publishing their prolific and sorely needed research in any great quantity. John Sells[46] in America was one notable writer, as was Graham Noble[47] in England, but in those pre-Internet days the acquisition of good, reliable information was hard to come by. Terry O'Neill's *Fighting Arts Magazine*[48] was the one serious periodical available to the British martial artist back then, and I soon began to savor its bi-monthly appearance on the shelves of my local magazine shop. There were plenty of "how-to" books and publications with dim-witted titles like *Karate's 100 Deadliest Techniques*, but such things did not interest me. So I looked to the writings of those few individuals who had written about their experiences, such as Gichin Funakoshi in his little book *Karate-do: My Way of Life*, published in 1975, and the Welshman C. W. Nicol's classic, *Moving Zen*, first published in England in 1975. Later I found a second-hand copy of *Zen in the Martial Arts* by Joe Hyams, published in 1982. Inside the cover, I discovered the following hand-written note: "Bill … Please, my friend, all I ask is that you read this book. The final interpretation is only for you." It was signed … "Marilyn." I also bought and read books that shone more of an academic light on karate: *The Medical Implications of Karate Blows*, written by Brian C. Adams, in 1969, and the landmark *Karate's History and Traditions*, by Bruce A. Haines, 1968. These and other books began to open up the rather limited understanding I had of karate at that time, and I would recommend them to anyone who has not yet read them. But reading was only one small part of the changes going on within me. I no longer felt that training three or four times each week was enough. I didn't want to become a fanatic either, but I did want to achieve, if I could, a greater sense of balance between my training and my other responsibilities. What I was searching for was a way to integrate karate into my everyday life in the way I had witnessed many Okinawans incorporate it into theirs.

Morio Higaonna was a rare exception in Okinawa, but not because of his exceptional skills in the dojo, for there were others on the island with such skills. He was unusual, and remains so to this day, because he has always made his living by teaching karate. Apart from a short stint working in a bank when he was a young man, he has never supported himself by any other means. He has written several books over the years and appeared in a number of instructional video and DVD productions; nevertheless, it is as head of a vast karate empire, operating in over sixty countries, that he has drawn the wealth that sustains him and his family. Enjoying almost god-like status among some of his followers these days, when I was training at his dojo his fame had yet to impact with quite so much force upon the karate world. That happened only after his move to Carlsbad, California, in September 1987. Once there he, and those around him, began to take full advantage of the "American Dream." In this respect, he was not a good role model for me. I saw first-hand the political infighting and the less than dignified behavior some people were quick to resort to in Higaonna sensei's name, in order to keep the "empire" alive and growing. This was not at all the role I wanted karate to play in my life. I returned to Japan again in the summer of 1986, this time to Tokyo, to train with Higaonna sensei before his move to America the following year. I was also making plans to move to Australia and had no idea when I would get the opportunity to see him again. The political tentacles that stretched out from England to disrupt my training at this time convinced me that my way forward in karate could no longer happen in association with Morio Higaonna. Several phone calls were made to Japan from those in England who felt I needed their endorsement for my progress; they were wrong of course, as I had no interest in their opinion of my karate. Higaonna sensei took me for lunch one morning after training, and having explained the situation, asked me for my understanding. I'll never forget the look on his face as he did so. For me it was a clear case of the tail wagging the dog. The writing was on the wall; it was time to begin looking elsewhere for inspiration. Higaonna sensei was, for whatever reason, simply unable to put the morals of budo ahead of the demands made by those who were supporting him financially. I was reminded of something the English statesman and philosopher Edmund Burke (1729–1797) once said: "All it takes for evil to flourish is for good men to do nothing." Evil may be too strong a word to use when discussing the political infighting that plagues martial arts organizations. Even so, there is an obvious parallel here; people do get genuinely hurt, and lives are often severely disrupted, and all because focus continues to be placed more on the organization than the activity it was set up to preserve. As breathtaking as Morio Higaonna was when he was in the dojo and as inspirational as he was as a decent human being outside of it, I was going to have to look elsewhere to find an example of the balance I was searching for in life.

I had no name in mind for the process that began in me during my time in Okinawa; back then, I was unaware of the concept of *shinjin* and even if I were, I'm not sure I would have known how to make use of it. But a series of events had taken place, leading me to believe my present direction in karate was heading toward a dead end. I harbored no ambition to achieve titles or status within a particular organization; my relationship with karate had nothing to do with such aspirations. What I was looking for was a way of making karate a natural part of my everyday life instead of something I did extra, or out of consideration for financial reward. Karate for money seemed to make life more complicated for those who pursued it that way. I knew, although I don't know how, that karate could help simplify my life. Eventually I began to think of ways to let go rather than hold on, to lose in order to gain, and in doing so attain a clearer picture of what karate could be beyond the often brutal techniques practiced during training. Gichin Funakoshi famously wrote the maxim: "Part the clouds, and seek the way," a copy of which hangs on the wall of my dojo. Realizing there were better ways to live and better ways to make use of karate in my life other than as a method of fighting, I was determined to take practical steps to better myself. I was going to train in karate every day from now on—not with fanatical conviction or with the mind of a zealot, but calmly and quietly and without fuss, just me and the challenge of training, regardless of the weather or my commitments at work or at home. I wanted to be like the Okinawans who found time in their busy lives to visit the dojo and do their training. Calling out "Onagaishimasu!" as they entered the door, this was their time to practice. I wanted to see if it was possible to practice my karate as I saw the Okinawans practice theirs: naturally and with purpose.

Hosshin: Making a Start

My return to England was marred by sickness. The journey home passed through the Middle East and during the brief stopover I was bitten by an insect. The resulting infection left me with a dangerously high fever and saw me locked away in isolation in the local hospital. It took two weeks to recover enough for the health authorities to allow me to leave and a further couple of months to recover the level of fitness I had enjoyed prior to my encounter with the mysterious Arabian bug. During that time,

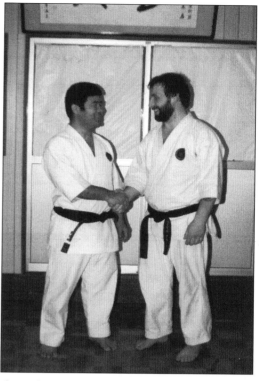

The author and Higaonna sensei just after the Tokyo grading test.

I continued to read as much as I could and do what physical training my body would tolerate. I also began to run. Kathy and I had moved to a small coastal town in England's southwest, and running the cliff paths with the wind blowing in off the Atlantic Ocean had a way of restoring a very real sense of being alive. Each morning my run ended in a local park, and there, I found a secluded spot to practice my karate. I was never comfortable training in public though, not that many caught a glimpse of me kicking and punching my way through the kata of Goju ryu. So I began to explore the possibility of creating my own dojo, and over the following months, did just that. I found an unused workshop over a row of lock-up garages and with the meager resources available, transformed the space into a dojo. It was a huge investment in both time and money; the time I had, but the money was in short supply as it took me around six weeks to find work. Throughout this time, Kathy supported me in my efforts, and within a few weeks of taking on the building, I had a small but entirely adequate dojo in which to pursue my exploration of karatedo. I gave the dojo a name: Jin Sei Do (Way of Life). It was here that my morning run along the coastal paths now ended each day, and my exploration of Okinawan training methods began in earnest. However, I soon discovered it is one thing to train hard when pushed by a sensei, such as Morio Higaonna, and quite another

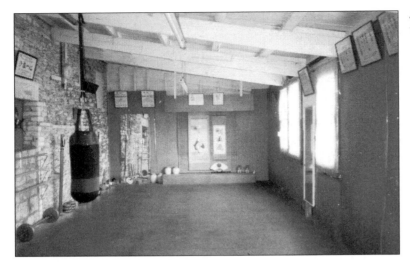

Jin Sei Do, the author's first dojo.

to bring about such levels of intensity from the realms of self-motivation. I must confess, on some days, training hardly came close to the intensity of the training in Okinawa, but then on others, I found myself literally exhausted from my marathon efforts. In my own rather naïve way, I was attempting to find a kind of clarity that I now understand does not exist. I was expecting to see the way ahead make itself known to me, as if through all my hard work and sweat, the clouds would part and somehow "reveal," a la Funakoshi, what to do and how to do it. Unfortunately, budo does not give up its treasures quite so easily. If all that were required was 'hard work', then progress would have been assured, but no, to understand budo and to reap the rewards of its true worth would require much more than simple physical exertion. I was going to have to find a sense of direction. The trouble is, when you are lost it is better to know where you are going than where you have been. When I was in Okinawa training with Higaonna sensei, I thought I knew where I was going; now, I was beginning to doubt myself.

I had this small idea in the back of my mind that wanting something too much might be the very thing that would keep me from getting it. I'm not sure if this idea came from something I read or something someone told me; nevertheless, the idea began to geminate and grow and before too long it was at the forefront of my thinking when it came to making progress. There was plenty about Goju ryu I did not know back then, including several of the kata as handed down and preserved by Morio Higaonna. Returning to England in 1984, I made contact with a group that was affiliated with Higaonna sensei's organization and through that connection, hoped to learn more. Within a relatively short time, however, this connection would prove to be less than fruitful. I understood instinctively that if progress were to be made, I had to make it myself, from within, and through my own discoveries and experiences. So began the changes to my daily training; sometimes it lasted only forty-five minutes or an hour, sometimes much longer. It all depended on what other commitments I had that day. My idea was to have karate find its natural place in my daily life and not to force it into a strictly defined time when all else was required to yield. In Okinawa, I discovered that quite a lot of older people had been going to their dojo each day for decades. No one in the West knew their names; they had no global organizations behind them, and yet they were in fact senior to many of the "celebrity" sensei that the West thought of as Okinawa's finest. I was introduced to people like Seiko Kina,[49] a man whose karate pedigree was second to none, and yet had a dojo no larger than an average-sized bedroom. He had few students apart from his son and a number of older gentlemen who I saw training on each of my three visits to his dojo, the Junkokan. I needed to find a sense of balance and began to think of Kina sensei's approach as an example of how to achieve it. So over the next four years, as I endeavored to establish and consolidate the place karate training was going to have in the rest of my life, I read more, trained a little less, and learned to live a whole lot happier.

Bussho: Doing Something Every Day

Climbing into my do-gi[50] each day was one thing, but I also had to find ways of changing how I felt on various matters too, and this was achieved by arguing with myself. If anything, this is where the real ground was covered. Now, as strange as this may seem at first (arguing with myself), it was in fact nothing more than listening carefully to my own thoughts and then putting those thoughts to the test, taking an opposing view to see where it got me. It was like a one-man debating society going on in my head: first, training hard in the techniques of karate and then spending time silently working my way through my thoughts. I did try to engage others in these conversations, but other karateka were not interested in the things I was thinking about. My mind was full of ideas of how to achieve a sense of balance in life and how to see beyond the obvious. For example, one day, after a particularly strenuous hour of kata training, I asked myself this question: How many techniques are there in a kata? The simple answer came by counting how many punches, blocks, strikes, and kicks were performed. But then, what about my breathing? Surely, the correct method of breathing is vital to the integrity of

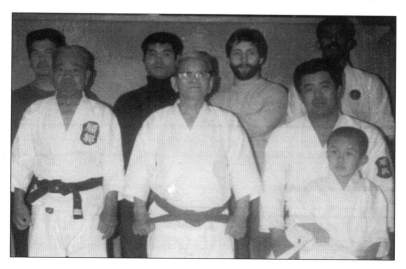

After training at the Junkokan. The author is behind and to the right of Seiko Kina sensei (center).

each technique, is it not? So where should I be inhaling and exhaling? And was there anywhere in the kata where my breath should be held? Consideration was also given to how I moved from one posture to the next, and if the prescribed method of movement was being used, *tai sabaki, suri ashi, chakuchi*,[51] or just a series of controlled falls to get into the next position. I also wondered if bringing all these things together on demand was a technique in itself.

It was my habit back then, as indeed it is today, to play some Okinawan or Japanese music quietly while getting changed, following my morning practice. I liked the feeling of connection it gave to the activity I had a moment ago engaged in, and it stirred pleasant memories of my time on the island. One morning while listening to a tape of the *shakuhachi*[52] being played, a thought came to mind. The music was slow and soft, and full of mood and atmosphere. It dawned on me that the silence between the notes was as necessary for creating the mood as the notes themselves. Music was not made just from a collection of notes, but from the gaps between each note too! Get the length and inclination of the gaps wrong, and you end up with just as awful a noise as if the notes were flat. It was the same with kata. Move from one posture to the next poorly, and the reliability of the technique is lost. It became apparent there were far more techniques in a kata than the obvious kicking, punching, and blocking. If I wanted to appreciate the lessons locked away within each kata, I was going to have to look at them differently and pay a lot more attention to what I was doing and how I was doing it. Returning home that morning I began to see the world in a different way and noticed for the first time that the doorways in my house were in effect pieces of nothing in the walls allowing movement from one room to another. The windows too, were smaller bits of nothing that let the light in from outside. Even the tea I was drinking was occupying the previously empty space in the cup. All the useful solid objects in my home used space, and the nothingness of the space was as useful and important as the surrounding solidness of the object. You could say it is the space within and between objects that gave them their significance, just as the gaps between these words allow you to read my thoughts long after I have written them:

Imagineiftherewerenone!

During my early years of training in karate, I became very judgmental of others. However, there was an emerging awareness of how negative an activity this was and how such negativity only served to divert me from making progress. I made a conscious choice to stop looking at what others were doing and to focus instead on my own training, and its shortcomings. It was no easy task; I was young and very opinionated, and to tell the truth, not altogether sure if what I was attempting was something fanciful and perhaps even misguided. Time would tell. At the time, I was content to continue with my efforts to change and to do at least one thing each day that allowed karate to permeate into other aspects of my life. Vivid memories still linger from that time, of walking away from people whose behavior toward me would have booked them a trip to the hospital only a few short years earlier. Now I was learning when to speak out and when to hold my tongue, when to make my point and when to let the moment pass. None of this behavior came easily to me, and I understand now that significant changes in the way we deal with life are always achieved through struggle; my frustrations were taken out on the kick bag and the makiwara[53] and in that way I left the dojo ready to continue toward a better way of life.

Jikaku: Self-realization

When the concept of *jikaku* is first introduced to the students at my dojo, it is often mistaken for something more important than it is; people have their own opinion of what jikaku really means, but usually they over-engineer the idea. For self-realization is nothing more than developing a particular level of clarity in the way you see your situation in life. Problems with your ability to do this arise from a common human error that many of us make, the mistaken belief that we are in some way more important than others! We come to such beliefs by many paths: racial, religious, political, financial, academic, and social, to name but a few, all or any of which can lead you to believe you are somehow better or more deserving than other human beings. First-world societies actually encourage us to feel this way. Wealthy people are held up to be more valuable to society than people with less wealth. University graduates are considered automatically more intelligent than non-graduates. And perhaps the saddest and most erroneous belief of all, many individuals feel that fair-skinned people are somehow superior to dark-skinned people. All these assumptions and beliefs stem from the depths of ignorance, of course, but for all that, they are opinions that are widely held in many parts of the world. It takes no more than a split-second to dispel such nonsense, but for that to happen you must be prepared to listen and to accept what may be more than one inconvenient truth. Is it not worth taking a moment to consider this: given that your life is finite, what should you do with it? How can you pass through your existence in a meaningful way, a way that brings contentment to you while causing as little negative impact upon others as possible? I do not have the answers for you. What works for me may not work for you. We are not clones and therefore we all come to *shinjin*—an awakening of the senses—with our own unique perspective. You choose the circumstance of *hosshin*—how you make a start for yourself—and follow through with *bussho*—the things you choose to do each day—that will eventually bring you closer to *jikaku*—a deeper level of self-realization. When you achieve jikaku and arrive at a new level of self-realization, you come to appreciate that the way of karate is endless,[54] and in that awakening you recognize the need to make a fresh start and to do things every day that will eventually deliver an even clearer sense of self-realization.

The cycle of shinjin, hosshin, bussho, and jikaku flows through the lives of all who practice their karate with budo in mind. It is a cycle of learning and progression that was so elegantly described in the words of the poet T. S. Eliot (1888–1965) when he wrote: "We shall not cease from exploration, and the end of all our exploring will be to arrive where we started and to know the place for the first time." Each time you return, you are different, changed by the journey. Those changes allow you to envisage a finer and more balanced way to live. So you begin again. In the Jundokan, my late teacher's dojo in Okinawa, a banner on the shomen written in the most wonderful hand proclaims, *Kyu Do Mu Gen*, i.e., "Investigating the Way is Endless." As I write this book, I am in my thirty-seventh year of training in karate; the longer I continue to practice, the more deeply I appreciate the meaning of that proverb.

Unraveling Knots in The Thread of Life

Over a period of about eight years, beginning in the early 1990s, I began taking a closer look around the world at the various religious and philosophical beliefs people held, and saw in many of them much to be admired. I also noticed there was quite a lot of common ground. I was initially astonished to discover, for example, how the sacred text of Judeism, the Torah, tells the same story as the first five books of the Bible, known to Christians as the books of the Old Testament. And far from teaching a radically different doctrine, as I had assumed, I was surprised how much the Christian Bible and the Koran (Quran) of Islam have in common. Often the same names came up again and again in all three books, Abraham, for example. Jesus too is mentioned by name many times in the Koran. That the god of the Christians was a Jew, who in turn is revered in the teachings of Islam as a prophet, only served to make me wonder if what I was discovering here was a basic human need for comfort. Also, I began to see why the notion of faith is so important in religion, as without faith many religious teachings become confusing and even contradictory.

The doctrine of the Roman Catholic Church I endured as a child did little to prepare me for tolerance of those who were different from me, and as soon as I was able I left its teachings behind. Growing older, I have come to appreciate that the concept of god is not a puzzle wrapped in an enigma as I was taught as a five-year-old child, but a deeply rooted need in some to believe in a better existence than their present one. At any rate, I discovered nothing within the teachings of the world's most popular religions to convince me they had anything unique to say, just the opposite. Many remarkable teachers from history have given the world enormously powerful gifts of thought and of action. They have left behind words of profound philosophical wisdom, and in the displays of compassion for others during their lives, examples of the way mankind might live if only it had the desire to do so. How poignant that for all our technological sophistication these days, mankind as a whole continually fails to understand the value of simplicity.

Zen: The Way Unseen

Within the martial arts much is made of a supposed connection between the philosophy of Zen (Chinese: *Cha'an*) and karate. I would argue, but only politely of course, that such a connection has more to do with the Japanese psyche than the mindset of the average karateka today. For the overwhelming majority of the estimated forty million plus karate and *kobudoka* in the world these days,[55] karate is just a hobby and they neither search for nor aspire to the same frame of mind as the samurai warriors of old Japan. Had karate spread across the globe directly from Okinawa, and not filtered through the Japanese desire to hold on to their undoubted military prowess of long ago, then I have no doubt you would hear less of karate's connection with Zen and see fewer images of karateka posing with samurai swords. Parallel themes and ideas are found in Zen and Japanese karate because Japanese karate schools have borrowed much of their philosophical ideas from Zen. As I mentioned earlier, overlapping ideas are as common throughout the world's major religions and philosophies as they are in all of man's great endeavors. In many religions, the importance of particular historical characters and the significance of certain dates throughout the year are easily found once you take the time to look, as are stories of virgin births and visitations from angels, particularly the angel Gabriel: coincidence? I think the nature of faith and the essence of Zen share a common thread. If you have faith in a god or can grasp the concept of Zen, you have no need for proof or explanations; if, on the other hand, you do not have faith in a god and do not grasp the concept of Zen, then no explanation will be adequate or proof suffice. Such is the dilemma when you try to fathom the unfathomable. Still, it would be a mistake to ponder too long on such things, for far less weighty matters in life, like balance and a sense of humor also share these characteristics; but no one worries too much if you fall off your bike or you don't get a joke.

By hitching the philosophy of Zen onto their karate, it allowed the Japanese to ignore Okinawan culture altogether and make karate their own. This they did with the help of some Okinawan karate teachers who resided in Japan; they willingly collaborated with the push to absorb their native method of self-protection into the pantheon of Japanese fighting arts. By changing the names of several kata to make them sound more Japanese, *passai* became *bassai*, *naifanchin* became *tekki*, and so on; the kata were stripped of their cultural links to Okinawa and China. At a time when the Okinawan language (*Uchinaguchi*) was being purged from the population through the school system and replaced by standard Japanese (*Nihongo*), it should come as no surprise to find the same pressure to conform was being applied within karate. It never ceases to amaze me how humanity can take something that is essentially good, twist it, bend it, and stretch it into something unrecognizable from the original, and yet still claim to respect it. With the resurgence of fundamentalism in the world's major religions, we have done this with ancient wisdom of great spiritual import. With politics we have done this with democracy and the concept of leadership; and even ecologically, we have done this with the very planet we all depend upon for life. If indeed there is a primal need for man to have faith in something, it is a pity that faith is seldom placed in his fellow man.

I read somewhere that Zen was a finger, pointing directly to clarity. My first thought when I read this was "Whose finger?" In the building of temples and in the industry of commercial expansion, humankind has taken Zen, a concept that defies packaging, and wrapped it in his own self-importance. The idea that one human being can be more "enlightened" simply by adhering to a particular set of rituals and reciting words written by another human being is an absurdity, and I'm reminded of a parable from Zen that points to the fallacy of "attachment" to rituals:

> One day a young monk was sitting in zazen, the traditional kneeling posture familiar to students of both Zen and karate; he was deep in meditation. The master passed by and seeing the young monk, stopped and asked: "What are you doing?"
> The young monk opened his eyes and said, "I'm practicing zazen so that I may gain enlightenment."
> The master then picked up a piece of broken roof tile lying nearby and began to rub it with his sleeve.
> "What are you doing?" said the young monk.
> "I'm making a mirror," said the master.
> "But you can't make a mirror like that!" said the monk.
> To which the master replied, "And you can't gain enlightenment like that either!"

Zen, like religious piety, grows from within or it does not grow at all. It germinates inside an individual and expands unreservedly outward toward others, or it does not develop at all. It cannot be owned by some and dispensed to others deemed less knowing. There is a kind of institutionalized arrogance sometimes found within philosophies like Zen. Such an approach to the understanding and acceptance of our fellow man is, I believe, ultimately unhealthy for the human spirit. There is nothing unique to be found in Zen, nothing that cannot be found in other sources of wisdom: no profound knowledge that will help the martial artist gain a level of clarity he could not gain by other means. I believe the claims made by some on behalf of Zen speak more to the earthly desires of a few and the misguided faith of others who truly want to believe, than to anything based on a wholesome truth. If you understand the concept of Zen to any degree at all, you will also understand the error of trying to claim anything. The more you try to hold on to Zen the less chance you have of appreciating what it has to offer. Zen, as I understand it, is a secret hidden in plain view, it is the oxygen in the air and the 'common' in common sense, and yet for all its simplicity it seems beyond the reach of many, a condition touched upon by the English poet Alexander Pope (1688–1744) when he noted, "Some people never learn anything because they understand everything too quickly."

Bunbu ryo do: The Way of The Martial Scholar

In the early part of the twentieth century, when Okinawan karate teachers were first asked to provide names for their karate by the Butokukai in Japan, they struggled to come up with a name that did justice to the martial art they practiced. Many of those from the royal capital, Shuri, settled on poetic sounding names that conjured up the spirit of their homeland; Choshin Chibana (1886–1969) chose the name Kobayashi ryu, the small forest school. While other teachers with a similar lineage later chose comparable names like the young forest school, and the pine forest school, Shobayashi ryu

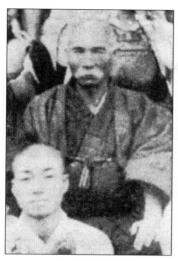

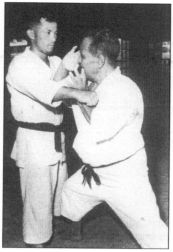

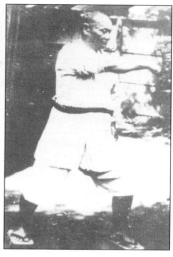

Anko Itosu (1831–1915), one of Funakoshi's main teachers.

The author's teacher, Eiichi Miyazato, training with his sensei, Chojun Miyagi, ca. 1951.

Choki Motobu training on the makiwara. Note the lack of hikite being used.

and Matsubayashi ryu respectively, others chose to honor their teacher, or teachers, and in doing so took kanji from their names to give a name to their karate. Juhatsu Kyoda (1887–1968), for example, called his karate Tou'on ryu by simply using an alternative reading of the kanji used to write his teacher's family name: pronounced Higashionna in the Okinawan language, Uchinaguchi. Others struggled a little with what to do for the best, like Kenwa Mabuni (1893–1957) who at first called his karate Hanko ryu, meaning the 'half-hard school' of karate. Later however he changed his mind and renamed it Shito ryu, a name he arrived at by using the first kanji from the family name of each of his two principal teachers, Kanryo Higashionna and Anko Itosu. The first Okinawan to name his karate in accordance with the Butokukai's request was Chojun Miyagi (1888–1953) who registered the name Goju ryu, the strong and gentle school, in 1930.

My own belief as far as attaching names to the various schools of karate is concerned is echoed in a line from Romeo and Juliet, written by the great Bard himself, William Shakespeare: "What's in a name? That which we call a rose by any other name would smell as sweet." Karate, like every other martial art, is nothing more than the personal expression of an individual's physical skills combined with his intellectual understanding and depth of feeling for what he knows. It is not fixed nor is there an end to it; the study of karate is quite literally endless! Packaging, branding, distributing, and franchising are all terms I have heard applied to karate by individuals and groups intent on selling karate to others. But karate is not for sale. If you wish to have ownership of your karate, you start by taking responsibility for it. The first act in doing that involves finding a good teacher. The second act is to devote yourself to being a good student. The third act is to be honest with yourself. The fourth act is to become independent, not when being a

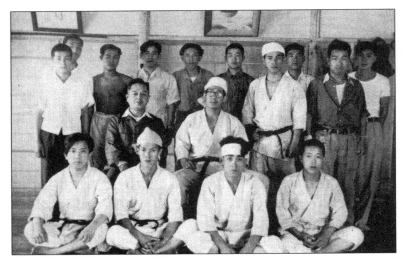

Kenwa Mabuni with his first generation of Japanese students, Chojiro Tani is sitting in the center of the group, next to his teacher, ca. 1948.

student becomes difficult, but when the time is right. In the teachings of budo there is the concept of *musei jinko*, of calling people without using the voice; in other words, a good person will attract others by his example. If you can approach your karate in this way, you will give yourself a chance to find what you are searching for. Accepting guidance from your teacher while making your own way, you display genuine gratitude while remaining unattached, you celebrate your accomplishments while remaining humble; and by continuing to be mindful of your thoughts and actions, you maintain the steady and methodical development of who you are.

Bunbu ryo do, the way of the martial scholar, speaks of living a balanced lifestyle free from the price other people pay for their lack of self-discipline, the 'wheel of suffering' as it is referred to in Hinduism and Buddhism. That so many aspire to extreme wealth or celebrity these days is a sign, to me at any rate, that modern society may have already lost the balance that is vital for individual contentment. Modern culture teaches us to want more, and the concept of "enough" has, for many, now slipped from general use. In karate too, people desire to wear a black belt only to discover upon acquiring it, that it has no value. Rather than learn from this discovery, they simply shift their desire to acquiring extra dan ranks and titles. The results of course are the same. There is simply no value in such desires; they are unnecessary and serve you poorly. Meanwhile, your desires continue to damage your integrity, waste your money, and may even take years off your life by way of dubious physical practices. A person who adopts the way of Bunbu ryo do is said to be training his body for war and his mind for peace. In the Okinawa of old, such men were known as bushi, gentlemen warriors. Revered by all in their community, the best of them lived dignified and cultured lives. You too can live this way if you choose, ready and able to interact with others of whatever station in life, as equals. By blending the parallel paths of the body and the mind, such desires as you do have can become investments in the growth of your spirit and the development of you as a human being.

The Author's Ten Precepts: The Way of One

Men occasionally stumble over the truth, but most of them pick themselves up and hurry off as if nothing happened...
—Sir Winston Churchill

Truths abound. They are all around us like radio waves carrying music through the air; the trick is to discover how to tune into them. For over three and a half decades, I have been guilty of stumbling over more than a few truths and, as Churchill said, hurried off as if nothing had happened. Now, however, I am less likely to distance myself so quickly when I stumble. Taking ownership and personal responsibility for my karate has taught me to linger when my life reveals an awkward truth; and in doing so, I am able to find something to be grateful for. In times past I not only missed the signpost, but I often missed the turning altogether. Is it any wonder that I became hopelessly lost? These days I am more accepting of others and myself. Wisdom and truth have been discovered in many places and from many sources, often when I was not looking and so least expected to find them. As this book is pointing to the development of the body and mind, through the practice of karate techniques, I want to speak about ten important guidelines. These guidelines have helped steer me to a better appreciation of life, and of karate too. But even now, I occasionally glance at others and see in them more progress than my own. Still, I gain solace in the knowledge that in budo there is no contest, just an acceptance of the struggle going on inside and of doing your best to deal with it. So here are ten maxims that you may find of value. None of them originated with me, and you may well have come across a number of them before; but in the order I have placed them you may find, just as I did, a route to a better understanding of your life, and your karate. I would ask only that you ponder each of them for as long as it takes to gain some insight into how, if at all, each relates to you. You may want to take a break from time to time, have a cup of tea, or take the dog for a walk. If you do, you might be surprised at how much clearer your thoughts become.

1. KARATE NI SENTE NASHI
   No first attack in karate
2. KI KEN TAI NO ICHI
   Harmonize your spirit, fist, and body
3. GAI JU NAI GO
   Gentle looking but strong
4. BUNBU RYO DO
   The Way of the martial scholar
5. IKKYO ISSHIN
   One heart, one mind
6. KATA WA SO TOKU E NO MICHI TAI
   Study kata to make progress in the Way
7. KYU DO MU GEN
   Investigating the Way is endless
8. BUTSU KOJO NO HOMON
   Do not become attached to things
9. KOKORO WO TAGAYASU
   Plough your spirit
10. KAI UN
    Develop your own fate

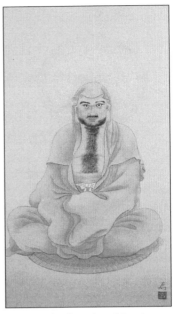

Daruma, the founder of Zen in Japanese popular culture. From the author's private collection.

The concept of "no first attack" in karate has kept karateka bewildered for generations; so what exactly does it mean? For me it points to karate being a defensive art rather than an offensive one. In fact, all the classical kata I practice begin with the premise of being attacked first, and then provide ideas and strategies of how I might best defend myself. But *karate ni sente nashi* also speaks to the intention of others. If I perceive an attack is imminent, then, as far as I am concerned, the first move has already been made and I feel justified in reacting with an appropriate physical response. That physical response would, I trust, express the second precept, *ki ken tai no ichi*, in the blending of my body's movement, the technique(s) I use, and the spirit in which I use them. Dynamic and effective, and always with control, this is how karate should be applied in circumstances where self-protection is necessary. To witness a well-trained karateka in action is an impressive sight; indeed, he can make personal combat look effortless. So we should be mindful of the third precept, *gai ju nai go*, and how things done well always look easy, just as techniques that look gentle are capable of unleashing great strength. Thinking about the martial art you practice and how and why you practice it is the beginning of the fourth precept, *bunbu ryo do*, the way of the martial scholar. Researching the past in order to better understand the present, you are rediscovering the old, making it new once again. By using your intellect as well as your muscles in the pursuit of personal development, you discover the importance of the fifth precept, *ikkyo isshin*, and how your heart and mind must be equally engaged in such a quest, while appreciating that the gift of kata, left to us by our predecessors, are there to be studied and not treated like museum pieces to be handled with kid gloves. The sixth precept, *kata wa sho toku e no michi tai*, clearly reminds you that your progress depends on study, not on clinical preservation. Kata are there to be learned, mastered, dismantled, and rebuilt in the image of the individual making the study, not some long dead master. Knowing this, it is perhaps easier to understand why Okinawan karate schools teach less kata than schools found elsewhere. For the study of kata is continuous and is about developing the depth of your understanding of the kata you practice, rather than your capacity to remember as many as possible. The seventh precept, *kyu do mu gen*, reminds you of an important distinction with this advice: investigating the way is endless. As time passes, those of you who study kata, as opposed to just remembering them, learn to unlock the principles encoded within the patterns. You learn to let go of the rigid form and appreciate more the strategies involved; by doing this you learn the meaning of the eighth precept, *butsu kojo no homon*, of not becoming too attached to things. When you remove your karate from the box marked "use for fighting only" and separate it from the idea of doing battle with another, you have already begun to cultivate your nature. Appreciating that your training is less about fighting others and more about the mêlée going on within you, you begin to see more clearly the need for the ninth concept, *kokoro wo tagayasu*, ploughing the spirit. Ploughing the spirit, like ploughing the land, is done in preparation for what is to come. Eventually, if you enter deeply into your investigation of the "way," you will become skilled not only in your martial art, but more importantly, in the art of living; this is why the tenth and last guideline, *kai un*, is a final *aide memoire* reminding you to develop your own fate.

Austere Training: Shugyo—Kangeiko—Gasshuku

> *He who has exhausted all his mental constitution knows his nature.*
> *Knowing his nature, he knows heaven.*
> —Mencius (371–289 B.C.)

Regular training in karate is a challenge, or at least it should be. Unfortunately, these days this is not always the case as those who join a commercial karate club often face challenges quite unlike those practicing karate in a traditional dojo. This is because the psychological impact upon the person pursuing karate is different from the demands made upon the follower of a sporting activity. When speaking of karate, I'm speaking of budo karate, not commercial karate. I'm speaking of a type of training that prepares the body for combat and guides the mind toward peace. Individuals who are engaged in karate as a sport to keep fit, or for purely commercial reasons have other considerations. The yearly calendar in budo karate contains annual events designed to test not only your physical resolve, but your mental tenacity too; such schooling is known as austere training: *shugyo*. What differentiates shugyo from normal training is the intensity of the physical workout and the resulting state of mind that emerges in the student as a consequence of being pushed to exhaustion. Achieving a state of mind, where what I call 'meeting one's true self' occurs, can be accomplished in a number of ways. However, I would not recommend this type of training be attempted by people with less than three or four years of serious karate training already behind them, and even then, the teachers conducting shugyo training must always have personal experience of undergoing shugyo themselves. To impose shugyo on a student without personal experience is not only dangerous, but also cowardly. In the pursuit of karate no amount of imagined empathy can compensate for personal experience, and this is especially true when it comes to shugyo, for the very nature of the training will take the student to his physical limits and then, hold him there. The benefit derived from such training is long lasting, if not always immediately obvious. We are, among other things, a product of our combined experiences; and those who have learned to successfully negotiate extraordinary hardships tend to go on to live extraordinary lives. Not heroes, but instead, people of whom it might be said follow an approach to life advocated by President Theodore Roosevelt (1858–1919) when he advised: "Speak softly and carry a big stick; you will go far." When you endure the rigors of shugyo you get to look deeply into yourself, and in doing so catch a glimpse of your true nature. Because of this experience your appreciation of karate and of life, too, is irrevocably altered. You learn to move quietly through life, to speak softly and, although remaining empty handed, carry within you a big stick.

At the Shinseidokan dojo, students approaching shodan must first undergo shugyo. This involves two consecutive days of solitary training over a weekend designed to test the student physically and mentally. The student is able to call a halt to the training at any time; he simply has to ask for it to end and it's over. When this happens, the training is brought to a close just like any regular training session; the student cleans the dojo, gets changed, and returns home. Nothing more is said about the shugyo and the student returns to the dojo during normal training times to continue his training as usual. Time passes, and when I think he is ready, the student is once again invited to experience shugyo. Until such time as a student has successfully navigated his way through this trial, he remains ineligible to test for shodan. My thinking behind this is clear; when I issue a dan rank to someone, I am primarily concerned about the kind of person he is. Of course an appropriate level of skill and knowledge has to be demonstrated too, but my main concern remains a person's character. Shugyo, when conducted with all due diligence, will establish this. One-on-one with your sensei a student has no place to hide, and you must rely on your own resources to get you through the challenges set by your teacher. These take the form of exhaustive physical training, coupled with simple mental tasks like decision making. In fact, a student's success or failure with shugyo hangs on his ability to make the final choice given to him at the end of the first day of training. Although he does not appreciate it at the time, the entire weekend is designed to bring the student to this point; what he does here will decide the course of his karate for the following year at least, and perhaps even longer. Successful students are invited to test for shodan one month after shugyo. This allows the student time to recover from the training and to polish his technique for the display ahead. The actual test for shodan at the Shinseidokan dojo is no more demanding than an average training session; I have already tested the student's character under extreme conditions and he has not been found wanting. The shodan grading exam itself merely offers the student one last chance to fail, but this will only happen if he displays too strong an attachment to the color of the belt. Not all shugyo is as severe or demanding as the pre-dan shugyo students undergo at the Shinseidokan. Throughout the year there are other challenges awaiting the student, challenges like *kangeiko*, mid-winter training. Although not a part of Okinawan karate tradition per se, due to the island's sub-tropical climate, kangeiko is nevertheless a useful tool to help a student gain some measure of his own progress. It is conducted in the colder months of the year, in the depth of winter when the days are short, the nights are long, and the air is very cold. At the Shinseidokan, kangeiko training begins at 5:00 A.M. each morning for one week. During this time, the normal evening training is suspended and attendance at the dojo is voluntary. If I made the kangeiko compulsory, the test facing the student would change. It would no longer be a matter of challenging himself to get out of a warm bed in the pre-dawn darkness of winter and go to a cold dojo; instead it would simply be the student doing as he was told. The student's state of mind creates the nature of the challenges he faces; altering perception lies at the heart of all forms of shugyo training, for both the student and the sensei alike.

The word *gasshuku* actually implies lodging together, that is to say, students come together for a time to live and train; forsaking all other considerations, they live and train karate for the length of the gasshuku, which can last from as short as two or three days to as long as a couple of weeks. As well as the kangeiko training, which continues to take place each winter, in the past I held two gasshuku at the Shinseidokan each year, one in spring and the other in autumn. At these times the students gathered for training that ran from Friday evening through to Sunday afternoon, and immersed themselves in karate: training, eating, and sleeping in the dojo. In between training, they prepared food and learned to get along with people they usually only interacted with when they were trying to hit them. It was a chance for students to see if their understanding of karate could develop beyond the realms of kicking and punching. First time participants were often surprised to discover the most difficult part of a gasshuku was not the long hours of training, but the social skills they realized they lacked. For some, the concept of sharing and of being considerate of others proved a steep learning curve. Of all the stories I have been able to coax from students over the years, how they dealt with the seven-minute showers were perhaps the most enlightening. Let me explain. Not having shower facilities in the dojo, at the end of each day's training the students would use the shower in my home. The most senior student went first and the most junior student went last. From entering the bathroom, undressing, taking a shower, drying off, getting dressed again, and leaving the room exactly as he found it, each student had no longer than seven minutes. For that was the amount of time, multiplied by the number of students, allotted to the water. If students lingered in the shower it meant those who came after them would suffer and perhaps miss out on a shower altogether. I did this, not to save on water, but to teach consideration for others, and to remind the students that whenever they indulged themselves, in this case by taking a long hot shower after a hard day's training, it was always at the expense of someone else. I am pleased to say that in all the years I held a gasshuku at the dojo no one ever missed out on his shower, nor did I ever have to clean up afterward. Apart from the clearing steam still hanging to the surface of my shaving mirror, the room was always left as it was found: clean and tidy. What proved so edifying to me was that even though there were no children involved here, this was often the first time a small number of the students had ever consciously, as young adults, considered the needs of others over their own, let alone did something about it. This was a little test I gave the students each gasshuku and one I am happy to say they passed each time. If you think seven minutes is ample time to take a shower, why not try it. Set the clock and take your shower as I have described here, and don't forget to leave the room as you found it: neat and tidy. I no longer hold a gasshuku at the Shinseidokan, but I do continue to commemorate the birth and death of Chojun Miyagi each April and October with special training, which runs over a weekend and equals the amount of training, both in time and intensity, done on the gasshuku: typically around fourteen hours. Now, however, students return home at the end of each day's training, the hardship of sleeping on a cold and hard dojo floor no longer a challenge they have to face. But the experience is no easier, training still begins at 5:00 A.M., and students still have to be there, changed, warmed up, and ready to go when I walk through the door exactly one minute before training commences. Now the challenge has become one of getting out of a warm and comfortable bed at 4:00 A.M. in the morning, when you're stiff and sore from the previous day's hard training. Like so many things in life, if you wish to succeed in your endeavors, you find there is usually a certain level of sacrifice involved. I am not sure if the students understand the lesson here, or indeed if they are even aware of a lesson being taught, yet I think it is a lesson worth the giving.

Shugyo training is not a test of super-human strength or testosterone-fueled toughness. It is a challenge to step out of your comfort zone for a time and handle whatever comes your way, or as Mencius pointed out, "To know your own nature." It is an opportunity during group shugyo, to give of yourself by supporting and encouraging those who are weaker than you, those who may be struggling either physically or mentally. It is also a chance to see if you have what it takes to work hard and stay calm, to deal with the inconvenient, and overcome the petty. When you learn to be gentle from a position of strength, then you become truly powerful, and for those of us who align our karate training with the memory and name of Chojun Miyagi, this is particularly important. For at the core of Miyagi sensei's teachings lies this very message, the balance of strength and gentleness, the *go* and the *ju*, the harmony of opposites to see you through the challenges of life; get this balance right, and life starts to line up a whole lot closer to the way you want it.

Shugyo, in all its many forms, lies at the heart of budo training. In January 1991 when I established the Shinseidokan dojo in Perth, Western Australia, the notion of shugyo was at the forefront of my thoughts when deciding upon the name Shinseidokan, which is made up of four kanji (真誠道館) that together direct your thoughts to the nature of the challenges that lay ahead when you train there. They not only give a name to the dojo but also express my underlying belief in the need to be truthful to ourselves and sincere in our dealings with others, to become a *genuine* person in a world where authenticity is often thin on the ground. Briefly speaking, Shin (真) means to be truthful—with yourself and with others. Sei (誠) implies sincerity—not only in your dealings with others, but also in your pursuit of karate. Do (道) refers to the "way"—how to conduct yourself in your daily life. Kan (館) is the building itself—the place where you come to study karate, and in doing so, discover what kind of person you really are. The Shinseidokan dojo is not a karate 'club', nor is it a home for elitist views held by arrogant individuals; it is an Okinawan-inspired karate dojo inhabited by non-Okinawans, and anybody who approaches the dojo with a sincere attitude will always find a welcome.

What is Balance: Change versus Stability

Balance: just what does that word mean? On the face of it, you might think it is that which keeps you upright while kicking, or stops you from falling over when trying to move quickly from one position to another. Those who are new to karate can be forgiven for thinking of balance in this way, but hopefully, karateka who have been training for four or five years will have reached a better understanding and realize there is more to balance than not falling over. At some point, although this will happen only to individuals who dive enthusiastically into their training, the word 'balance' will take on a whole new meaning. It will come to apply less to the physical aspects of training and more to the way in which that training begins to fit, and even shape, the life of a karateka. My teacher, the late Eiichi Miyazato sensei, told me to try to find a balance in life between family, work, and training. He also said this was the order of importance each should be given if I wanted to achieve a sense of harmony and contentment. I agreed with him completely, having already learned this lesson some years earlier. Almost forty years ago, when I was new to karate, my sense of balance was woefully inadequate. At least four nights each week and three weekends out of every four were given over to training in karate. If not at the Shito ryu dojo I was a member of, then at the dojo of friends who trained in either Shotokan or Goju ryu. It made little difference at the time what kind of karate I was training in, just so long as I was training. For a single person with no one else to consider, such a way of life might be fine, a little hectic maybe, but fine. Unfortunately, I was not single; I had a wife at home. Looking back on these circumstances now, I can only wonder how she put up with my behavior for as long as she did. My situation was by no means unique. Others too were busy making the same mistake I was making, and, just like me, they were failing miserably when it came to achieving a sense of balance in life. I was failing to see the 'bigger picture', focusing only on the short-term gains I seemed to be making in karate. Sadly, but perhaps not surprisingly, the acute imbalance in my life at that time led to a divorce; and like many others who found themselves in a similar situation, I never saw it coming! I was, after all, as I saw it, pursuing a noble cause, one of self-development leading to self-improvement. Like so many, though, I had failed to recognize the simple truth that all such improvements come from within; concentrating on the external, the physical training, was only developing my body.

Thankfully, for me, my first wife and I separated in amity thus saving me from some of the deeper wounds that such a situation might have inflicted. Today I see karateka making the same mistakes I did, and not all of them are new to karate. Many of them are individuals who should, quite frankly, know better. Instructors who spend their weekends away from home teaching seminars month after month may well be catering to the needs of their followers, but what about their families? In such a lifestyle, where is the balance that the study of karate challenges us to achieve? Individuals may be making a lot of money and receiving a lot of praise, even adulation, but are they making progress toward a balanced and contented life? This is a question I cannot answer. So much depends on the individual and his idea of what being balanced and contented is. If, however, folks were completely honest, I suspect that for most who travel around teaching groups of karateka they don't know things they won't remember, their lives are just as unfulfilled today as they ever were. When you focus on your training to such an extent that it creates problems in your life outside the dojo, then clearly you are making a mistake. Progress evolves from effort, and some part of that effort will entail sacrifice, not the fatted calf variety, but sacrifice all the same. Balance is the key to being successful when it comes to personal development. What goes on inside the dojo should support what is happening outside of it, and vice-versa; your life should not be a continuous question of either/or. If it is, you can be sure your situation in life needs attention. Realizing the importance of having a broader perception of balance opens the door for the making of real growth. For in reality there seems little point in achieving the skills necessary to blend effortlessly with your training partner in the dojo when your life outside the dojo is at odds with the world. Our ego, that false friend to us all, is usually lurking somewhere in the background at times like this. Whispering in your ear about the virtues of training hard, it forgets to mention that your neglect of partners, work, family, and friends can all lead to overwhelming pain and suffering. You have to ask: for what? So that you might move up a rank or two in karate, an activity by the way that the vast majority in the world has absolutely no interest in. Surely, this is a huge price to pay for such a small prize.

The connection between your training and your ego cannot be denied, although some do try. They convince themselves that life is driven by a noble desire to find the deeper and more meaningful aspects of karate; but in truth, their inability to find a sense of balance is enough to keep them from ever acquiring such wisdom. Some karate students are more inclined to make progress than others. Those who continue to base their training on forceful exchanges with an attacker tend to stop making progress once the intermediate ranks of sandan or yondan (third and fourth dan respectively) are reached. By then, they have spent many years training to achieve a certain kind of attitude: usually an aggressive one. This was, after all, exactly what was needed for the kind of tough physical training they were doing; it was forceful and full of power, and it was constant. It was not, however, well balanced. Whereas a strong attack that is met with an equally powerful defense so often fails, a subtle attack frequently finds an open pathway to the target. A better sense of balance can result in people being able to deal with a softer, though potentially no less deadly, kind of attack. But such is the rush in some karateka to be fast, hard, and strong that the notion of balance is often buried or lost altogether. When students are training in karate and their sole aim is to learn methods of defeating another person, they can sometimes forget the need to defeat their own ego first. An old adage comes to mind: "There are no shortcuts in karate." Undoubtedly, then, a path must be traveled before a destination can be reached, with experience being the journey and understanding the destination. So, just as clearly, attempts to avoid taking the necessary steps we need to take along the "way" are futile and will, rather predictably, lead to disappointment and frustration or even worse: a life of delusion. Regretfully, the karate world is full of self-proclaimed 'masters' leading their followers along the road to nowhere.

The responsibility for our progress lies with each of us; I know this now. A teacher can teach and a sensei can guide, but in the end, it is always up to the individual student to find within himself the attributes required to advance and grow. One of those attributes is a well-developed sense of balance. We all know that trying to do a job without the proper knowledge or the right tools inevitably leads to a poor result: a hodgepodge of ideas, principles, and techniques, holding things together. As the study and investigation of karate is, ultimately, addressing your life, surely you owe it to yourself to obtain the best 'tool box' you can. How much better if you learn to make your own tools instead of relying on those found on sale at seminars and workshops and sold to an unsuspecting public by karate salesmen. How much more value and appreciation for karate would you gain from the learning of your art apprenticed to a sensei, as opposed to simply purchasing training time from an instructor. Standing in a hall with dozens of others is not the ideal way to either pursue your personal training or learn the psychological skills needed to understand the essence of the karate you are training in. When the late Gichin Funakoshi sensei wrote "Part the clouds and seek the way," he did not advocate getting someone else to part the clouds for you. His advice was, and still is, pointing the student of karate toward self-discovery. Personal realization is brought about by personal experience, by seeing things clearly for what they are, and looking beyond the imagery projected by individuals and groups that make a living peddling the physical skills of karate. A sensei teaches largely by example, not by talking.

From Miyazato sensei I learned 'kokoro wo tagayasu', to cultivate my spirit, and 'kai un', to develop my own fate. His concern for me was that I become the kind of person who could grasp the essence of karate rather than execute perfect techniques. Believing that if he could help his students help themselves, this would ensure the preservation of Chojun Miyagi's philosophy and fighting principles. In 1942, Miyagi sensei wrote down some of his thoughts on karate; later, they appeared as a short article in the journal *Bunka Okinawa*, volume 3, number 6, on August 15 of that year. Since the death of his teacher, Kanryo Higaonna almost thirty years earlier, Miyagi had harbored a sense of loss

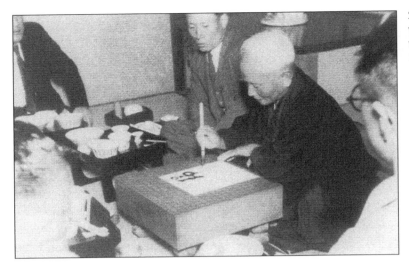
Students gather to watch Funakoshi write words of wisdom, ca. 1955.

he never quite got over. Although seen by many today as a great innovator in karate, he clearly viewed himself in a different, more humble light. Here is some of what he wrote:

> "I have been practicing karate for a long time, but I have not yet mastered the core or truth of karate. I feel as if I am walking alone on a distant path in the darkness, the further I travel, the longer the path becomes. But this is the way truth is, precious! If we move forward to find the truth of karate by our own strength of mind and body, we will be rewarded, little by little, day by day. The truth is near, but hard to reach."

Miyazato sensei counseled me many times, "Anyone can learn to kick and punch," and reminded me that such skills had limited value in life. Some years after my sensei passed away I came across the work of the Brazilian writer Paolo Coelho and discovered in one of his books, *The Pilgrimage*, published in 1986, a wonderful account of the role teachers play in their students' education.

In the book, he tells the story of following his teacher along the lengthy and arduous pilgrim route to Santiago de Compostella across northern Spain. Since medieval times, pilgrims had walked this way and now he found himself walking in their shadow. From the outset he knew the master would lead and he would follow; however, the nature of the journey turned out to be far more exigent than he had ever imagined. His teacher warned him that he would have to make his own journey, by his own efforts, and in doing so find his own way. One particular lesson takes place when they come upon a high waterfall. Together they stand at the base of the wall of water and look up. Suddenly, the teacher dives into the water and disappears for a while before emerging again at the top of the waterfall. He had made his way there by climbing the rock face at the back of the curtain of fast-flowing water; so even though Paolo had seen his teacher making progress he could not see clearly how he was achieving it. The water obscured all the important details of exactly where his teacher gripped the rocks and found secure footholds. It was now the student's turn to make the climb, and Paolo soon discovers the force of the water is much stronger than he imagined. He describes the doubts threatening to overwhelm him at that moment as "the sense that weakens us at the moment we most need to have faith in our powers." Passing behind the cascade to get away from the full force of the falling water he finds the climb becoming a little easier than anticipated in those first few worrying moments. It is only when he reaches the top of the climb and once again must find a way to get through the violent flow that his doubts return. The force of the water and the thundering noise it made once again threaten to overpower him. Like so many, when faced with a seemingly impossible obstacle in life, he started to look for ways out instead of ways through. Close to giving up, his mind began to drift and he starts to dream of reaching a place where … "there would no longer be any need for the superhuman effort it took; there would only be rest and peace." In his struggle to make progress he pushes his head up through the water but sees nothing he can hold on to. He looks about, searching both sides of the river for his teacher, but he is nowhere to be seen. This is the moment he understands that if he slips and falls, his teacher will not save him. He is on his own, making his own choices, alive, and experiencing his own journey. He decides to stop fighting his situation and begins to go with it instead. Letting his hand become … "like a fish," it finds its way through the water to a rock on which he is able to lever himself through the torrent and climb to the top. Finally free of the struggle with the water, he crawls his way on to dry land and drops into an exhausted heap on the grassy bank of the river, where he falls asleep.

Before his teacher jumped into the water at the bottom of the waterfall, he said … "I will make the climb without you being able to see where I place my hands and feet. In the same way a disciple such as you can never imitate his master's steps. You have your own way of living your life, of dealing with problems, and of winning. Teaching is only demonstrating that it is possible, learning is making it possible for you."

I was reminded, when I first read this story, of an old Chinese proverb, which states: "Tell me, I will forget. Show me, I may remember. But involve me and I will understand." Like Paolo's story of the waterfall, this too, captures the difference between a sensei and an instructor. My late father would sometimes say, "You can't teach what you don't know," hardly original, but nonetheless truthful for all that. It is also said that the Buddha once wrote, "We are what we think. All that we are arises with our thoughts. With our thoughts we make our world." By training diligently in karate, you cultivate your spirit and learn to develop your fate. With such tools at your disposal, it becomes clear why choosing to fight someone to solve a problem appears small and even somewhat childish. You may well carry the big stick that Roosevelt spoke of, but using it should always be a last resort.

Sitting with the late karate master Shoshin Nagamine sensei in a small room off to one side of his Kodokan dojo in Naha, Okinawa, back in 1992, he told me karate could be thought of by dividing it into three main parts. He used the term, Shin Gi Tai, a quick translation of which would be Spirit, Technique, and Body. He explained that as a youth learning karate—he was 86 years old at the time of our conversation and had been training in karate for 70 of them—he and his fellow students were encouraged to find and capture the spirit of karate. Whereas, he noted, the modern approach to learning directed the student of karate to copy exact postures and strive for perfect techniques. The problem with this modern approach is obvious; no one ever achieves perfection. Nevertheless, an untold number of people around the world continue to practice their karate with this as their goal. For my part I know that the pursuit of perfection with regard to technique is a false god if ever there was one. Shin gi tai asks students of karate to balance their mind and spirit (*shin*) with their physical techniques (*gi*) and the way they use their bodies (*tai*), this final part relating to the use of the breath also. Nagamine sensei told me it was no accident the first thing a student needed to understand was that executing powerful techniques came from having the correct spirit. "This comes first, in order to achieve a balance." Since then I have witnessed for myself the truth of his statement, many times. Karateka who have failed to appreciate this sense of "spirit" also fail to develop, and for many this leads to a departure from karate altogether. Often, in spite of their excellent physical skills and fitness levels, they have failed to make the connection between making progress and the development of their spirit. Some people leave karate for legitimate reasons and, ironically enough, in doing so display a well-developed sense of balance, by understanding that training in karate should always come third to family and work commitments. It is a well-established concept within karate that the mind leads and the body follows. So when you first enter a dojo you are, or should be, encouraged to maintain an open mind, that is to say, a mind that is open and inquiring, a beginner's mind (*shoshin*). Ready to, as Funakoshi said, "Part the clouds and seek the way." Without a keen sense of balance in your training and in the way you live your life, I believe such an endeavor will

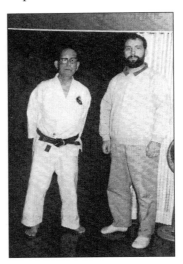

The author with Shoshin Nagamine sensei at the Kodokan dojo in Kume, Okinawa, in 1992.

prove to be impossible. Knowing when to change direction in life and when to remain on course is a talent a long time in the making. Such insights are crafted over many years; there are no shortcuts. Sincere and consistent training in the dojo cultivates the spirit, which in turn, facilitates problem solving in your life outside the dojo.

4 GI—TECHNIQUE

The Purpose of Training: Karate Renshu

So far I have looked at concepts that may or may not be familiar to karateka. What follows in the next two chapters is, in many ways, the counterpoint to that truth-seeking discussion. While it is important to appreciate the significance of such philosophical underpinning, as karate without the maturing of your spirit leads to brutality, it is also important to note that karate must never be allowed to polarize in the opposite direction and become a solely theoretical exercise. In the dojo you foster a strong body and an even stronger mind; you lubricate the techniques of your karate with your sweat and strengthen your resolve by focusing on the problems at hand. In doing this, then karate, if taught and studied correctly, is ideal for the personal development of individuals whose sense of balance in life may not be all it could be.

In 1961, the late Shoshin Nagamine posted a large sign on the side wall of his dojo to help direct the minds of the growing number of American military personnel looking for instruction. Under the heading, "Ethics of the dojo: Courtesy—Cleanliness—Diligence," it continues,

> First of all, purify your mind. Cultivate the power of perseverance by strengthening your body and overcoming the difficulties that arise during training. The dojo is a special place where guts are fostered and superior human natures are bred through the ecstasy of sweating in hard work. The dojo is a sacred place where the human spirit is polished ...

Polishing the spirit (*sen ren shin*) is the term used to point the student of traditional karate toward the idea of developing fortitude. This is achieved through diligent training conducted frequently over a protracted period of time. Those who insist on looking for shortcuts or a quick fix in karate never cleanse their spirit; the very act of looking for such things ensures your spirit remains tainted. It is to some of the methods used in the polishing of your spirit that I turn now, and in doing so, hopefully, I will illustrate the way karate training (*renshu*) is merely the outward, physical expression of a deeper and more meaningful internal struggle. I hope to lay siege to the myth that the purpose of karate is purely one of learning how to fight. Indeed, if there is any sense of fighting at all in your training, then it is against the negative aspects of your own ego that you must look in order to find an adversary worth the trouble.

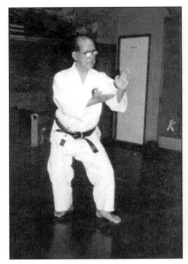

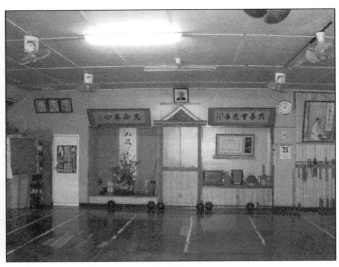

Shoshin Nagamine sensei
(1907–1997)

Inside the Kodokan dojo, Kume, Okinawa.

Fighting Strategies

When people think of fighting it would be fair to say they are usually thinking of some kind of clash between two or more individuals, with everyone involved hell bent on inflicting as much damage as possible to each other: karate takes a different view. If a disagreement turns physical and the need to protect yourself becomes necessary, karate's core message is to control the situation. This is done by dominating the other person, or persons, involved and then bringing the conflict to as speedy a conclusion as possible. The concept of 'sparring' plays no role in traditional karate training. Why? Because it encourages you to keep boxing. It gives you a false impression of what a real fight is like and allows you to gain a sense of confidence in your fighting ability that, in reality, could prove fatal. In his excellent book, *Meditations on Violence: A Comparison of Martial Arts Training & Real World Violence*, (page 30), Rory Miller had this to say regarding strategy training:

> Goals differ in different situations. Real violence is a very broad subject and no two encounters are the same. What is a "win" in one situation may not be in the next. The *goal* is how to define the win in that particular encounter. Sometimes it will reflect your martial arts training. An incapacitating blow may be what you need. But sometimes the goal is to break away or to create enough space to access a weapon or just get enough air to scream for help. If the goal changes, so does everything else. If you have only trained for one goal, (e.g., the submission), you will be hampered when the goal is different.

He heads up this section of the book with the following maxim: "*Goals dictate strategy. Strategy dictates tactics. Tactics dictate techniques.*" Now, while it may look at first glance like Rory's book has little to do with traditional karate training, I think otherwise. His attitude toward dealing with conflict is no different to the underlying principles found in the karate of Okinawa: assess the situation as best you can, adopt an appropriate attitude, posture, and distance, and above all, endeavor to dominate the situation as quickly as possible and by all means at your disposal. When you spar you do so governed by guidelines that would, in a real situation, leave you exposed to more danger than you may already be in. As Rory said, "Goals differ in different situations … If the goal changes, so does everything else." When you engage in sparring, you change the goal because sparring is not motivated by violence. In karate, the goal is to stop the fight as soon as possible, and to this end, we often hear the term *ikken hisatsu*—one blow, one kill—being used. If you followed that maxim to the letter, it would of course lead to even more conflict, this time with the law. However, the ikken hisatsu adage is useful in that it reminds you yet again to bring the fight to a close with the minimum of techniques, an impossible goal when engaged in sparring. With sparring, there is no intention to stop the fight, only a desire to continue 'boxing' and to tag your partner in specifically designated, safe areas of the body, such as the chest or stomach. Unless the goal is to break the sternum, in a real fight punches are better placed elsewhere: in the face, on the jaw, to the kidneys, in the bladder, or under the arms on the side of the ribcage. Kicks too would be better placed in soft targets—like the groin, kidneys, spleen, bladder, or against the side of the knees, rather than higher up the torso as practiced in sparring where points are awarded for a "theoretically" successful hit.

There are a number of ways traditional karate training allows you to gain insight into sound fighting strategies that will help you overcome a stronger aggressor. At the risk of sounding somewhat 'hippie-like' here, it is better to blend and move with an attack, a little, than try to stand where you are and stop it. Okay, so the obvious needs to be mentioned here; attacks rarely happen in isolation. Unless the first strike was a knock-out blow, no fighter I ever came across on the street threw one punch or one kick and then stopped. The tactics I want to discuss here address strategies employed either in the split second immediately before 'first contact', or immediately after contact has already been made, if you have been grabbed, for example.

Irimi

This means 'to enter'; in other words, move in on a person, closing the gap to either deny an opportunity to kick or punch or allow your own strike to be thrown from its optimum range. It takes some courage to move toward a person you know is trying to hurt you; natural instinct would tell most people to back off, but karate requires you to develop courage, and in doing so presents a natural barrier to all those who would shy away from such daring behavior. The two examples given here (figs. 4-1, 4-2, and figs. 4-3, 4-4) serve only to illustrate ways students are introduced to the idea of moving toward an attacker. These images, as well as all the other sequential photographs, are not intended to represent anything other than the concepts and training drills being discussed. Let me make it very clear: throughout this entire book, the importance lies in the ideas being discussed, not the precise formalization of physical movements. You can stick rigidly to one way of doing things if you like, but if you do, you'll miss the whole point of karate training. The irimi tactic is found within many of the kata of Okinawan karate that I practice; kata, such as *saifa, seiyunchin, shisochin, sanseiru, seipai, kururunfa, seisan,* and *suparinpei,* all contain examples of entering into, moving around or moving under, an attack. Some kata deal more with being kicked at, some with being punched at, and others with ways to move in on an attacker who has already managed to lay his hands on you. Should the last of these circumstances be the case, then it is time to employ another strategy, *kuzushi.*

But before addressing the notion of destroying an attacker's balance, I want to remind you of the importance of bringing a confrontation, any confrontation, to a positive and speedy conclusion as soon as possible. Imagining yourself going head to head with someone trying to inflict serious damage on you, as if it's a scene from *Kill Bill,* is as likely to see you lying on a slab in the local mortuary as it is walking away with an interesting story to tell. Even in the dojo, training with a partner can result in serious injury if the two people involved are not focused on the job in hand. You go to the dojo for a reason, not for a 'fun' time, but to learn skills and develop certain feelings that in times of danger may make all the difference between life and death.

Both examples represent a very sound doctrine in combat: keep it simple! In the first example of irimi on display here, the attacking punch to the body is shut down by a rapid move forward, checking the punch with one hand and striking hard to the face with the other (fig. 4-2). The second example deals with attempted grabs or chokes; when the attack is made, the defender steps in rapidly, punching the attacker in the throat or face. Both examples are quick, simple, and, with good timing, very effective.

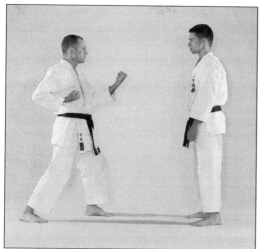

Figure 4-1

Figure 4-2

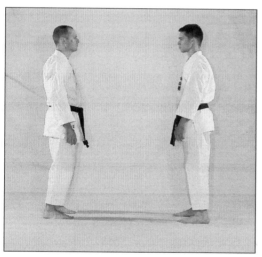

Figure 4-3

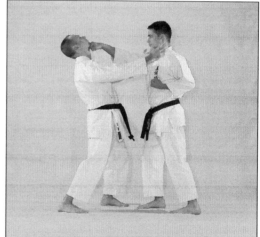

Figure 4-4

Kuzushi

This principle is best understood as 'destroying a person's balance'. It is a tactic used to give the other person something to deal with while you make your move and establish control of the situation. At the Shinseidokan dojo, the classic kuzushi/irimi combination at the start of the kata saifa is usually a student's first serious introduction to this strategy. Students quickly learn it is not simply a matter of moving from point A to point B in the kata, followed by a block and counterstrike. The movement itself is a technique; in fact, I would argue that the block and the *uraken uchi* (back-fist strike to the face) counterstrike

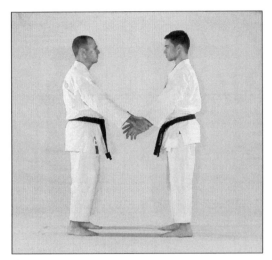

Figure 4-5

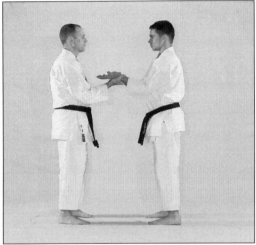

Figure 4-6

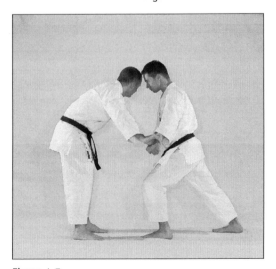

Figure 4-7

would not be possible at all if the opponent's balance is not first destabilized and the gap rapidly closed by means of *tai sabaki* (body shifting). Here are two examples of kuzushi in action taken from the kata of Goju ryu: the first example (figs. 4-5, 4-6, and 4-7) is found in shisochin, the second (figs. 4-8, 4-9, 4-10, and 4-11) in saifa.

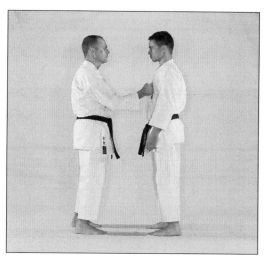

Figure 4-8

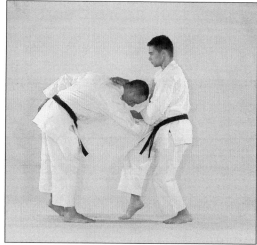

Figure 4-9

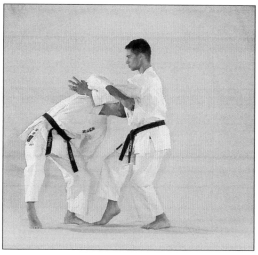

Figure 4-10

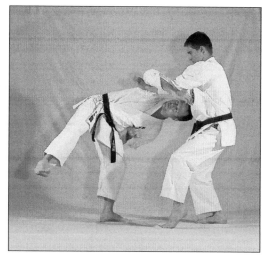

Figure 4-11

Sen No Sen

Sen no sen means 'taking the initiative'. Whereas kuzushi looks at physical ways to regain control when you are already being held and irimi looks at ways of closing the gap in order to engage an attacker on terms more favorable to you, the concept of sen no sen points more to an attitude. It is an attitude that should be adopted the instant the need arises. Sen no sen, in karate terms, means to quickly observe the opponent and, from his posture and overall behavior, anticipate his attack. In the fraction of a second it takes for him to think and then act on his attack, you try, by means of sen no sen, to take advantage of your attacker's fixation on his commitment to the imminent assault and execute your own pre-emptive attack. In layman's terms, it is a bit like the 'quick-draw' gunfighters in old Western movies. The good guy never makes his move until the bad guy commits and then, quick as a flash, the good guy beats him to the draw and it's all over. Sen no sen takes intuition and courage and forges them into action. For there can be no hesitation whatsoever in the execution of sen no sen, just an explosion of energy projecting you from a position of comparative calm to ballistic velocity in an instant, taking advantage of the aggressor's preoccupation with launching his own attack.

Here (figs. 4-12, 4-13, and 4-14, 4-15) are just two of the ways students at the Shinseidokan are introduced to the concept of sen no sen, the first against a punching attack, the second against a kick.

As you can see, the students face off against each other in a less formal way than before. Although karate training must always be wrapped in a strong sense of discipline and etiquette, these considerations should not act to keep your practice locked into rigid methods of movement. In spite of all the time spent learning how to stand correctly, move properly, and make good postures, at the end of the day, you are trying to make your karate natural. Natural to you that is! So at some point, perhaps after several years of continual training, you should step out of the strict conformity of "style," and begin making your responses to an attack as natural to you as the way you drive your car.

Sen no sen is as much an exercise in good timing as it is in technique and has as much to do with developing a good sense of distance and the setting up of appropriate angles as it does being the first to the punch. A big part of sen no sen is invisible and springs into action long before a physical move is made on either side. Developing an ability to "read" your opponent by the way he moves and the postures he adopts enables you to anticipate not only what he is likely to attack you with, but when he is likely to do it. When karate is being used as intended, its strength lies more in the mind, your mind, than it does in the powerful physical techniques that draw so many to it. With your mind, you have the power of choice. When standing opposite someone who is about to attack you, sen no sen can be a very valuable option.

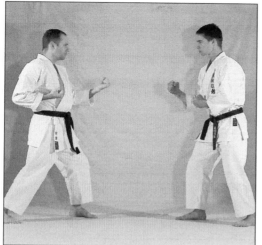

Figure 4-12

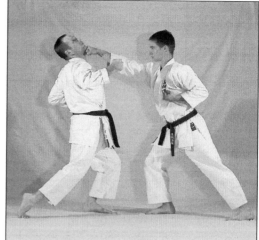

Figure 4-13

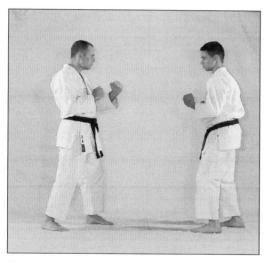

Figure 4-14

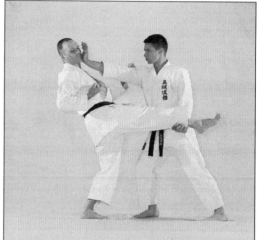

Figure 4-15

Go No Sen

The principle of *go no sen* requires a little more patience. This tactic allows the aggressor to make the first move, so it carries more risk than sen no sen; but given the opportunity (as sen no sen has been lost) it is nonetheless a very useful 'next best' option. Go no sen requires an immediate counterattack once the aggressor's initial attack has been deflected and while his mind is still committed to his attack. If this strategy is to work as intended, your counterattack must be driven home with complete conviction. The danger in any confrontation arises from the loss of control. Put simply, if you are not the one in control in a fight, then you are the one in trouble. So regardless of why the fight is happening or who threw the first punch, the aim of karate as an art of self-protection is to improve the odds of your taking control; once that has been achieved, the situation can be brought to a safe conclusion, and by safe, I mean you're still alive.

Again, the examples shown here are by way of introduction to the concept of go no sen. What you are looking at should not be taken as examples of how karate is applied in a real life situation. You go to the dojo to train and to practice the principles

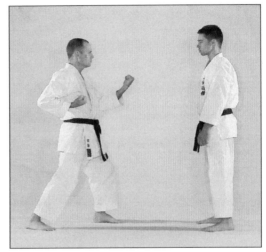

Figure 4-16

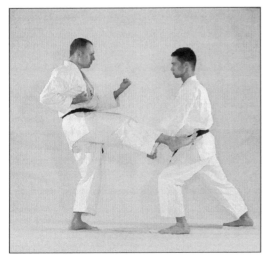

Figure 4-17

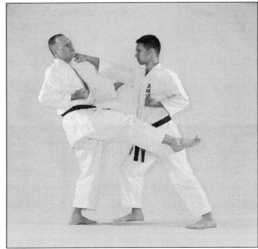

Figure 4-18

of your karate, not to apply them. Had my teachers applied their karate to its fullest extent on me, I would have died many years ago. What is on display in all the sequences is nothing more than an attempt to capture an image of an idea.

In the first example of go no sen (figs. 4-16, 4-17, and 4-18), two students face off against each other, the kick is blocked and immediately countered with a punch to the face. The second example (figs. 4-19, 4-20, and 4-21) shows a high punch being deflect-ed away and the blocking arm being immediately transformed into the counterattack.

In the Shinseidokan dojo, students practice one attack (*ippon*) and repeated attack (*renzoku*) fighting (*kumite*) drills, as well as spending a considerable amount of time investigating the twelve kata found in the Goju ryu tradition. Rather confusingly, the kata have taken on a different appear-ance, depending on which school of Goju ryu you visit in Okinawa, and I strongly doubt any school teaching Goju ryu today is teaching the kata exactly as Chojun Mi-yagi taught them. Still, it is worth remind-ing ourselves that the tradition of karate is not limited to, nor can it be judged by, aes-thetics alone. The principles being handed down from one generation to the next are important here, not the particular order or

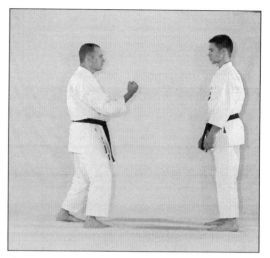

Figure 4-19

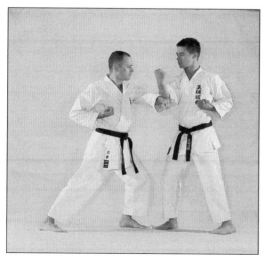

Figure 4-20

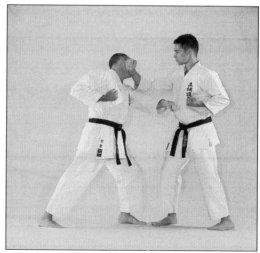

Figure 4-21

look of one kata over another. Keeping a low center of gravity and the body upright, the armpits closed down, and the attacker directly in front of you are all core ideas in the karate of Chojun Miyagi, as is the concept of harmonious breathing and movement to maximize the effect of the technique. How an individual goes about employing these principles is up to him. The karate found around Naha, even as recently as 30 years ago, had few kicks; people favored hand techniques and preferred to keep their feet on the ground. When kicks were used, they were always low and to soft or vulnerable targets, such as the groin, bladder, or skeletal weak points on the lower body, like the feet, ankles, knees, and hip joints. For a fighting system that relied on striking to win the day, Goju ryu karate has always been heavily dependent on grappling to establish control prior to the strike. Understanding the core principles involved in the karate you practice is vital. If such a thing as 'style' exists, then it is in the way you exhibit your understanding of the principles you have studied. To say you practice a particular 'style' of karate while remaining unable to display the principles that style is based upon makes a mockery of the statement and casts doubt upon your maturity as a karateka.

Sabaki

Sabaki, shifting the body, is important because it not only moves you away from danger, but toward a place where you can take advantage of the changes that now exist between you and your attacker. When his assault began, he knew where you were; now he doesn't, but you know exactly where he is. *Tai sabaki,* body shifting, is a generic term used to describe movement. There are several methods of *tai sabaki,* and depending on the circumstances and the outcome you are trying to achieve, the kind of body shifting used also changes. Sliding, stepping, dropping, and turning, all come under the banner of *tai sabaki.* The examples looked at here cover some of the most obvious, i.e.,

those found in the kata studied by students with no more than a year or two of karate training behind them. Therefore, there is nothing 'advanced' about them in terms of ability or understanding.

The first example of *sabaki* comes from the kata saifa. Facing off against each other (fig. 4-22), the defender avoids being hit

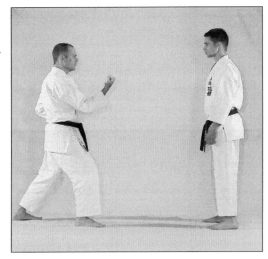

Figure 4-22

by shifting quickly off the line of attack (fig. 4-23) where the blocking technique continues through the blocking action to become a counterstrike (figs. 4-24, 4-25) before following up with a much stronger blow to the ribs (fig. 4-26).

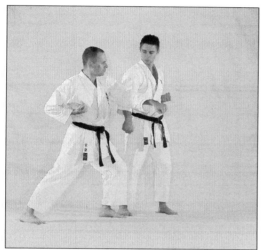

Figure 4-23

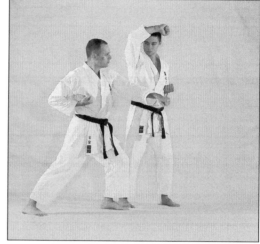

Figure 4-24

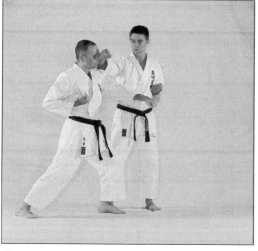

Figure 4-25

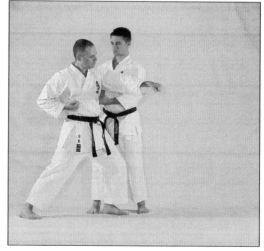

Figure 4-26

The second example of *sabaki* is taken from the beginning of the kata kururunfa. The control of the attacker's grip (fig. 4-27) is lessened considerably by the defender moving sharply to the right, while at the same time pushing the attacker's elbow to the left (fig. 4-28). Because the defender's elbow is wrapped over the top of the attacker's arm (fig. 4-29), trapping him, the defender has now taken control, and from here he counterattacks to the knee joint, forcing it hard into the ground (fig. 4-30).

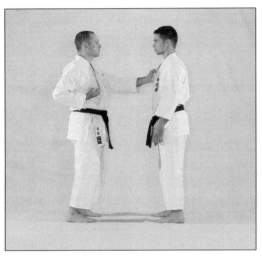

Figure 4-27

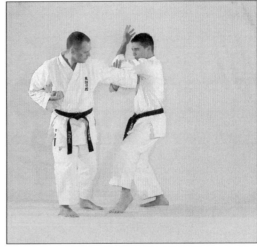

Figure 4-28

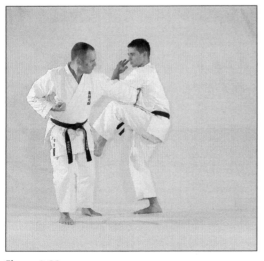

Figure 4-29

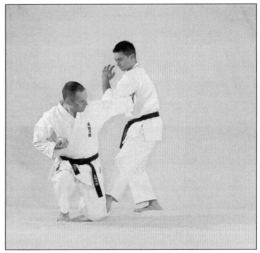

Figure 4-30

This is, I believe, an appropriate time to offer a brief opinion on the whole notion of 'advanced' techniques over those practiced by 'beginners', so I want to make my opinion on this topic completely unequivocal here; there is no such thing as an advanced karate technique! All karate techniques are 'advanced' if you don't know how to apply them. Every technique will do what it is meant to do, but only if the user is skilled enough and has the correct attitude to employ them. It is not the individual techniques that are important, but the person using them. Simply remembering how to move and in what order is not the same as knowing a technique, and knowing a technique is not the same as having a strong feeling for it. Ability with karate will not come from a list of techniques committed to memory and regurgitated on demand. Like balance, or even humor, it is something you can feel or you simply do not have it. No amount of explanation or demonstrations from your teacher will change the fact that knowledge is always a poor substitute for understanding. Although I can see how it might apply to the young and inexperienced, I do not hold with George Bernard Shaw's view, "Our lives are shaped not as much by our experience, as by our expectations," and can only believe he was choosing to display his capacity to be the unreasonable man he once indicated was responsible for all progress in the world. I believe the nature of learning is to be taught by your own experiences, for only by experience do you gain both the knowledge of, and a feeling for, that which you are trying to understand. The Greek philosopher Pyrrho (360–270 B.C.) believed it was the *nature* of man to hold strong opinions on everything. But he argued it was impossible to really know anything for certain; to his way of thinking everything had an element of uncertainty with which humans would always struggle. Pyrrho was among the first Skeptics, who, like other philosophers in ancient Greece, often challenged the so-called *knowledge* of the established schools of thinking. He stated that individuals can only know how things *appear* to be to them. Identical events, words, and even ideas, can all appear differently to different people; therefore it is impossible to know which *opinion* is correct, only how things apply to you. A contemporary example of this might be the notion that one man's terrorist is another man's freedom fighter. Pyrrho supported his philosophical standpoint by pointing out that the phenomenon of relevant opinion is prevalent "among the wise and the vulgar." He believed an individual's ultimate achievement in life should be 'inner peace', a state of mind he called '*ataraxia*'. Others have used the same word, (*ataraxia*), to mean 'apathy'. Are the two states of consciousness the same? According to Pyrrho, that all depends on you! Karate is no different from any other activity we humans engage in, so even when you walk a similar path to others you will come to understand karate in your own unique way. To paraphrase Pyrrho, since nothing can be known for certain and nothing can be right or wrong, being right is a matter of opinion. If there is no good reason to prefer one way over another perhaps you should withhold your assent from all doctrines regarding what is correct and what is incorrect. A sage will renounce all desires based on untenable opinions and live with undisturbed tranquility in his soul, free from delusion. I accept many of the ideas attributed to Pyrrho, in particular his idea that at best, what you know 'for sure' applies to you, and only to you. However, I part company with him when he casts doubt upon the very nature of knowledge with his suggestion that we cannot trust our own senses; for insomuch as Pyrrho's thinking makes for interesting debate, I have no inclination to spend my life questioning, in an ever-descending and muti-layered way, the validity of what I *know*. However, if the need to question what you *know* about karate and how you came to know it resonates with you, then perhaps you should consider Gichin Funakoshi's advice, and look to the past to understand the future. Whatever the empirical nature of your knowledge might be, it's all you've got!

With all the apparent advancement mankind has made over recent millennia, it would be a mistake to think you can rely on anything other than your most primeval resources when engaged in the real and immediate dangers of a fight. Even a brief altercation over something trivial can turn bad quickly and lead to death. A push leads to a head coming into contact with the pavement, and before you know it someone lies dying on the street. It happens, and it is real. There are people in the world willing to do much more than push you if they can; and dealing with them cannot be learned in the warm, family-friendly atmosphere of a commercial karate club. As I mentioned earlier, going to the dojo should be challenging every time you go; if this is not the case, then I would question the activity you are doing there. By all means, enjoy the physicality of sport and the benefits of good health that training in karate can bring, but do not mistake either kyogi or kenko for budo. An ability to physically defend yourself will only come about by an ability to use the techniques of karate in unison with the appropriate attitude, and in doing so advance your chances of walking away from a serious fight with your life intact.

Fighting Applications

So much has been written elsewhere about how to apply karate in a 'real' fight, I am reluctant to add to that particular discussion here; safe to say I have never been aware of any fight that was not 'real' to the loser. Even an exchange of words can often leave one party feeling deeply hurt. To them, their pain is real: it hurts. Physical confrontation also inflicts pain on an emotional level, and with it comes the added impact of physical injury, reminding you you're not good enough to defend yourself. Even if you emerge from an altercation dominant and in control, you may well suffer from the psychological after-effects of having to deal with a fight you did not choose to enter into. As a youth I often fought on the streets of inner-city Manchester; afterward, I would sometimes suffer uncontrollable shaking as I came down from the highly charged state my mind and body entered prior to and during the fight. It was not unusual to batter one opponent into bloody submission, only to have a relative or friend step up and decide to extract revenge then and there. Weapons had to be dealt with too, as on occasion, knives and broken bottles were not that uncommon. During one fight, I was stabbed in the stomach with a car wiper blade. It was ripped off the vehicle as I held my opponent over the hood doing my best to rearrange his facial features. In the heat of the battle, I felt nothing.

The fight ended soon afterward when the stabber was dragged off the car and kicked into unconsciousness. I have always believed the use of weapons on an unarmed opponent to be a cowardly act and always felt obliged to press home this opinion whenever one was used against me. Thankfully, the life I was leading back then, and such encounters, is long gone. Nevertheless, I have on occasion had to call upon that same mentality during karate training. The techniques changed, as there was no real desire to hurt the person standing opposite me, but the tactics and the attitude returned once it became clear my training partner was out to prove a point. Whenever this happened, I made it as clear as I could there was going to be a price to pay for his attitude; kick bags hang from the wall in a dojo; they don't wear a gi. If ever I took what I considered to be an unfairly hard blow, I always did my best to return the same and in good measure. For me, such situations always became as much a mental game as a physical contest. I am just not happy with the thought of being dominated by another human being. I strongly believe the only way to train for a so-called 'real' fight is to have one, and then another, and then another, and keep having them until your mind and body become accustomed to the toll such activities extort from your humanity. For make no mistake about it; if you fight with people on a regular basis, the violence will change you. When this happens you had better be happy with the 'new' you, and hope those you hold most dear are happy too. Personally, I have never met a happy or contented person who was also a committed fighter. In a traditional karate dojo, the aim of the training is to avoid fighting and to resort to it only in the most extreme of circumstances. Fighting should always be the last best hope of walking away from an incident that might otherwise leave you damaged.

Since olden times, the question of fighting in Okinawan karate has been addressed by pre-arranged training methods. While some see this as a fatal flaw in bringing the training closer to 'reality', you do well to remember the two things necessary for success in a fight: control and conclusion; if you fail to gain the first, the second is up for grabs. If this happens, then you had better pray your grab is quicker than your opponent's. When students spar, they adopt a mindset that encourages a continuation of the fight, leading to the abandonment of a core principle in any brawl: bring it to a conclusion. Okinawan karate has always looked to the kata for the answers to fighting. Within them are tactics and strategies handed down over many generations. In a reversal of today's approach to training, it should be understood the fighting strategies were developed first, and the kata were planned and calculated later to allow the tactics to be remembered, practiced, and transmitted to others. Eiichi Miyazato sensei, my teacher, always told me, "Bunkai came first, then kata!" The word 'bunkai' is best understood as 'component parts', the bits that go together to make something. By accepting this point of view, that bunkai came first and kata came later, the way you study and practice kata will alter from those who adhere to the common misconception that bunkai are merely an offshoot of kata. Trying to extract the information contained within each kata by simply repeating the movements over and over again is a mistake born of ignorance. These days, Japanese karate is busy trying to reverse-engineer its drastically altered kata to extract sensible fighting strategies that in many cases have been irrevocably lost in the constant remodeling of the kata, which they began a little under a hundred years ago. The redirection of karate, away from self-protection toward sport and commerce, changed the nature of the activity people were engaged in, and as Rory Miller reminds us, "If the goal changes, so does everything else." Vertical sidekicks, overly-exaggerated stances, and postures that offer you little real protection may seem impressive to a receptive audience of fans, but this "Hollywood" approach to karate leaves much to be desired when reality taps you on the shoulder and invites you outside.

Bunkai

The bunkai of each kata can, and should, vary according to the person studying the kata. You are not a clone! Just as you learned to speak, you speak in a unique way, and just as you learned to write, you write in your own way. Each kata is a collection of strategies based on principles that have been proven to work, not by samurai on some long forgotten battlefield in Japan, but by civilians who used such methods to survive attacks upon their person. Handed down through successive generations in China and crossing over to the people of Okinawa within the past few hundred years, these training drills (kata) remain vital to the transmission of various proven self-protection strategies. Later, I will go into more detail concerning the symbiosis between kata and bunkai, but for now, I want to take a closer look at the purpose of ippon and renzoku kumite.

Ippon Kumite: One Attack—One Response

Far from being a beginner's introduction to fighting in karate, ippon kumite (one attack fighting) represents the ultimate solution to personal combat. It echoes the maxim mentioned earlier, ikken hisatsu, one hit—one kill, and epitomizes the skill of the karateka, a person able to bring a confrontation to an immediate conclusion with the minimum of fuss. What makes this form of training so worthwhile is the attitude it helps to develop in those who use it over a protracted period of time; and it is this particular mentality, of dealing with an attack quickly and decisively, which brings about success. Some years ago, on the wooden cover of my makiwara I carved the Japanese proverb: "In budo it takes one thousand days to learn a technique, ten thousand days to polish it; the difference between victory and defeat is measured in the fraction of a second." I did it to remind myself, each time I face the makiwara, why I'm standing there. My punch was strengthened fairly quickly once I began to use the tool regularly, one thousand days; my method of delivery and the conditioning of my fists took a little longer to perfect, ten thousand days; but I have come to understand that even with such training, a split second's lack of concentration can bring with it certain defeat. How have I come to understand this? Through the injuries suffered over the years when I have failed to focus my attitude correctly, and landed poorly executed punches into the makiwara at high speed and with full force. In those fractions of a second between the start and finish of my punch, its success or failure was inextricably linked to my thinking; because my mind was not clearly focused, my punch was not focused either. The result of such 'lessons' have ranged from as little as split skin that caused an impressive amount of bleeding but did little harm, to damaged finger joints and knuckles that took some time to heal. Those who say the makiwara cannot hit back have, in my opinion, never trained with the tool seriously.

To begin with, ippon kumite is best kept formal, which is to say, during training, classical karate attacks are met by classical karate responses. I think this is wise until students have developed a certain level of control. Kumite, in all its forms, has the potential to over-excite some people, so I always keep a close eye on students when they face each other. That is, until I trust their judgment. Once that has been established I leave students to develop their own responses.

The three examples of ippon kumite shown here are simple and straightforward reactions to common attacks. Keeping a good distance from the attacker to begin with (fig. 4-31), a swinging punch to the head is met by checking the blow with the left elbow (*empi*) as the defender moves in (fig. 4-32). The block continues over the punching arm, trapping it, while the defender's right elbow impacts the attacker's jaw (fig. 4-33).

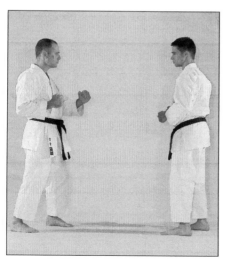

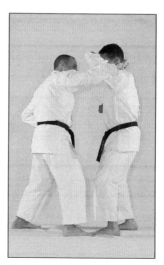

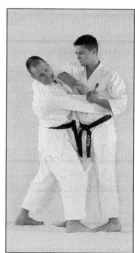

Figure 4-31

Figure 4-32

Figure 4-33

In the second example (fig. 4-34), a low swinging punch to the body (fig. 4-35) is checked with a low block (*gedan barai*), and immediately followed up with a short jab (*ura zuki*) to the attacker's body (fig. 4-36).

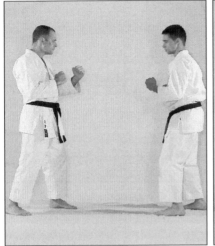 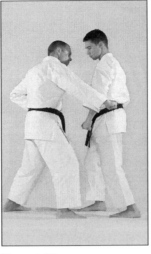 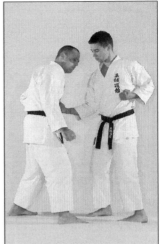

Figure 4-34   Figure 4-35   Figure 4-36

In the final example of ippon kumite (fig. 4-37), the kick is caught in a sweeping block as the defender uses *sabaki* to close the gap (fig 4-38) and from close in, counter-attacks using the elbow. The attack is driven home by the momentum of continuing to move forward, while lifting the leg higher (fig. 4-39), sending the attacker crashing to the ground.

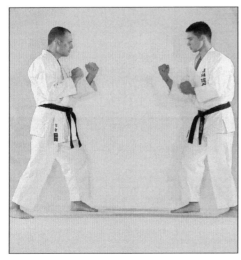 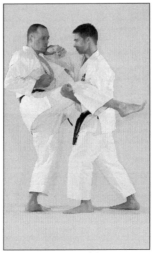 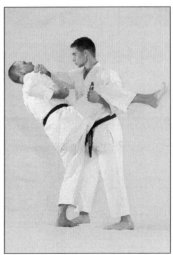

Figure 4-37   Figure 4-38   Figure 4-39

Let me stress this point once again before moving on: ippon kumite is practiced more to develop an attitude than it is to develop specific responses to specific attacks. It begins with the attacker and the defender both using classical karate techniques to attack, defend, and counterattack. However, as you gain skill and make progress this type of training needs to change. At some point you should begin using more common 'street' techniques: swinging punches, grabs, and kicks that sweep up from the ground without the knee being lifted first in classical karate fashion. These kinds of attack are what the eminent karate researcher and teacher, Patrick McCarthy, has labeled, "Habitual Acts of Physical Violence." The coining of this phrase is an apt description indeed. Under pressure, we tend to do what we know; what is habitual, and what street fighters know, or more accurately, what they don't know, is how to be effective fighters using classical karate stances and techniques such as straight punches. As the defender too, you must learn to respond using the principles of your karate rather than the textbook postures found in your classical training. Above all, your attitude, when you are being attacked, must be tuned in to the person doing the attacking, and you must be ready to respond instantly. This is, after all, the whole point of the exercise.

Renzoku: Multiple Attack—Multiple Response

Okay, so you have not been able to bring the fight to a close in one move; it is not the end of the world, but the longer a fight continues the greater the chance of your getting seriously hurt. In reality, it is better never to fight, but once you're in a fight it is better to win. You do this by bringing it to an end without trading one more blow than is necessary. One decisive strike is ideal, but if this is not an option, renzoku training will help you deal with a continuous attack. Familiarity is once again the main point of this type of training, getting used to people throwing not one but two, three, and four punches at you in quick succession. Kicks too, but not fancy jumping, spinning, back roundhouse kicks, more the front kicks coming up from the ground kind. Combination attacks of punches and kicks are the last form of renzoku I teach. At this stage, the training can begin to look less 'karate' like and to my mind this is exactly as it should be. The classical training is done to teach us ways to understand the principles and strategies involved in fighting, not 'how' to fight. In a real altercation, no one should consider standing in *nekoashi dachi*, cat stance, and yet this is how many people train all the time without ever moving on to use the principles involved in such a posture. Instead, they cling to the dream of making a 'perfect' stance. I will say it again here; the purpose of traditional karate training is not to accomplish perfect techniques, but to achieve workable techniques that improve your chances of survival when used for personal self-protection. During the life-long effort to attain workable techniques, we polish our spirit and find out exactly who we are.

Keeping the training close to the kata we practice is a good place to start. It not only reinforces the lesson learned during solo practice of the kata, but also links with the bunkai and other two-person drills done in the dojo. If a case can be made for 'styles' within karate, then it is found in a body of thought and practice where the things we do and the feelings we develop enhance each other. The idea that we can take the best techniques from various styles is a myth; for in truth there is no such thing as 'best techniques', and style is nothing more than your personal interpretation of what you have understood. So you can copy my way of doing something, but you cannot say you took it from Goju ryu, only that you took it from me. Had you copied the technique from another person holding the rank of 7th dan in Goju ryu karate, you would no doubt have ended up with something different. The question of 'best technique' is meaningless. The only requirement a technique has, any technique, is that it works for you! If it does then you gain some value from it; if the technique does not work the way you do it, then either learn to do it better or throw it away! Traditional karate presents students with a body of techniques and principles, and challenges them to make them their own. In doing this, traditional karate training has a habit of sorting out the weak-minded and the lazy. It shines a spotlight on those who have the will to continue and those who find an excuse for everything. In a traditional karate dojo, you stand alone, surrounded by others, and walk a steady path toward yourself.

I'm showing two examples of renzoku kumite, both taken directly from the same kata, *seiyunchin*. Facing off against a training partner (fig. 4-40), the first attack takes

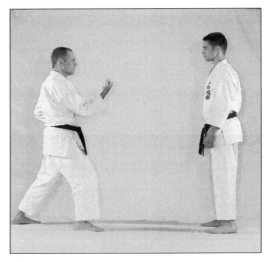

Figure 4-40

the form of a kick to the body (fig. 4-41) followed quickly afterward by a punch to the face (fig. 4-42). The defender has once again moved into the attack, using his forward momentum to catch the attacker off balance. Having hooked the kick in his arm and dodged the punch using his elbow as a shield, the defender now uses another fundamental idea found in Goju ryu, the application of opposites. As the attacker's head and shoulders are swung downward in one direction, his leg is lifted higher in the other direction (fig. 4-43). This flips the attacker over and sends him sprawling to the ground (fig. 4-44).

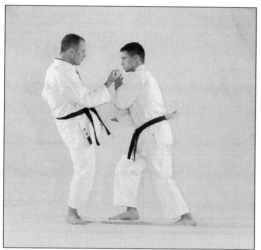

Figure 4-41

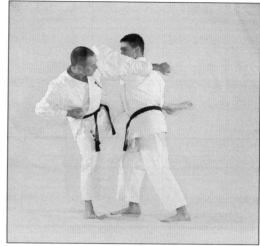

Figure 4-42

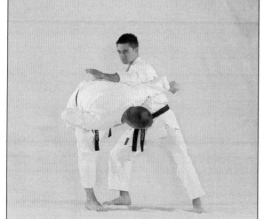

Figure 4-43

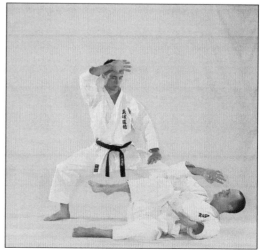

Figure 4-44

The second example of renzoku kumite (fig. 4-45) begins with a mid-level punch to the defender's chest, which is deflected by moving off the line of attack while covering with a *chudan uke*, supported by the other hand (fig. 4-46). This type of 'supported' blocking is known as *morote uke*. From this position, the defender goes on the offense and steps in to deliver a strike to the attacker's groin, but is stopped by the attacker grabbing the defender's arm (fig. 4-47). Before another attack can be launched, the defender changes stance (fig. 4-48) and begins to unbalance the attacker. As the defender's right arm continues to pull the attacker off balance, his left elbow is pushed hard into the attacker's arm (fig. 4-49) before he lowers his body weight (fig. 4-50), forcing the attacker to the ground.

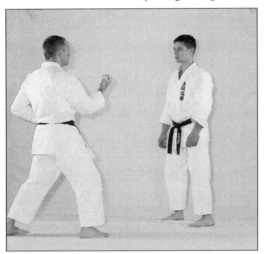

Figure 4-45

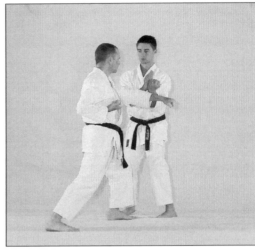

Figure 4-46

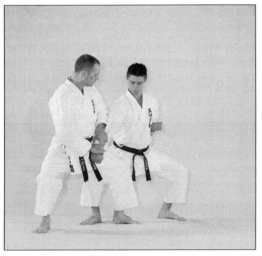

Figure 4-47

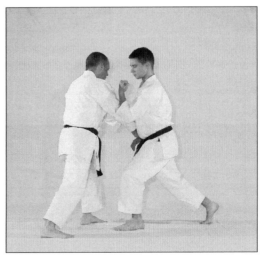

Figure 4-48

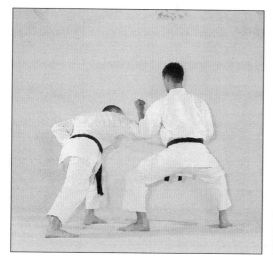

Figure 4-49

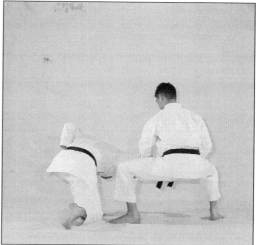

Figure 4-50

Kakie: The Application of Subtlety

I was told once while in Okinawa that Chojun Miyagi thought of kakie in much the same way as some modern karate people think of sparring; that is to say, it was practiced in order to grasp an understanding of how techniques work. I have to admit this confused me at first; my understanding of sparring did not tally with the way I saw kakie training: the first having more to do with a sporting approach to karate, while the latter was more in tune with self-protection. Looking back now I can see I had fallen into the old trap of believing I already knew what I was looking at when it came to kakie. I mean, how hard could it be to understand; it was just two people connected at the wrist, pushing each other around … right? Well, I was subsequently proven wrong about that, and quite happily so. Over the years since my introduction to kakie at the Higaonna dojo in Okinawa, I have come to appreciate the subtle strength and endless possibilities that come with training this way. If indeed Chojun Miyagi saw this type of training as a way to develop a fighter's mind in his students, as some assert is the purpose of dojo sparring, then his insight was correct. I now understand much more about controlling the distances involved in a fight and the importance of the advice given by the great Chinese general and strategist Sun-Tzu, who lived between 500 and 400 B.C., when he suggested we "keep our friends close, and our enemies even closer!"

When training in kakie, contact is already made with your opponent; what you do with this contact is at the heart of the training. To begin with, it's a simple matter of learning how to disrupt your training partner's balance (*kuzushi*). If he pushes hard, you gently pull; if he pulls hard, you go with him and strike. After a while, the tactics become a little more involved with the focus shifting to timing. When this happens, the response to being pushed or pulled depends entirely upon your sense of timing. Too soon or too late and you find your response collapsing around you; so now you must give some thought to how you might best achieve your aim, which is, of course, to subdue your opponent. Hidden within your search to find the correct sense of timing is the principle of harmony, and by harmonizing your movements with that of your attacker, you can learn to render his movements ineffective. Now, this is a lot easier to write about than it is to achieve on the dojo floor, so please remember I am as much a student of karate today as I was when I began. I see the way forward a little clearer these days, but I still have problems making progress.

In an attempt to get across this idea of blending with an opponent's action in order to render him inert, I sometimes use the following metaphor. Imagine you are standing on the back of a flat truck doing fifty miles per hour (80 km) along a straight road. Another truck pulls up alongside and remains only an inch (2.5 cm) away from the truck you are standing on. Would you be able to step from one truck to the other? Given a little encouragement, or the right incentive, I think most people could in spite of the speed the trucks are moving at. Now, imagine for a moment that the truck beside you continually changes speed, not by much, just a few miles an hour, slowing down then speeding back up again. Would you be as willing to step across? The point I am trying to make with this story is one of harmony. When the two trucks are evenly matched in speed (timing), there appears to be no motion between the two, even though they are hurtling along at fifty miles an hour, but as soon as one truck moves in a different way from the other the harmony between them is lost, as is the perception of being able to step safely across from one to the other.

When we fail to harmonize with an attack, we fail to grasp an opportunity to control the situation. In a fight, such opportunities may come only once, and often this will be at the very beginning as the attacker gears up to make his first move. Far from being a fanciful notion advocated by many senior martial artists, most commonly by teachers of *aikido*, establishing a sense of harmony with an opponent is vital to a weaker person overcoming a stronger person. The principles of timing, irimi, kuzushi, and sen no sen, all come into play during kakie training. It is a test of subtlety not strength, as anyone who has had the pleasure as I have, many times, of engaging in this type of training with senior Okinawan karateka who have mastered those subtleties will tell you. I'm showing four examples of kakie here, two very simple and direct, and two that require a little more subtlety, but they hardly scratch the surface when it comes to ways to manipulate a training partner. Only time and hours spent practicing will bring you an ability to read your partner's intentions through the subtle shifts in the body. Like every other aspect in the learning of karate, there are no shortcuts.

All kakie applications are done from the continuous exchange of pushing going on between training partners (figs. 4-51, 4-52, and 4-53). It is important to note there is no pulling involved in the basic exchange of hands. Your hand returns to your chest only because your partner has pushed it there. Some applications are executed on your push, while others come about as a result of your partner's push; all the examples shown here are done against a push by your partner. Kakie is an exchange between training partners;

there is no attacker and defender, as the roles cross from one to the other constantly. Here you will see each student in turn attempts to apply his ability to manipulate his training partner with nothing more than a good sense of timing, distance, and the subtle use of angles. Both arms are used in kakie training, and you should change from one arm to the other, about every two or three minutes.

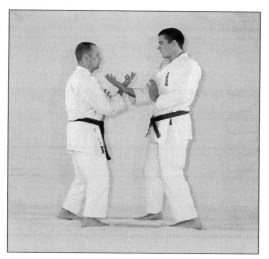

Figure 4-51

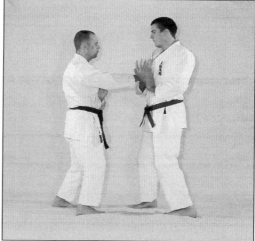

Figure 4-52

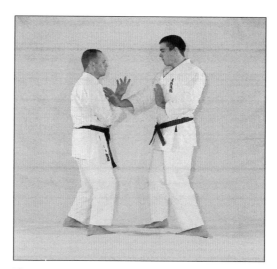

Figure 4-53

In the first example (fig. 4-54), the pushing hand of the opponent is guided toward your other hand, where it is waiting to trap the fingers (fig. 4-55, and the close-up image, fig. 4-56).

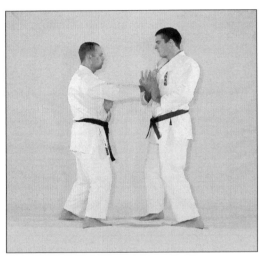

Figure 4-54

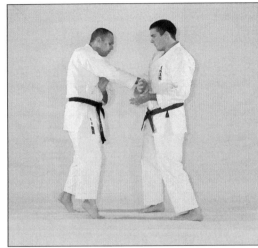

Figure 4-55

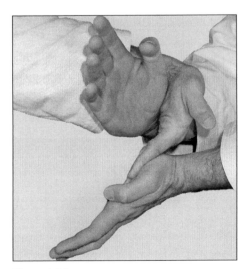

Figure 4-56

Next, in the second example, as the pushing hand comes in, it is redirected upward while the body drops into a low stance and strikes to the groin (figs. 4-57, 4-58).

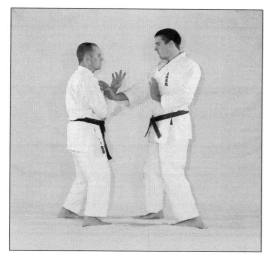

Figure 4-57

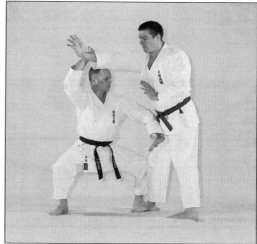

Figure 4-58

In the third example (fig. 4-59), the pushing hand is directed past the body while at the same time a punch is directed into the face of your training partner (fig. 4-60). The elbow is dropped down in front of the pushing arm, breaking your partner's balance (fig. 4-61), and from there continues on, under the arm. Your hand is placed on the back of

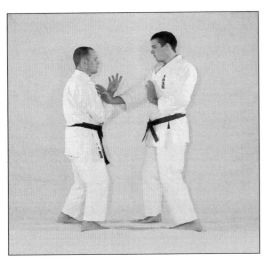

Figure 4-59

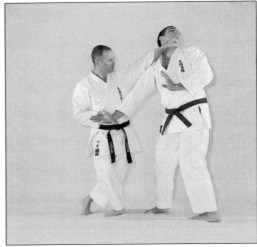

Figure 4-60

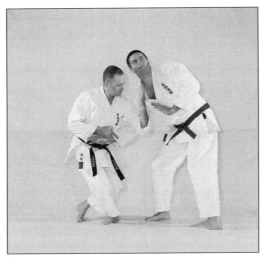

Figure 4-61

your training partner, pulling him in toward you, trapping his arm (fig. 4-62), and from there a strike to the jaw is accompanied by dropping your body into *shiko dachi* (fig. 4-63) to collapse your training partner to the ground.

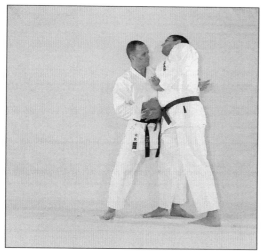

Figure 4-62

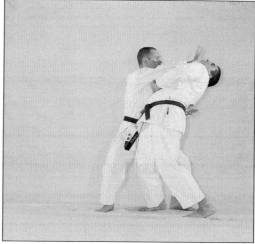

Figure 4-63

The final example of kakie draws on knowledge of the kata *shisochin.* Having started on the right, the students have switched arms, and are now working with their left arms. As the push comes in, the arm is directed past the body while an elbow is driven into it (fig. 4-64). The attempt to retract the trapped arm is exploited by twisting back around, now facing toward your training partner (fig. 4-65). What was an arm-bar using the elbow, now becomes an arm-lock (fig. 4-66) as the arm is pushed into the elbow joint and a tight spin is used to continue the momentum backward and down (fig. 4-67), resulting in a painful wrist lock (fig. 4-68).

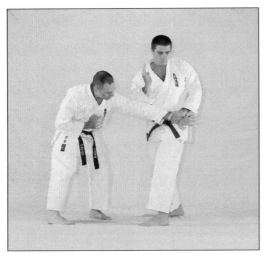

Figure 4-64

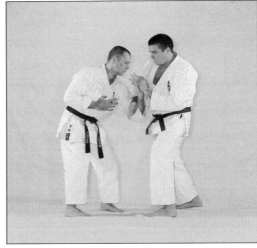

Figure 4-65

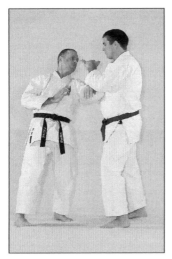

Figure 4-66

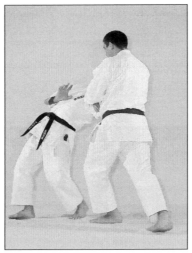

Figure 4-67

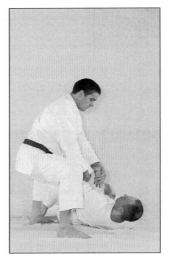

Figure 4-68

Kata: Focus on Gekisai Dai Ichi

In 1940, Chojun Miyagi and Shoshin Nagamine, working in collaboration, created the *gekisai* kata. *Gekisai ichi* reflects the karate of Shoshin Nagamine, while Chojun Miyagi is thought to have devised *gekisai ni,* incorporating within it his ideas about moving backward during combat. Some years later, my teacher, Eiichi Miyazato, added the 'great' (*dai*) suffix. In the Matsubayashi school of karate founded by Shoshin Nagamine, the kata *gekisai dai ichi* is known as *fukyugata ni.*[56] Regardless of the name given to a kata, remember, it is the fighting principles and strategies contained within each of them that gives them value. Simply committing the movements and postures to memory is not the same as 'knowing' a kata. Learning the classical moves provides only a common template by which each generation of karateka is introduced to the strategies locked away in

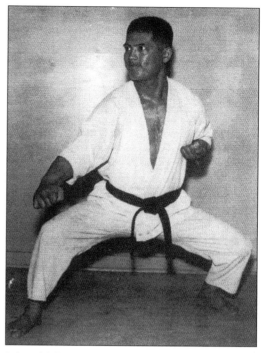

Seiyu Shinjo sensei's face reflects the intensity of his kata training.

the kata; without further personal investigation, kata offer little to those hoping to improve their self-protection skills. The idea that there was only one 'real' meaning behind each technique found in a kata is silly and shows a complete lack of understanding when it comes to the purpose of kata as a training aid. In Okinawa the personal investigation and study of kata is not only understood by students, but also insisted upon by their sensei. In Japan, however, this is not the case. As with almost everything in Japan, there is a correct way to do something, and countless wrong ways. The correct way is achieved by strict adherence to the kata, the formal, and more importantly, the approved method of accomplishing any number of tasks. In his excellent book, *Kata: The Key to Understanding & Dealing with the Japanese*, the author, Boyé Lafayette De Mente, explains in great detail the role of kata in Japanese society. I suspect the majority of karateka around the world think the word applies only to the set of patterns they are required to learn and commit to memory in order to pass their next promotion test. Nothing could be further from the truth, for kata can be found in every aspect of Japanese life, and those who do not understand this will find doors of opportunity not only closing before them, but also disappearing altogether. Under the heading, "The Feeling of Rightness," on page 10, the author has this to say:

Born and raised in a cultural environment that was the result of centuries of conditioning in the art of living Japanese style and in the use of arts and crafts that were products of rigidly controlled kata, each Japanese naturally developed a sixth sense that told him when things were "right"—that is, when they were designed, made, assembled, packaged or whatever in accordance with Japanese concepts of aesthetics.

On page 54, when the author is discussing the Japanese martial arts, he remarks:

It is interesting to note that several hundred thousand Westerners have undergone intensive conditioning in Japanese kata since the 1960s, some of them without ever realizing the cultural significance, and the number continues to grow each year. These partly kata-ized Westerners are students of Japan's famed karate-do (kah-rah-tay-doh)—and most of them are good examples of the positive aspects of the kata system.

On page 56, he goes on to write:

Karate is thus a perfect example of Japanese kata in action, an ideal situation based on total control of the mind and body, absolute adherence to minutely prescribed behavior, the mastery of techniques designed to mount a perfect defense or demolish an opponent, and a moral philosophy that integrates peace and power.

Note the author describes 'karate' as a perfect example of 'kata', and not the other way around, as the majority of Westerners might imagine being the case. Regardless of which school of Japanese karate you join, you will soon discover there is only one way to do each technique and each stance, to sit down or stand up, and a correct way to perform each and every kata. That is of course until someone at the top decides to make changes; then everyone is expected to forget the way they once did things and adopt the new method with as much enthusiasm as they once practiced the old. The redundancy rate for techniques in certain schools of karate is surprisingly high. Usually explained away as 'progress' or 'development', in truth it shows a lack of depth and understanding regarding the role of kata in karate. If you train in karate for long enough, you will discover an interesting phenomenon within many schools: techniques and methods that were abandoned long ago amazingly come back into fashion; once again restored and given credibility, they are shamelessly (re)introduced to students under the pretext of progress or development, the very same explanation that saw them abandoned years earlier. The turnover of students within karate schools being so numerous, the majority fail to recognize the new techniques for what they are, and so the cycle of shallowness continues for another turn. That your karate changes is not in dispute here; in fact, I would think it very strange indeed if you had been training for fifteen or twenty years and your karate was the same now as at the time you started. With the passage of time comes experience;

your body, too, changes from youth to middle age, and eventually to old age. Training in your fifties the way you did in your twenties is not cause for celebration. It simply isn't possible. If it is, then you need to question why, as a twenty year old, you were training like a person in his fifties?

Eiichi Miyazato sensei spoke to me about training according to my age and my health. He had little time for macho-men who approached each training session as if they were trying out for the United States Marine Corps display team. At each age in your life, there is an appropriate way to train and ironically, it's the same: you train to the best of your abilities, taking into account your health and the well-being of your family, as well as the protection of your income. The classical kata handed down from the past are there to point you in the right direction; you need not study them all, nor work out intricate applications for every single movement. Instead, what is needed is an ability to dismantle your kata and reassemble them in ways that offer protection from aggression, for this is their purpose, i.e., not to deliver to you an arsenal of deadly techniques, but to provide an opportunity to discover what you are capable of. An ability to remember fifty kata will serve you poorly in comparison to a deep understanding of just one. As you age and mature so too should your karate. As it does, it will change: naturally. But the essence of what you do will not, for your karate should always be based on principles rather than techniques. A man who changes his principles to suit the fashion of the day is hardly a man at all.

Here, I am going to show a few ways the students at the Shinseidokan dojo work on kata. I have deliberately focused on one, gekisai dai ichi, as this is considered by most to be a beginner's kata. However, I want to reiterate my view regarding basic and advanced karate, which is, the difference lies not in the techniques being used but in the person using them. The name, gekisai—to smash and destroy—gives a clue to the strategy about to be employed. Although it may not look like a particularly brutal or aggressive set of techniques, how the techniques are used makes all the difference. I won't be looking at the solo practice of gekisai, as my aim here is to show a variety of ways you can investigate your kata other than in thin air; besides, as each school of karate has a different way of performing its kata, my kata would be meaningless. The point I'm making here is this: kata training is about more than remembering movements in thin air. Students are introduced to the fighting tactics of this and every other kata through a series of basic (*kihon*) kumite drills, which at this stage are designed to stay as close to the movements found in the kata as possible, thus placing little stress on either the attacker or the defender. Initially, all attacks are made using classical karate techniques to allow the attacker to practice his basic skills. As skill levels increase, applications take on a slightly more realistic flavor. However, please remember, what I'm doing here is planting a seed in your mind; if you want to grasp the essence of a kata, then you must investigate its hidden depths for yourself through various forms of kumite practice.

Ippon Kumite Bunkai

Number One:

   While facing off against each other (fig. 4-69), the attacker steps forward as quickly as possible, punching to the defender's face. The defender shifts to the right while covering the incoming punch with his left arm (fig. 4-70). He then throws a right-hand punch to the attacker's throat (fig. 4-71). With the drill over, both students move back to their original positions.

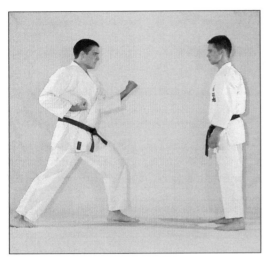

Figure 4-69

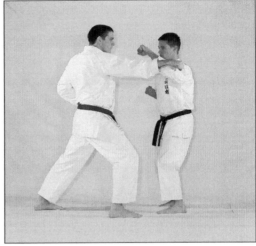

Figure 4-70

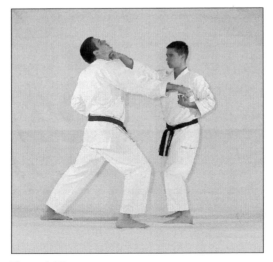

Figure 4-71

Number Two:

Facing off against each other (fig. 4-72), the attacker instigates his attack with a front kick to the bladder. The defender moves to the right and drops into *shiko dachi*, covering the kick as he does so with the left arm (fig. 4-73), before delivering a right punch into the stomach of the attacker (fig. 4-74). As before, both return to their original positions.

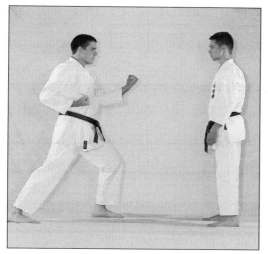

Figure 4-72

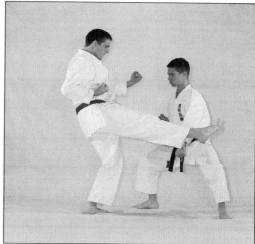

Figure 4-73

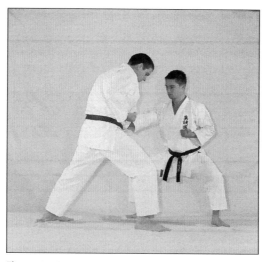

Figure 4-74

Number Three:

This drill introduces the idea of renzoku kumite, more than one attack. Facing off against each other (fig. 4-75), the attacker steps forward to throw a punch to the chest of the defender (fig. 4-76). The defender moves off to the right using *tai sabaki*—body shifting—to move off the line of attack. Blocking the punch with a *chudan uke*—mid-level block—he immediately counters with a kick to the groin or bladder[*] (fig. 4-77) before dropping forward to deliver *empi uchi*—elbow strike—to the chest (fig. 4-78),

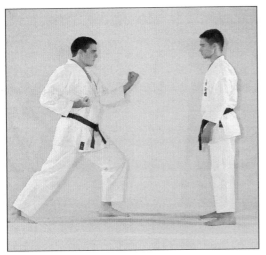

Figure 4-75

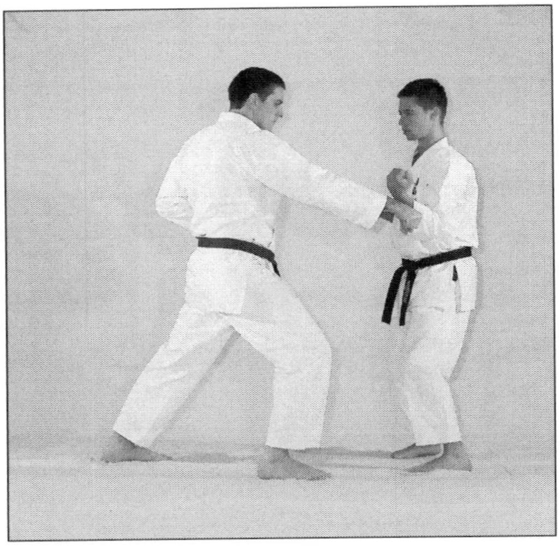

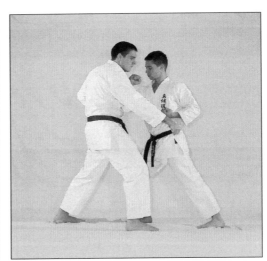

Figure 4-76

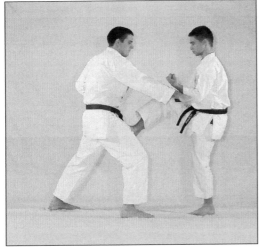

Figure 4-77

Figure 4-78

[*] In practice, this kick is aimed at the inside of the thigh.

followed in quick succession by *uraken*—back-fist strike—to the face (fig. 4-79). This motivates the attacker to shift backward before throwing a second punch into the body of the defender (fig. 4-80), who blocks with *gedan barai*—lower sweeping block—before countering for a second time with a body punch of his own (fig. 4-81).

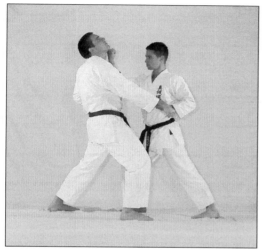

Figure 4-79

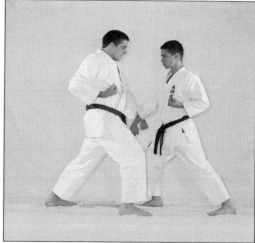

Figure 4-80

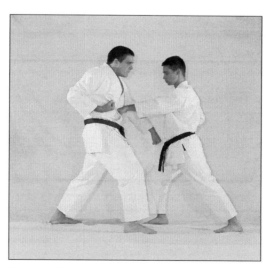

Figure 4-81

Number Four:

Facing off against each other (fig. 4-82), the attacker steps forward before throwing a mid-level punch to the chest of the defender. The defender moves sharply to the side, before grasping the attacker's arm and sweeping him with a simultaneous combination of a *jodan shuto uchi*—upper level open-handed strike—and an *ashi barai*—foot sweep (fig. 4-83). Controlling the attacker as he falls to the ground* (fig. 4-84), the defender turns his body and follows through with a *kakato geri*—heel-stamping kick—to the side of the ribs, just below the armpit of the attacker (fig. 4-85). Before releasing the arm, the defender throws it away from them and steps back, and from here, both return to their original positions.

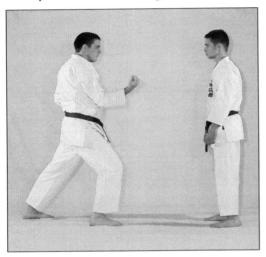

Figure 4-82

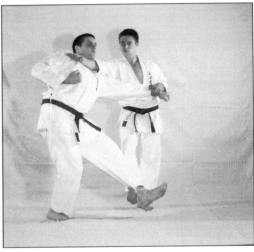

Figure 4-83

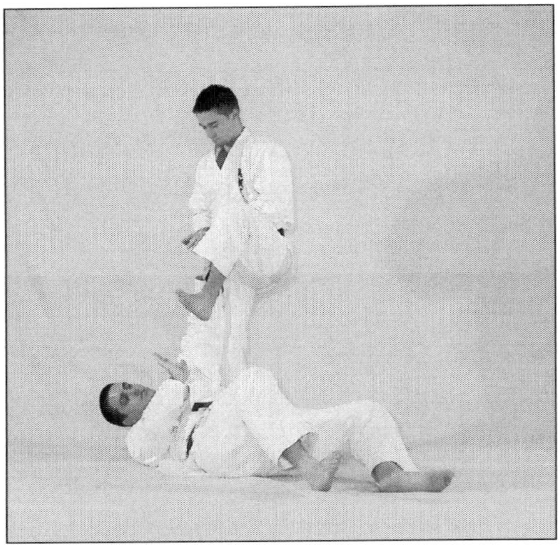

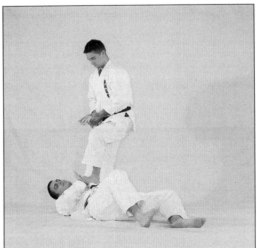

Figure 4-84

Figure 4-85

---

* This is achieved by holding on to the attacker's wrist as he starts to go down. The idea is to drop him to the floor under control so you can follow through with the stamping kick to the ribcage.

Number Five:

Facing off against each other (fig. 4-86), the attacker steps forward and throws a punch to the body. The defender has a choice here: he can move to the left or right. Shifting off the direct line of attack, he parries the punch (fig. 4-87) and without chambering his fists, continues through and throws a double punch (fig. 4-88), either into the attacker's side if he moved to the outside of the attack, or into the body, as seen here, if he moved to the inside of the attack.

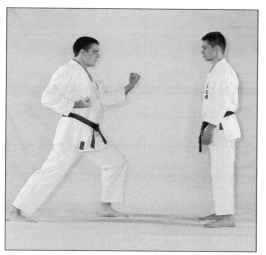

Figure 4-86

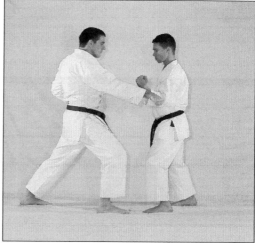

Figure 4-87

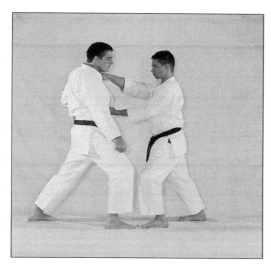

Figure 4-88

The five basic bunkai drills act only as an introduction to the combat strategies encoded within gekisai dai ichi kata. The student in the *attacker* role remains in character throughout. Only when the roles are reversed is he required to adopt a different attitude. The same is true for the student in the role of the *defender*. This is an important point, as the attitude you adopt, depending on which role you occupy, is entirely different due to the different outcomes you are trying to accomplish in each. As the attacker, you are trying to cover distance quickly, close the gap between you and your training partner, and strike him accurately. As the defender, your role is different; now you are trying to anticipate, blend, redirect, and control your training partner; you are trying to achieve a different outcome from the result the attacker is looking for. As Rory Miller points out, "If the goal changes, everything changes." A part of that 'everything' is your attitude. With *kihon ippon* kumite, basic one-strike fighting, the role you adopt is not only physical; inside your head, your mind should be working differently too. Get your attitude right, and the rest will follow.

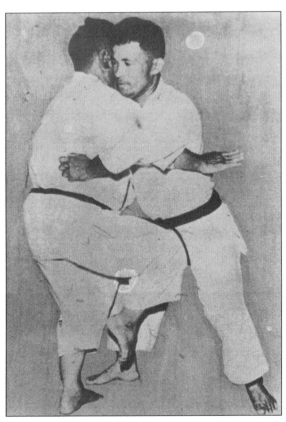

Chojun Miyagi practicing bunkai from seisan kata, with his student Eiichi Miyazato, ca. 1949.

Following on from this introduction to the application drills associated with gekisai dai ichi kata is another drill that requires the whole kata to be performed while under attack. Not only does this drill reinforce the solo training pattern, but also draws the student one step closer to the ever-changing mindset that exists in combat. Not being able to adapt to the physical changes going on in a fight can lead to disaster; that ability to adapt begins, like everything else, in your mind. Having the right attitude is therefore essential to gaining the upper hand. In this two-person version of the kata, the role of attacker and defender are constantly changing back and forth. Although the drill is still a long way from the reality of how the techniques might be used in a fight, the important point at this stage is for you to be able to switch your attitude quickly and yet maintain a sense of flow and rhythm. It is a two-person kata at this stage, not a highly choreographed fighting drill. Even when performed at high speed and with some force, it remains far too contrived to be thought of as fighting, so use the drill as intended. That way you will eventually absorb the lessons it has to give.

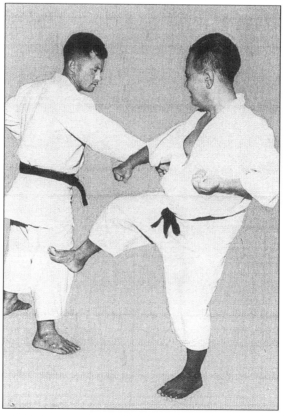

Here, Chojun Miyagi is working on a second application from seisan kata, with Eiichi Miyazato.

Two-Person Kata

Facing off against each other (fig. 4-89), the *attacker* (left) begins with his right leg forward and his right hand in *chudan kamae*. The *defender,* the student practicing the kata (right), stands in the *yoi* position, as if to perform the kata in thin air. The attacker steps forward and punches to the face; the defender steps backward on the right leg and blocks with the left arm (fig. 4-90). Now the defender counterattacks by stepping forward and attacking to the face, forcing the attacker to step back and defend (fig. 4-91). The attacker, in turn, makes the block and immediately steps forward again, dropping

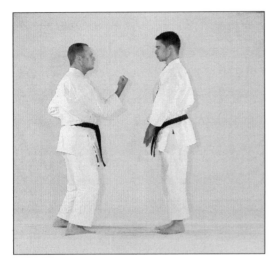

Figure 4-89

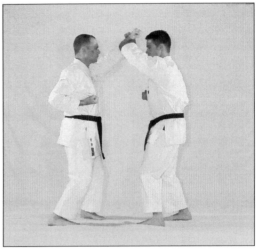

Figure 4-90

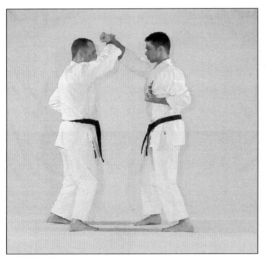

Figure 4-91

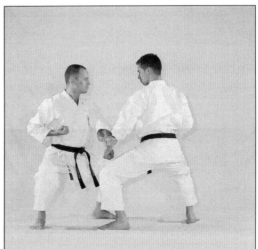

Figure 4-92

into *shiko dachi* and throws a low punch. At this point, the defender steps back, also into *shiko dachi*, and blocks the low punch with a *gedan barai* block (fig. 4-92). The attacker steps forward again, this time in *sanchin dachi*, and the same sequence is repeated, using the opposite side of the body (figs. 4-93, 4-94, and 4-95).

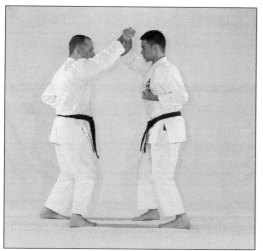
Figure 4-93

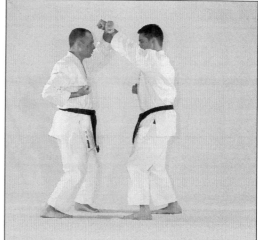
Figure 4-94

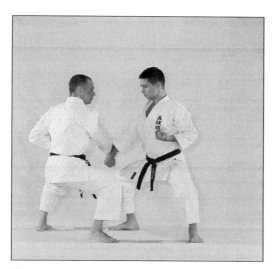
Figure 4-95

After the second low punch attack has been blocked, the attacker steps forward once again, in *sanchin dachi*, and punches to the midsection (fig. 4-96); the defender steps back, also into *sanchin dachi*, and blocks the punch. A second step forward and midsection punch from the attacker sees the defender step back and repeat the *chudan* block with his right arm (fig. 4-97), before moving forward with a low, left kick to the attacker's groin (fig. 4-98).

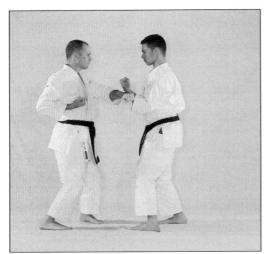

Figure 4-96

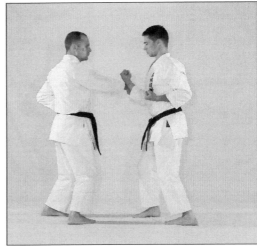

Figure 4-97

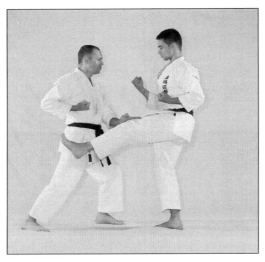

Figure 4-98

Dropping his weight down, the attacker parries the kick away with a sweeping block and immediately raises the same hand back up to parry away the incoming elbow strike (fig. 4-99), before using the wrist, *ko uke*, to check the back-fist strike, *uraken* (fig. 4-100). At that point, he counterattacks by throwing a mid-level punch into the ribs (fig. 4-101). The defender blocks the punch and straightaway throws the same punch with his right hand (fig. 4-102); the attacker checks this punch.

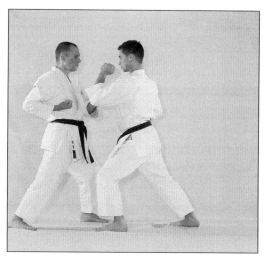

Figure 4-99

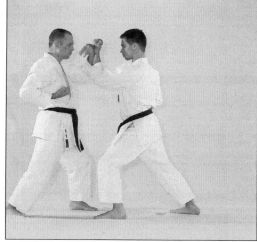

Figure 4-100

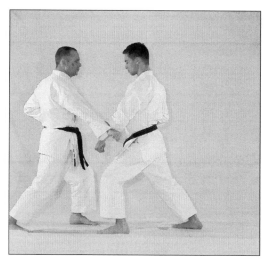

Figure 4-101

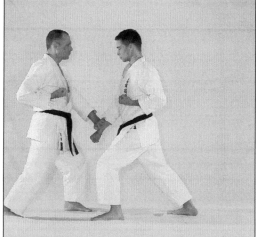

Figure 4-102

The defender presses home his assault by moving forward and following through with a leg sweep (fig. 4-103), *ashi barai,* and open hand strike to the face, *jodan shuto uchi* (fig. 4-104). The attacker is forced to avoid the sweep by lifting his front leg to escape and defend himself from the face strike with a second *ko uke* block, before turning the attack back on to the defender by quickly stepping forward and punching to the midsection (fig. 4-105).

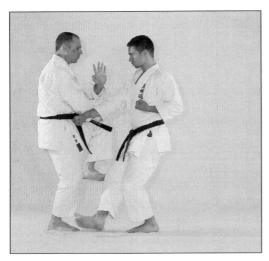

Figure 4-103

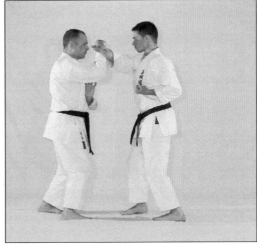

Figure 4-104

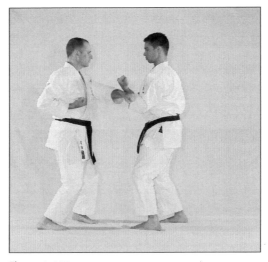

Figure 4-105

From here, the defender repeats his attacking sequence beginning, this time, with a right front kick to the attacker's groin (fig. 4-106), followed by an elbow strike to the body (fig. 4-107) and a back-fist strike to the face with the same arm (fig. 4-108). The attacker blocks in exactly the same way as before, prior to his left punch to the defender's body, which is blocked (fig. 4-109).

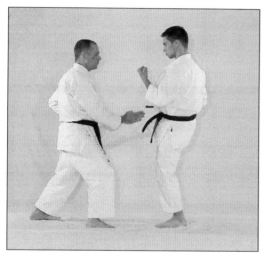

Figure 4-106

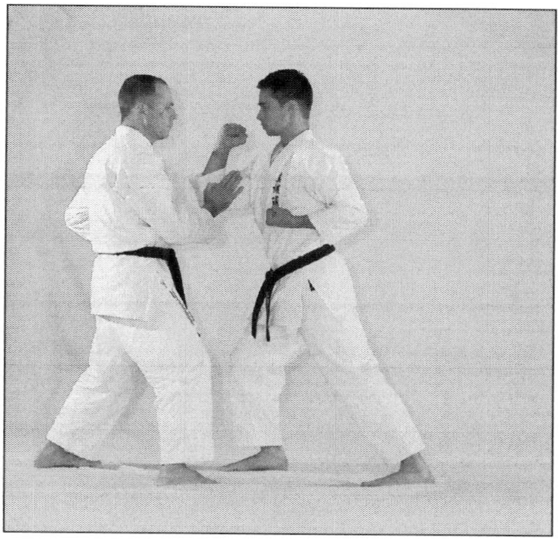

Figure 4-107

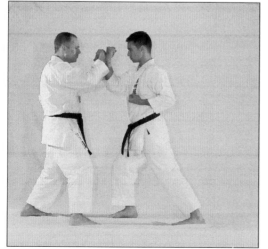

Figure 4-108

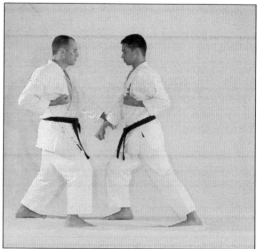

Figure 4-109

The defender finishes off this section of the kata by quickly following up on his block with a body punch of his own (fig. 4-110) followed by the same leg-sweep/knife-hand attack (figs. 4-111, 4-112), culminating in the attacker's final *ko uke* block before launching his closing assault with a lunging punch to the body (fig. 4-113).

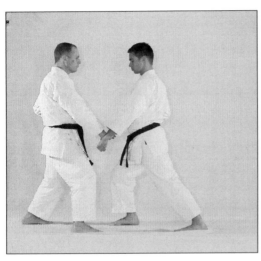

Figure 4-110

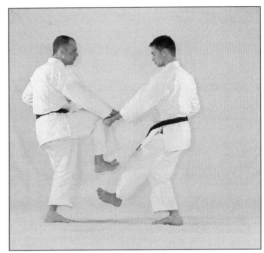

Figure 4-111

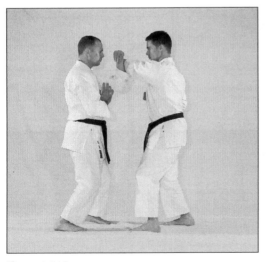

Figure 4-112

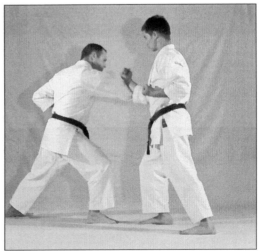

Figure 4-113

This, in turn, is deflected as the defender shifts quickly to the left before punching with both arms, with the left arm on top (figs. 4-114, 4-115). The final exchange takes place when the attacker turns sharply in toward the defender and throws his last punch. The defender avoids the punch by using *tai sabaki* once again, this time to the right, and repeats the double punch, only this time with the right arm on top (figs. 4-116, 4-117, and 4-118).

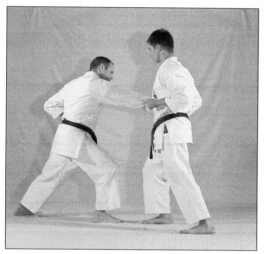

Figure 4-114

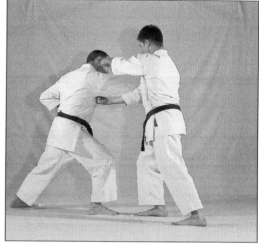

Figure 4-115

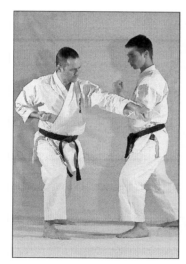

Figure 4-116

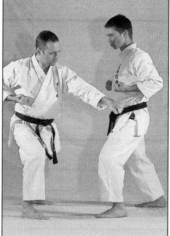

Figure 4-117

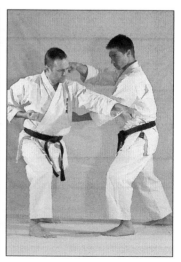

Figure 4-118

The drill is brought to a close with the attacker stepping forward onto his right foot, while at the same time, the defender steps backward onto his rear foot (fig. 4-119). As they do so they turn inward to face each other making a *yoi* (on guard) posture (fig. 4-120); both then sidestep to the left, which brings them back on line with the start position (fig. 4-121). From here, bow to your training partner: end of drill.

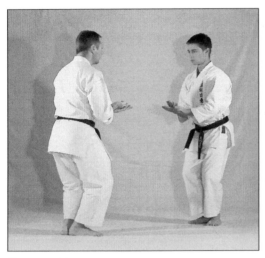

Figure 4-119

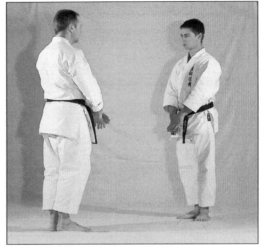

Figure 4-120

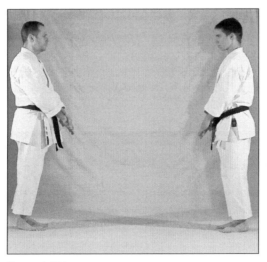

Figure 4-121

With the importance of a changing attitude now in place, the physical training can move on and take a step closer to the reality of application. Having powerful punches or kicks in isolation are of little use if you are unable to land them on target. The nature of physical violence is fluid and ever-changing; therefore, a sense of rhythm and flow, as well as an ever-adapting attitude, is necessary in order to deliver your techniques. But how do we practice this? Many schools of karate in Okinawa have come up with training drills designed to encourage a sense of flow. These flow drills, like the drills found in hojo undo are many and varied, and beyond the scope of this book; however, I am including a couple of flow drills that relate to both gekisai dai ichi and dai ni. Once again, you would do well to remember that these are not fighting drills per se; as with the earlier two-person kata drill, they stay too close to the classic single person form to be considered viable applications of the strategies found in the kata. They are, nevertheless, a good way to find a feeling of flow and of continuation; and for that reason, these are training drills worth practicing. There is a subtle difference in attitude here also. In ippon kumite training your attitude remains that of either the attacker or the defender throughout the drill. In the two-person kata, your attitude switched from one to the other as you worked your way through the kata. As the defender, flow drills ask you to steal your attacker's attitude; and you do that by switching instantly from a defensive mindset to an offensive one, pressing home your counterattack while continuing to move forward throughout the entire drill. Of course, these training drills, like all the others, are set up for the student doing the kata to triumph over his partner; even so, by working your kata in a variety of ways, you will begin to view the solo—thin air—training pattern in a more meaningful way.

With both of these drills, the students initiate their attack in ways more common to the street than the dojo. So instead of straight punches and kicks, punches are swung or hooked, and attacks sometimes begin with a grab. In the following two sequences, you will see how I have condensed the ideas found in the kata to deal with two common methods of attacks on the street, similar to what Patrick McCarthy so aptly calls his "Habitual Acts of Physical Violence" theory. When you consider the meaning behind the name given to these two kata, gekisai dai ichi and gekisai dai ni, you also begin to see the nature of the attitude you should adopt when you're training in them. The first part, *geki* (撃), means to fight or strike; the second, *sai* (砕), means to smash or break; the implication is therefore clear: if attacked, your response should be overwhelming. Far from being a paradigm for the novice, the gekisai kata, together, offer a decisive way of bringing an assault to a speedy conclusion.

Flow Drills

Facing off against a training partner, both students should adopt a natural but alert posture (fig. 4-122). The attacker, on the right, moves in quickly with a swinging punch to the head. The defender, on the left, also closes the gap and blocks the incoming punch closer to the elbow than the wrist of the attacker's arm (fig. 4-123); the block is immediately followed through with a punch to the throat or face of the attacker (fig.4-124) before dropping low while continuing to move forward, gathering momentum.

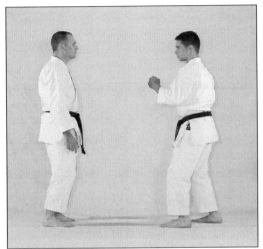

Figure 4-122

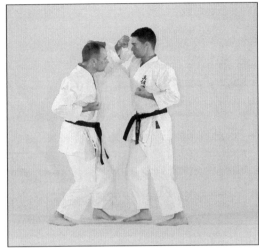

Figure 4-123

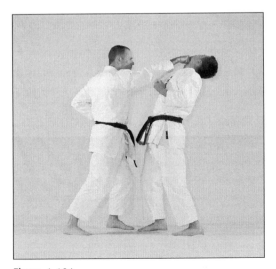

Figure 4-124

The strike to the attacker's groin with the left fist (fig. 4-125) is followed straightaway by rising up again, and with the right arm swinging in an arch to catch the attacker on the side or back of his head (fig. 4-126), tip his body forward and down (fig. 4-127). The attacker's crash to the floor is assisted by a leg sweep, followed immediately by a double punch (fig. 4-128). Depending on how the attacker lands, on his back or on his side, the defender's fists should land on targets that will do the maximum damage.

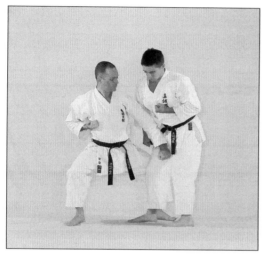

Figure 4-125

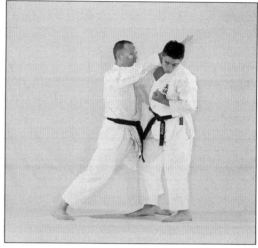

Figure 4-126

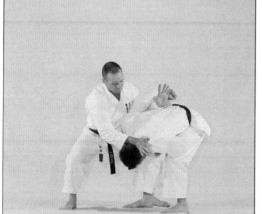

Figure 4-127

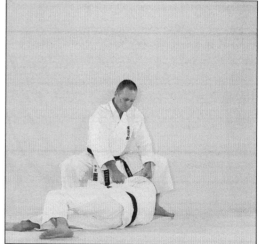

Figure 4-128

Obviously, even with all the 'attitude' in the world, you are only training here; this is not a real fight and so great care must be taken not to damage or injure your training partner. This is the shortfall in all martial arts and sports; you have to hold back to some degree or risk seriously hurting your training partners, which is something to think about the next time you hear the term "Full-Contact." I doubt there are many people in the world that could take a full contact kick to the groin or the head by someone out to do them harm. In this, and other two person drills, groin kicks are aimed at the inner thigh and great care is always taken when landing blows. A special mention is necessary here when it comes to grappling, in particular, the twists and pulls aimed at the neck. Throughout Goju ryu karate, there are many attacks aimed at the neck, and for good reason; it is a very vulnerable part of the human body. All the messages from your brain to your body travel through it, so any disruption here can have an immediate and catastrophic affect. Although disguised, or should I say, not obvious, students first come across this "target" in the gekisai kata. It is absolutely essential, in my opinion, that no adult under the rank of shodan—1st dan black belt—be introduced to such techniques. As for showing children this kind of thing, well that's just plain stupid!

The second drill begins with the attacker, on the right, grabbing the defender's arm (fig. 4-129). The defender responds by turning his hand upward to lessen the effectiveness of the attacker's grip, moving across and in front of his body to bring his elbow inward, adds to the weakness of the attacker's hold (fig. 4-130).

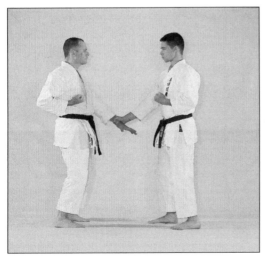

Figure 4-129

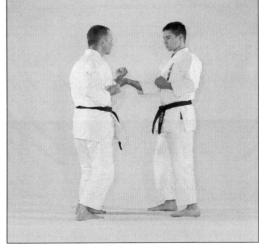

Figure 4-130

The defender then kicks the attacker's groin (fig. 4-131), landing with a stamp on the attacker's lead foot (fig. 4-132), following through with an elbow strike to the chest and a back-fist strike to the face (figs. 4-133, 4-134).

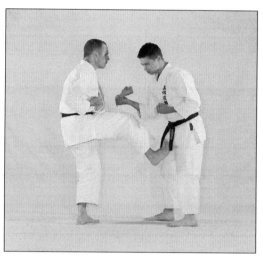

Figure 4-131

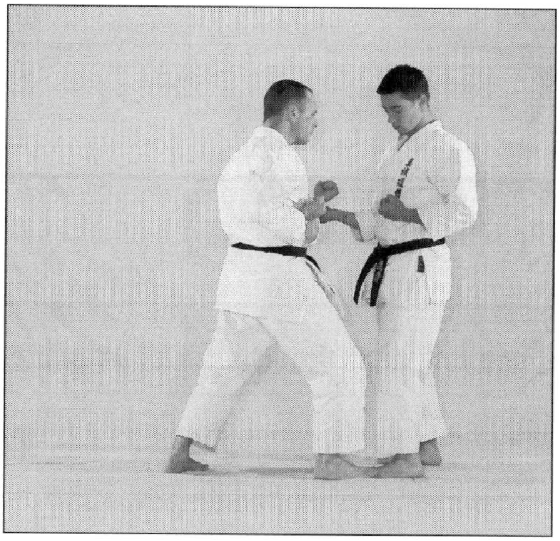

Figure 4-132

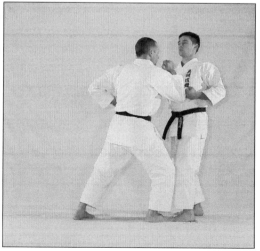

Figure 4-133

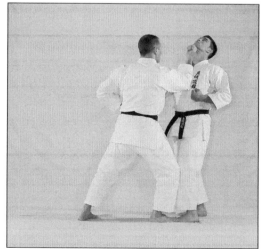

Figure 4-134

The shock induced in the attacker by the defender's rapid response, and the impact to the lower, middle, and now upper parts of the body in quick succession, gives the defender the time needed to bring the right arm over and break the attacker's already weakened grip (fig. 4-135). This response is then followed through with a strong left-hand punch to the attacker's ribs (fig. 4-136) before finishing him off in the same way as before, with an elbow/arm strike to the neck (fig. 4-137) and a leg sweep to bring him crashing to the ground, followed by a well-placed double punch to the appropriate targets (fig. 4-138).

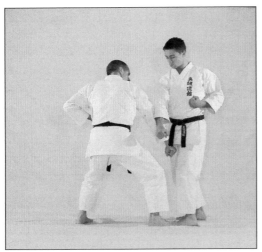

Figure 4-135

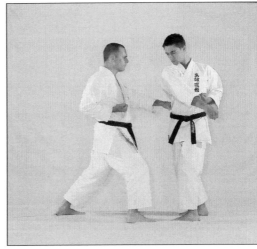

Figure 4-136

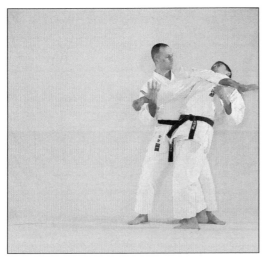

Figure 4-137

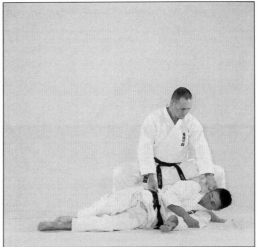

Figure 4-138

Finally, if you have no one to train with, you can still work on the fighting strategies by working your kata in thin air, by yourself. Keep in mind, as you do the possible applications, the purpose of the postures you are making and the techniques you are repeating, as you cultivate a profound feeling for what you're doing. It is said that prior to the Second World War, students of karate would spend a minimum of three years on one kata, and over the course of their lifetime of karate training study no more than two or three kata altogether. Chojun Miyagi is said to have taught all his students sanchin kata and would then introduce them to one or perhaps two other kata that he felt suited the individual student best. He selected which student studied what kata by taking into account a student's age, build, character, and personal situation. Back then there was no 'advanced' kata, no 'beginners' kata, and no kata practiced according to rank. Why? Because there were no ranks in karate back then.

The battle for Okinawa began on April 1, 1945, and lasted for three months, leaving over twelve thousand five hundred Americans dead, and ten times that number of Japanese and Okinawans. Witnessing the utter devastation of his homeland all around him, Chojun Miyagi had a change of mind regarding the passing on of his karate to a new generation. When the war was over and life on Okinawa gradually returned to some semblance of its pre-war normality, he began to educate what few students he had, in the complete list of kata. The pre-war students who returned to the backyard dojo around 1948 were only a small number, and for some time the full transmission of Miyagi sensei's Goju ryu was in doubt. I was told this by my sensei, Eiichi Miyazato, who was one of the few students to return after the war. As no one but Chojun Miyagi knew the entire collection of kata at that time, he began to teach his senior students the complete list. This was done relatively quickly over the remaining few years of his life. The war with Japan ended in August 1945 and Chojun Miyagi died in October 1953, a

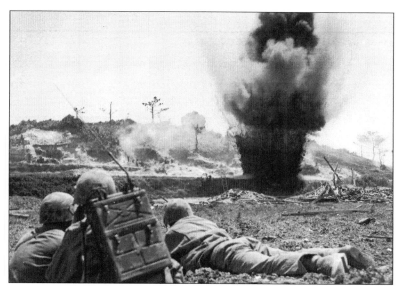

After a 'quiet' landing, the Battle for Okinawa got underway in earnest and lasted for three months.

period of just eight years and two months. After the war, he moved with his family from Naha to Gushikawa in central Okinawa and did not return to Naha nor re-establish his dojo until the end of 1947.[57] This means the students training with him during those post-war years had a little less than five years to learn all the kata and other information their teacher had to pass on. Chojun Miyagi died on October 8, 1953. By all accounts it was unexpected, although I have heard various stories from a number of Miyagi's sensei's students that the war had caused him to suffer a deep depression, a situation no doubt brought about by the loss of three of his children,[58] a number of his senior students, and countless neighbors and friends. It must be remembered, also, that learning a kata in those days did not mean simply committing the techniques and the pattern to memory; rather, it entailed understanding the strategies hidden within the kata, and a profound working knowledge of how to draw those strategies out through the use of bunkai and other training drills. Attempting to accomplish this with twelve kata over five years was a huge undertaking; and the suggestion made in some quarters, that this was a task Chojun Miyagi chose to take on with one of his junior students, simply defies belief. Much is made these days by the various schools of Goju ryu in Okinawa and elsewhere about which of Miyagi's students is his *true* successor. I want to make it plain that all such claims are nonsense! Each of his direct students who went on to open dojo of their own after the death of their teacher has contributed to the growth of ideas and fighting tactics known today as Goju ryu. For any one group or individual to claim exclusive inheritance of Chojun Miyagi's karate is disingenuous to say the least.

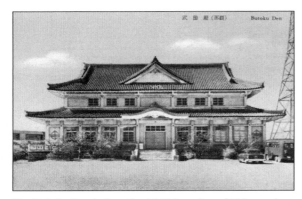

The Butoku Den before the 1945 invasion of Okinawa by American and Allied troops.

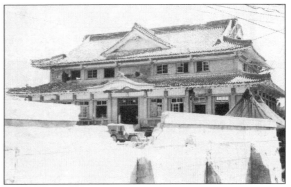

The Butoku Den after the WW II 1945 invasion of Okinawa.

5 TAI—BODY

Preparation Exercises: Junbi Undo

Before karate training proper begins, it is essential to prepare the mind and body; this is called junbi undo. While most karateka do some warm-up exercises, in traditional karate the method used is related to the fighting tradition being studied. Apart from preparing your body and mind for the training, the purpose of junbi undo is twofold: to enhance your overall flexibility and to improve your core strength. To do this, exercises include stretching and resistance, a combination that over time leads to both a greater flexibility and improved strength in all four limbs as well as the torso. The following junbi undo routine is performed before each training session at the Shinseidokan dojo, and is done for the reasons already stated, but also to bridge the divide between the life you live outside the dojo and the activity you engage in inside of it.

When you enter the dojo, you should leave your problems at the door. Training time is precious and should not become eroded by everyday matters that cannot be addressed during your training. Indeed, by applying yourself completely to the training at hand, you are often able to return to your daily life enriched by your efforts and better able to deal with your personal problems. It is for this reason, among others, that I say karate is as much a form of mental training as it is physical. For all you have done in life and all that you will do, everything begins in your mind. Without thought, you cannot have action. Balancing your conscious thought with an ability to act instinctively is the hallmark of someone who has not only mastered his martial art, but also the art of living. How or if you develop this sense of balance is a matter for you as an individual, and points to the way of karate being a personal journey; for in truth it can be nothing else. The appreciation of here and now, of being *in the moment*, although widely spoken of, remains an uncommon ability. When you are truly living in the moment, as in times of danger, then your poise and stability become evident. I know, from my own personal experience of being close to death on two separate occasions, when death draws near there can be an overwhelming sense of peace and acceptance; becoming completely aware of life as it edges close to ending seems ironic, and yet, I can think of nothing more capable of focusing your attention than the *finality* of your own demise. My survival from the abyss of death came in different ways, on two separate occasions; in 1978, I was saved from imminent multi-organ failure by the timely intervention of emergency surgery. On my recovery, the surgeon told me I was within half an hour of dying when I presented at the hospital; had all the operating theaters already been in use I would not have survived the transfer to another hospital. Startling news perhaps, but I wasn't shocked by it at all; instead I felt quite unmoved by the whole thing, experiencing no great fear at the prospect of death. If anything, I was slightly ashamed that my ego had stopped me from dealing with the problem earlier. The thought of making my young wife a widow was the notion that bothered me the most, for that would have been a truly selfish act on my part. The Legionnaires disease I contracted in 1982 was vanquished as a result of my exceptionally high level of fitness at the time. The medical world was still unsure of how to treat the condition back then, so they plied me with antibiotics and hoped for the best. Again, the possibility of death was very real and even though I was aware of it, still, I cannot say I was frightened by the prospect of my life ending. I didn't *want* to die of course, I was only in my twenties, but *if* death was coming I had no fear of it. Perhaps a violent demise is different, perhaps a lonely end is different too, but I have not faced either of these situations so I cannot say; I can only relate how I felt on the two occasions when death stood at the end of my hospital bed: waiting. The poet Dylan Thomas wrote:

> Do not go gentle into that good night,
> Old age should burn and rave at close of day.
> Rage, rage against the dying of the light.

I was not old when death came to visit but even if I am when it calls again, as call it must, I cannot say I fear its knock upon my door. I disagree with Thomas, if his counsel is to fight against nature; life is precious, no doubt, but as so many live lives without any great consciousness, it makes me wonder why they are so keen to hold onto it? It was my fitness that made the difference the second time I faced death; even so, my lungs were damaged by the illness and remain so to this day.

Some years ago, I had the privilege of meeting a master of *jujitsu*; his name was Jan de Jong. He died in April 2003, and in many respects his death was nothing unusual. He was in his eighties and had lived through many difficult and challenging times. Fighting against the German occupation forces in his native Holland during the Second World War, as a youthful member of the Dutch Resistance Movement, gave him a particular slant on life and the best way to live it. After the war he settled in Perth on Australia's West Coast and there raised a family. When de Jong sensei was diagnosed with a terminal condition, it came as a shock to everyone who knew him, especially his family. As you might expect, people close to him grew more and more sad as his health declined, and he entered a hospital to receive what comfort the medical world could offer. But for the man himself there was no sense of sadness, only acceptance. He spoke of having had a wonderful life and of being blessed by his wife, his children, and his many long-time students, some of whom had trained with him for well over thirty years. He laughed and joked and made light of the finality of the event about to take place, and when it came, he stepped away from this world as lightly as a butterfly lifting from a leaf. He not only lived well, but he had the great personal courage to die well. He was aware of what was

The late Jan de Jong sensei (1921–2003)

happening and faced it clearly, calmly, and with great dignity. As strange as this might seem to some, his example of being *present* at his own death displayed a level of almost unimaginable gallantry that I find truly inspirational.

It may seem unlikely that the exercises of junbi undo and the way you face your death are related, but consider this: budo teaches you to take responsibility, and to do that you need to be *present*. Being present is how you harmonize your mind and your body, your thoughts and your actions, and how you do everything in life while remaining fully aware of what you are doing: a condition the founder of analytical psychology Carl Jung (1875–1961) referred to as 'individuation'. Developing your nature and being fully present in the moment is important, whether you are warming up your body before karate, or facing the final act of your earthly existence. Zen philosophy points to this idea of 'being in the moment'. It reminds you that when you eat you should just eat, when you work you should just work, and when you relax you should just relax. It is not what you are doing but the way you are doing it that bestows the value. When you educate your body through the exercises of junbi undo, you should maximize the value and also train your mind; you do this by being fully present in the moment. At my dojo, junbi undo takes place at the beginning of every training session, and the following images have been included for illustrative purposes. I'm making no attempt to 'teach' the exercises here, only to show the type of preparation that is undertaken. If you are interested in performing any exercise you are unfamiliar with, I recommend you seek a qualified teacher to instruct you.

Working from the ground up, the feet are the first part of the body to be worked on, beginning with the toes (figs. 5-1, 5-2, 5-3, 5-4, and 5-5), before moving on to the

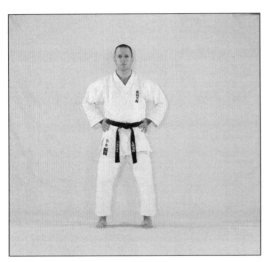

Figure 5-1

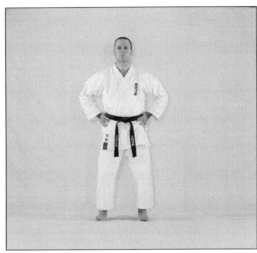

Figure 5-2

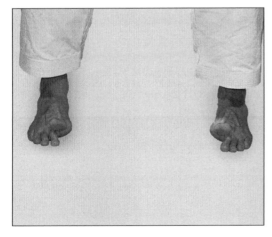

Figure 5-3

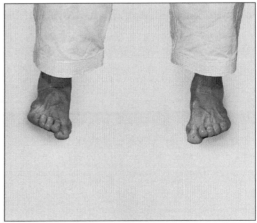

Figure 5-4

ankles (figs. 5-6, 5-7, and 5-8). The last of these exercises (fig. 5-8) involves springing the foot off the floor and driving the knee into the open palm of the hand.

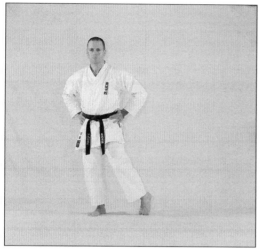

Figure 5-5

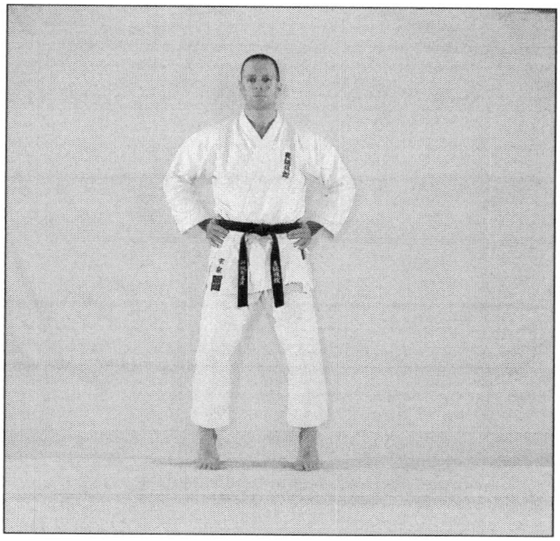

Figure 5-6

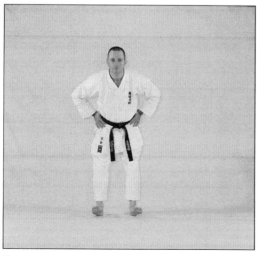

Figure 5-7

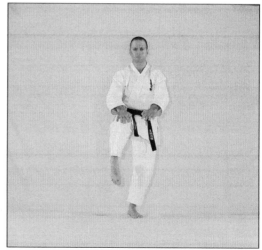

Figure 5-8

Next, the legs are warmed up individually, but with identical exercises. The lower leg is rotated, first clockwise and then counterclockwise (fig. 5-9), before the foot is kicked out in a snapping fashion (fig. 5-10). Here also, the focus is on acquiring a good sense of balance.

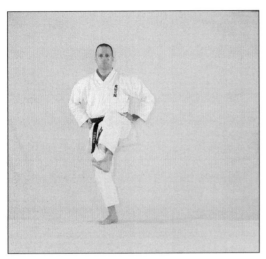

Figure 5-9

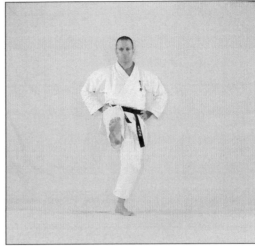

Figure 5-10

The legs continue to be worked on, and balance also, but now the main focus shifts to the knees. After several squats (figs. 5-11, 5-12) have been completed, the last squat is held for a moment. The eyes are closed during this time (fig. 5-13), which is done to help develop a good sense of balance.

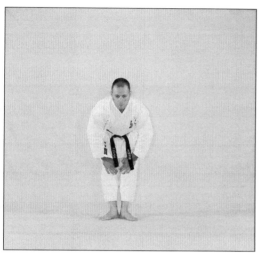

Figure 5-11

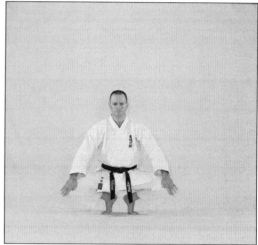

Figure 5-12

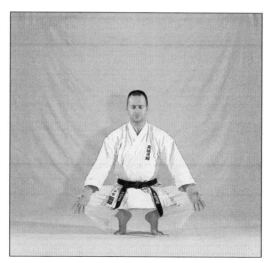

Figure 5-13

Moving into *shiko dachi* stance, each knee is pushed backward in turn while the feet grip the floor (figs. 5-14, 5-15), making sure the toes never leave the ground: this stretches the inner thigh. A final simultaneous push of both legs lasting around ten seconds (fig. 5-16) is completed before standing up.

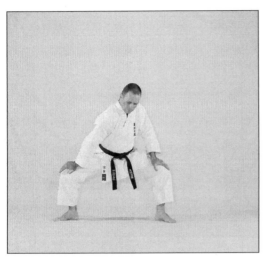

Figure 5-14

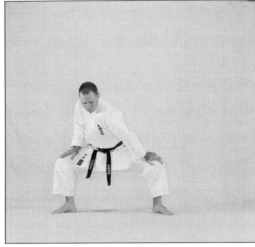

Figure 5-15

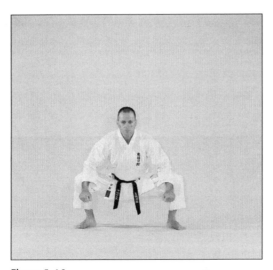

Figure 5-16

Dropping your weight onto one leg, the opposite leg is stretched with particular attention paid to keeping the toes in contact with the floor (fig. 5-17). This stretch isolates the calf muscles and tendons in the ankle and lower leg. When several of these stretches have been completed on both legs, the exercise is changed to a lower position as shown in figure 5-18. When moving from side to side to change legs, be careful not to rise and fall; rather, try to move across in as level a manner as possible. This will challenge the muscles in the legs and, over time, provide greater leg strength. The legs are stretched one more time, again for about ten seconds (fig. 5-19), before standing up.

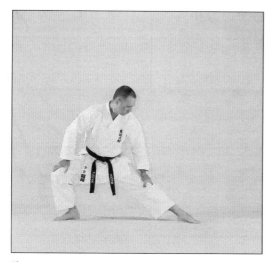

Figure 5-17

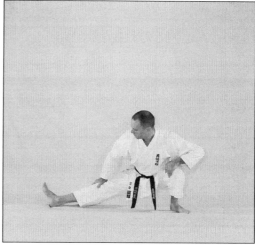

Figure 5-18

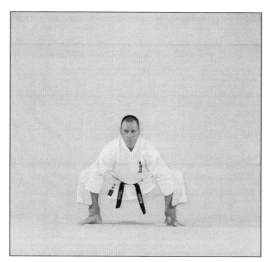

Figure 5-19

The hips and muscles at the side of the body (external oblique muscles), as well as the spine, are worked on next. A simple hip rotation (fig. 5-20), alternating in both directions, precedes the bigger stretches to the sides, the rear, and the front. Each of these stretches also changes from left to right and are each done following a *mawashi uke* (figs. 5-21, 5-22, and 5-23). The purpose here is to introduce the importance of harmony between breath and movement, as well as movement and intention. The *mawashi uke* is executed with a deep inhalation through the nose, while the stretches are accompanied by a strong exhalation (figs. 5-24, 5-25, and 5-26).

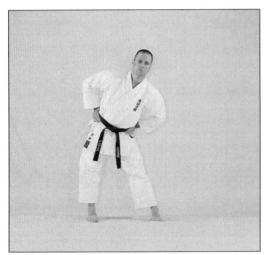

Figure 5-20

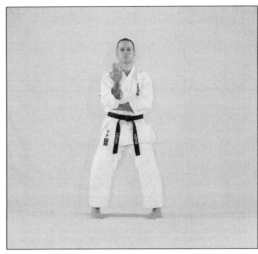

Figure 5-21

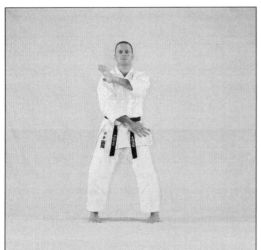

Figure 5-22

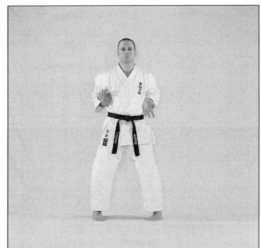

Figure 5-23

Next, move on to the arms. They are swung in large circles both forward and backward. As well, each arm is rotated in opposite directions at the same time (fig. 5-27), and these directions are switched too, so that the arm traveling one way is made to swing in the opposite direction. This builds dexterity as well as loosening up the shoulders. It also pushes blood toward the hands, the next part of the body to be worked on.

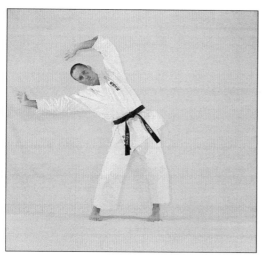

Figure 5-24

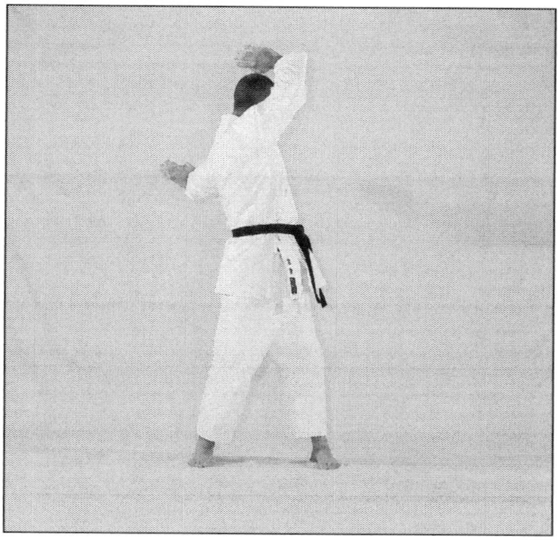

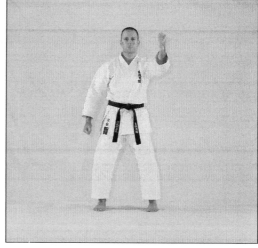

Figure 5-25

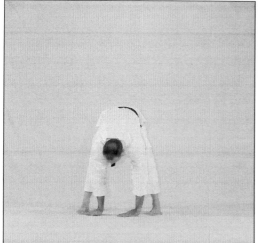

Figure 5-26

Figure 5-27

The fingers and wrists are the target of these stretches; first, begin by adopting the position shown in figure 5-28. From there, push the arm out and with the opposite hand pull the fingers of the outstretched hand backward (fig. 5-29). The hand being stretched is then returned to the starting position, the hand rotated so that the fingers now point downward and the arm extended once more (fig. 5-30). The grip is then changed as the outstretched arm is bent at the elbow (fig. 5-31) before the final change of grip, which brings downward pressure onto the wrist as seen in figure 5-32. This routine is then conducted on the other hand.

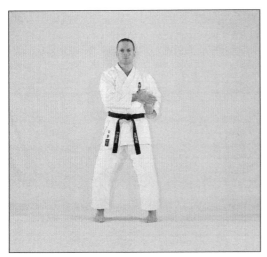

Figure 5-28

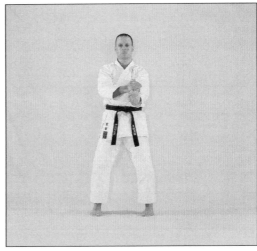

Figure 5-29

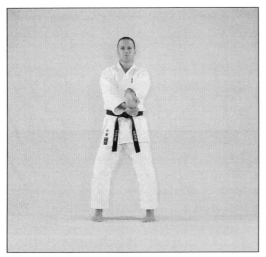

Figure 5-30

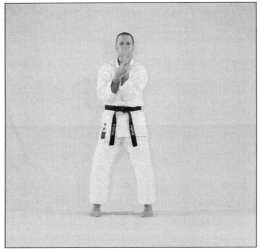

Figure 5-31

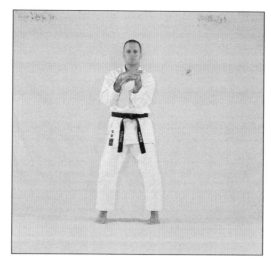

Figure 5-32

Staying with the hands, from *sanchin dachi* posture a deep inhalation is taken, and the hands and fingers are stretched out to their limit (fig. 5-33). A strong exhalation is then executed and the hands squeezed tightly into fists (fig. 5-34). Actually, the whole body is 'fixed' by the outward breath and held in that state for a couple of seconds before relaxing and repeating the exercise twice more.

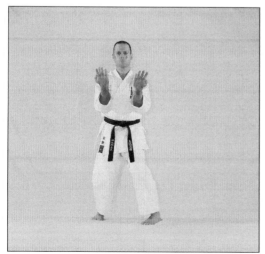

Figure 5-33

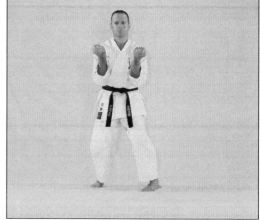

Figure 5-34

The final exercise for the wrists and fingers involves stretching the arms out in front of the body and pushing the hands together, as seen in figure 5-35. From this position, a deep inward breath is taken before the hands are brought back in toward the body and the emphasis moved to the fingers (figs. 5-36, 5-37).

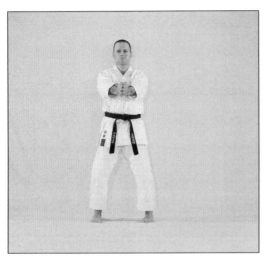

Figure 5-35

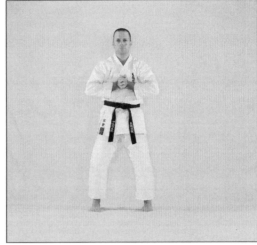

Figure 5-36

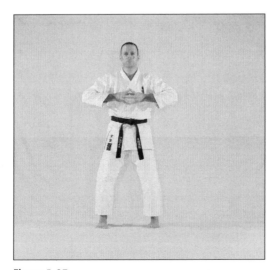

Figure 5-37

As well as stretching the arms out in front of the body, they are also stretched upward and downward (figs. 5-38, 5-39).

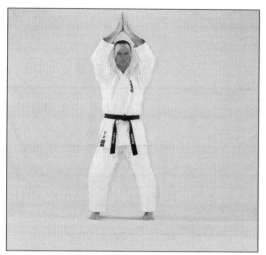

Figure 5-38

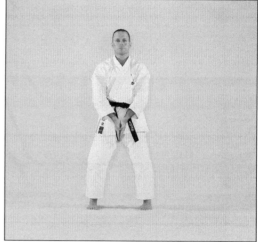

Figure 5-39

The neck is the last part of the body to be warmed up in this set of junbi undo exercises. It is considered unhealthy by health professionals to rotate the neck in a circular fashion, so that action is to be avoided. Beginning with a forward and backward tilt of the head (figs. 5-40, 5-41), take care not to lean the body, just move the head. With the sideways turn of the head (figs. 5-42, 5-43), the opposite shoulder is pulled backward to

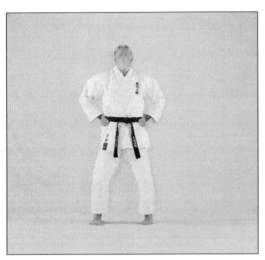

Figure 5-40

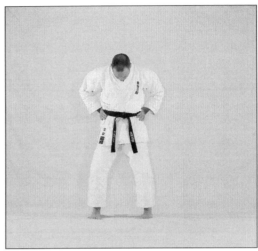

Figure 5-41

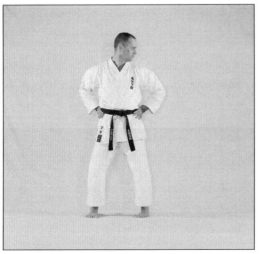

Figure 5-42

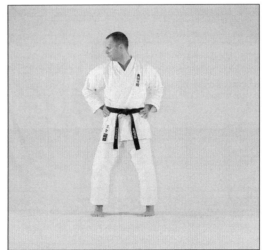

Figure 5-43

enhance the stretch, and this is also true when the head is dropped to the shoulder while facing to the front (figs. 5-44, 5-45). The last stretch, for the spine between the shoulder blades, is achieved by clasping the hands on the head and dropping the elbows forward as in figure 5-46. The arms should not 'pull' the neck, just allowed to become heavy. Again, care should be taken to keep the body upright.

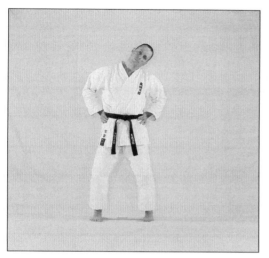

Figure 5-44

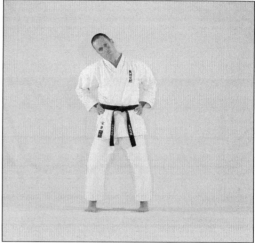

Figure 5-45

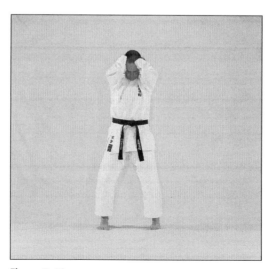

Figure 5-46

Apparatus Training: Kigu Undo

Training with various tools and pieces of apparatus and working against the resistance they provide has long been an integral part of Okinawan karate. The tools themselves constitute a part of training better known as hojo undo, supplementary training. In my book *The Art of Hojo Undo: Power Training for Traditional Karate*, I have explored in detail this particular aspect of karate training, and so do not intend to go as deeply into this topic again here. Those who wish to know more than this section presents may perhaps consider acquiring the book mentioned. That said, I believe this method of training to be vital in the overall learning and understanding of karate; without it, you cannot say you study karate, merely that you practice it. Kigu undo builds strength in specific tendons and muscle groups, improves breath control, and increases the 'feeling' for karate that you seek. An old karate proverb says, "Do karate with your whole body"; kigu undo brings this saying to life, as the smooth and constant manipulation of the tools is impossible without bringing the entire body, including the mind and the breath, into play.

Here I will present a sample of the tools used regularly by me for almost thirty years and offer only a small sample of the exercises you are able to perform with each of them. For a complete introduction into this aspect of Okinawan karate training, I recommend you read the book mentioned in the previous paragraph. Generally speaking, the tools used in kigu undo fall into two categories: those you lift and those you strike. While different tools offer different levels of stress, they all offer the same challenge, which is to find your limits and then to slowly push those limits further, and to expand the scope of your physical strength and your mental tenacity. As always, training in karate requires

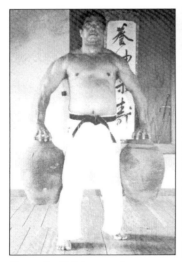

Masunobu Shinjo sensei strengthening his grip with a pair of gami (jars).

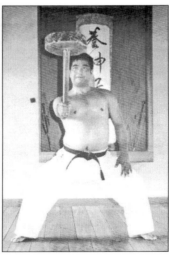

Masanobu Shinjo (1938–1993), working with the chiishi.

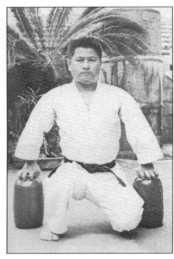

Ko Uehara sensei, ca. 1963, about to lift a heavy set of nigiri gami (gripping jars).

you to direct your mind to the question of safety and consideration for others. This is not only considered desirable in Okinawan karate, but essential, as without such reflection, training can quickly become dangerous, even life threatening.

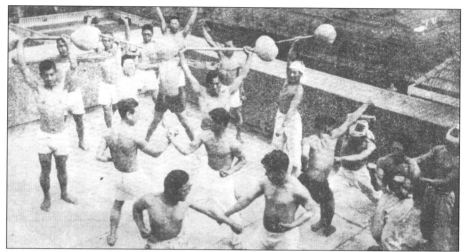

Kansai University students show off their karate training to the camera.

Of all the tools in the kigu undo arsenal the chiishi (figs. 5-47, 5-48) is, I think, the best. It is easily constructed, takes no space to store, and can be used to enhance many different aspects of your karate.

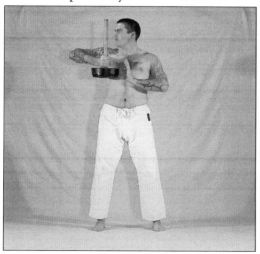

Figure 5-47   Figure 5-48

There is another version of the chiishi, a much heavier two-handled tool (figs. 5-49, 5-50), and this too can be used in various ways.

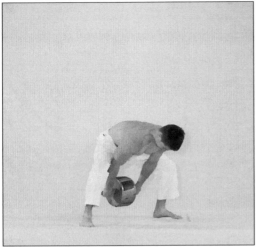

Figure 5-49

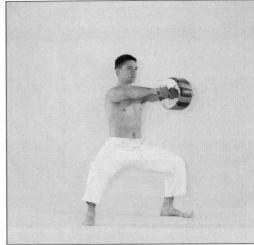

Figure 5-50

The tan (figs. 5-51, 5-52) is really just a homemade barbell; however, it is used in ways specific to karate, from enhancing the stability of your stances to conditioning your arms.

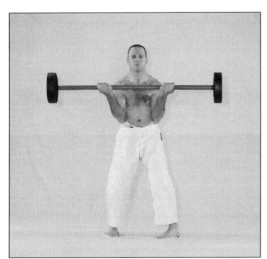

Figure 5-51

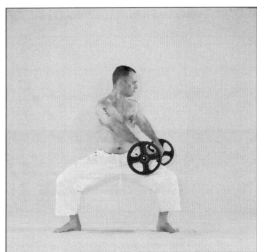

Figure 5-52

Nigiri gami, or gripping jars (figs. 5-53, 5-54), are another example of a simple tool that delivers tangible benefits, by promoting strength in the fingers and wrists.

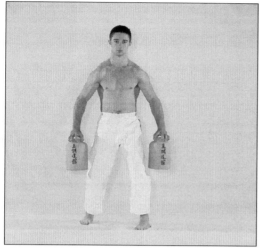

Figure 5-53

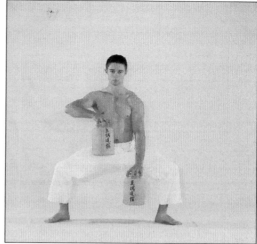

Figure 5-54

The ishi sashi, stone lock, promotes strength of grip and strong fingers and can be used in many different ways. The exercise shown here (figs. 5-55, 5-56) strengthens the grip as well as the wrists.

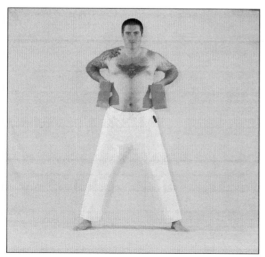

Figure 5-55

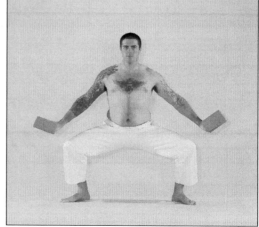

Figure 5-56

The kongoken, (figs. 5-57, 5-58), was brought to Okinawa by Chojun Miyagi on his return from Hawaii, where he witnessed it being used by the local wrestlers. As well as promoting overall strength in the arms and body, it is very useful for developing 'explosive' energy.

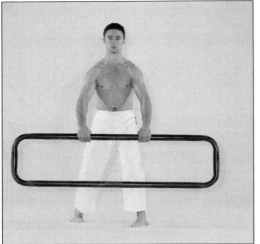 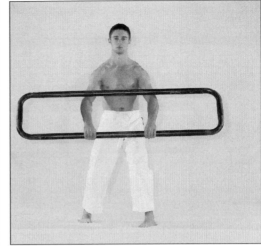

Figure 5-57   Figure 5-58

Rope has always been in abundance throughout the Ryukyu Kingdom due to the island nation's reliance on trade and shipping in particular. It comes as no surprise therefore to learn that Okinawan karateka have a number of innovative ways to use it. In this case, by simply pulling against your partner's resistance (figs. 5-59, 5-60) it is possible to develop an unyielding stance, a powerful grip, and increased strength in the muscles of the upper body, specifically, the *Latissimus dorsi*, the *Teres major*, and the *Infraspinatus*.

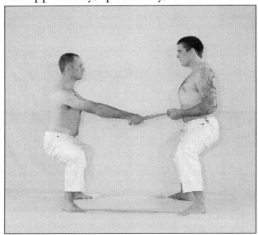 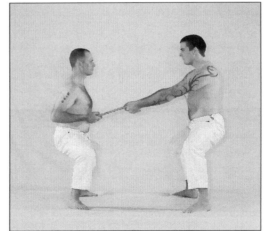

Figure 5-59   Figure 5-60

The tetsu geta, that is, the iron geta, is used to target the muscles of the legs, as well as improve your balance. Here, a basic leg lift to the side (figs. 5-61, 5-62) is made all the more challenging by the weight of the 12 lb (5 kg) geta.

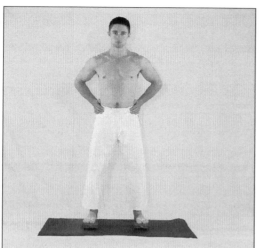

Figure 5-61

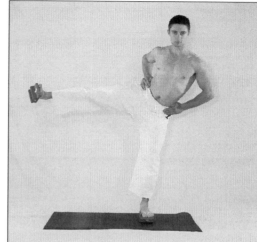

Figure 5-62

A simple container filled with sand or smooth stones, the jari bako (figs. 5-63, 5-64) has been used for centuries in Okinawa to toughen the fingers and improve the grip.

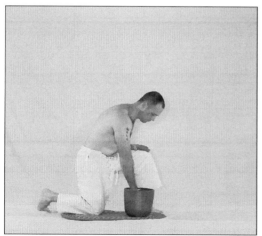

Figure 5-63

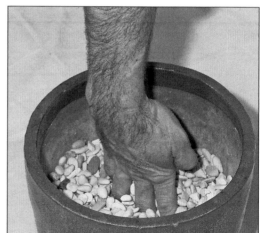

Figure 5-64

The tou (fig. 5-65) is nothing more than a roll of bamboo, or any type of cane, bundled together. Like the previous tool, the jari bako, the tou is used to develop powerful strikes with the fingers (fig. 5-66) as well as a strong grip. The thumb too is strengthened (fig. 5-67) with this tool and becomes a potent weapon when used against vulnerable targets like the groin, throat, and eyes.

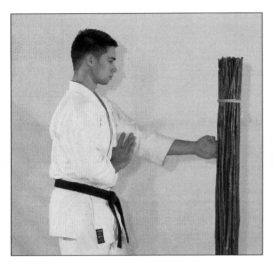

Figure 5-65

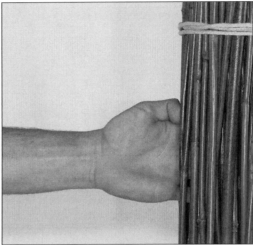

Figure 5-66

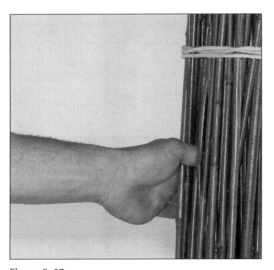

Figure 5-67

The ude kitae is used, as seen here (figs. 5-68, 5-69), to condition the legs and hands. It is also used extensively to toughen the arms and, in fact, any other part of the body used to strike an opponent.

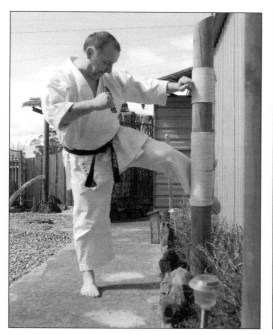

Figure 5-68

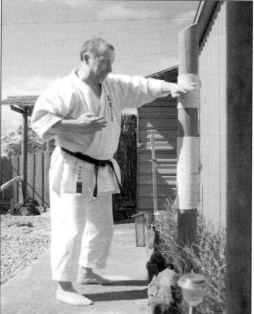

Figure 5-69

The makiwara (figs. 5-70, 5-71) is the best known of all the kigu undo tools used by karateka. Made by planting a sturdy post in the ground and topping it off with a target made of leather, this tool is used to condition the first two knuckles of the fist, used when punching. However, it goes further than that by strengthening the wrists and improving the penetrative power of your punch. Working with the tool should be natural and prolific. Counting how many punches you can do is counterproductive. Just stand and face the makiwara, give yourself a time limit, say twenty minutes at first, and then see who wins.

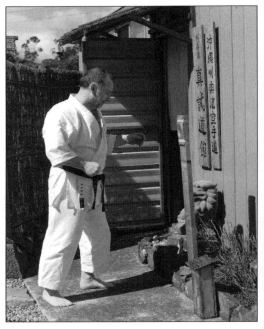

Figure 5-70

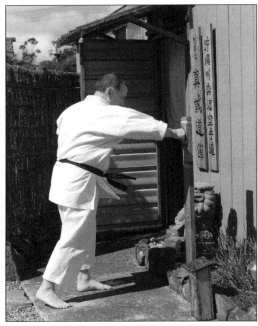

Figure 5-71

Supplementary Training: Hojo Undo

Apart from kigu undo, the kind of hojo undo done with tools, there are many other training methods used in karate dojo around the world where the traditional Okinawan methods are preserved. Without the tools to work with, a training partner is required who is, ideally, of similar build and experience; although not strictly essential, a partner with equal body mass and abilities allows the training to take on a more forceful approach. As with all forms of hojo undo the key is to build your strength slowly and to be patient in the learning and acquisition of your knowledge through dedication and an adherence to regular training. Simply being able to do the moves is not the same as understanding what you are doing; and without an understanding of karate, there is little value in obtaining knowledge of it.

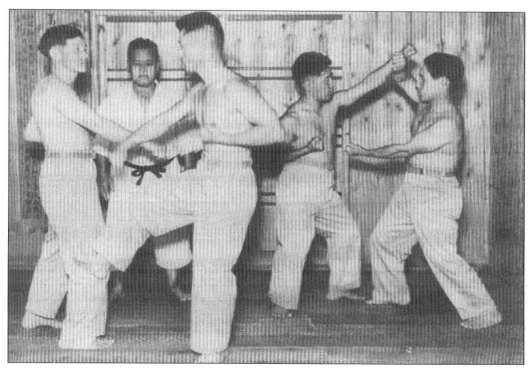

Miyagi Chojun training four of his post war senior students, L-R: Meitoku Yagi, Eiichi Miyazato, Seikichi Toguchi, and Eiko Miyazato.

Ude Tanren

Forearm conditioning is important in karate, as the arms are the part of the body expected to take most of the impact during a fight, whether blocking, being blocked, or when used to strike a blow; all of these situations rely on the arms. So if impact to your arms is going to cause you to wince in pain, you can forget having the wherewithal, mentally or physically, to strike a decisive blow and make good your escape. A good way to begin conditioning the arms is by working with a partner, rubbing your arms together as you practice alternate blocking and punching as seen in figures 5-72 and 5-73.

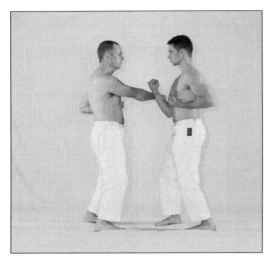

Figure 5-72

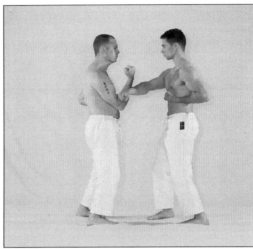

Figure 5-73

To introduce the sensation of impact into the training, the arms are swung loosely into each other, over and over. The position of the arms should be changed regularly to imitate the postures found in the basic blocking techniques of karate: *gedan barai* and *chudan uke*, as seen in figures 5-74 and 5-75.

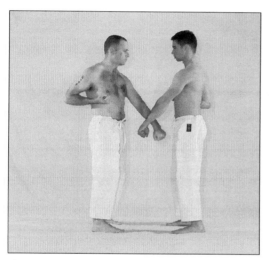

Figure 5-74

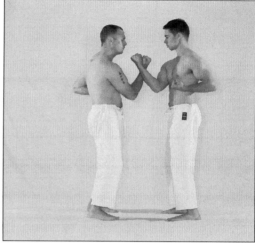

Figure 5-75

Ippon Uke Barai

A series of exercises stepping into the block are then added. This establishes the need for good timing and breath control, and encourages both as the speed increases and the blocks are driven home that much stronger. In this exercise you face off against a training partner as shown in figure 5-76. Both step forward with the right leg and block with a right high block (*jodan uke*) (fig. 5-77), before stepping back to the original position (fig. 5-78).

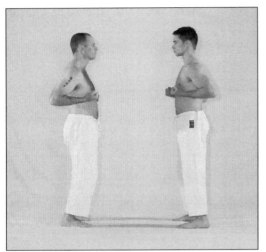

Figure 5-76

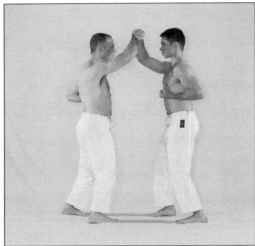

Figure 5-77

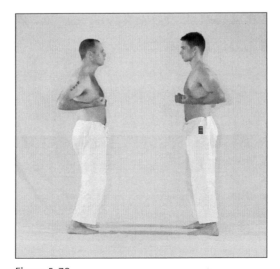

Figure 5-78

From there change sides, stepping in on the left and blocking with a left mid-level block (*chudan uke*) (fig. 5-79), before returning to the original position (fig. 5-80). Complete the exercise by stepping forward for a third time, this time with the right leg again, and both execute a low block (*gedan barai*) (fig. 5-81), before returning to the original position.

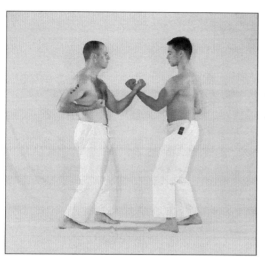

Figure 5-79

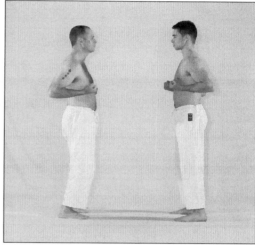

Figure 5-80

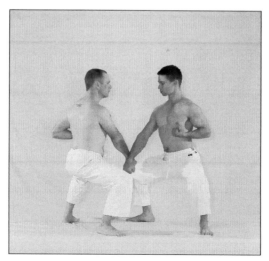

Figure 5-81

Sandan Uke Barai

With the feeling of contact now well and truly established, and the harmony of movement and breath understood—if not yet mastered—there is one more exercise I teach novice students at the Shinseidokan dojo. This involves one student attacking and one student defending and is known as three-step-blocking (*sandan uke barai*). I was introduced to this form of training on my first trip to Okinawa when I trained at the Higaonna dojo in the Makishi district of Naha. However, the students there only ever did the first of the five drills you are about see. Since then I have seen other versions. The four drills following the first were developed by me over twenty-five years ago. At the time I had just established my first dojo (see the section "Hosshin" in chapter three) and was spending several hours each day in the dojo; even so, I doubt these drills are unique. Over time everything everyone has ever thought of is thought of again and again; history has taught us that the source of human ingenuity is seldom limited to one individual or one location. In all these drills one student initiates the attacks while the other tries to catch his opponent's timing in order to defend himself without the use of gratuitous force. Once the drills you see here have been familiarized, it is possible to double up by continuing to attack after the first three, and this way students get to practice the three basic punches and blocks using both sides of their bodies. It is also possible to have the student defending himself, stepping forward after the last attack and reversing the roles by becoming the attacker.

For clarity here, all these drills are shown with the student on the right attacking the student on the left.

Number One:

Facing your training partner as shown in figure 5-82, the student on the right steps forward with the right leg and punches *jodan zuki* with his right hand; at the same time, the student on the left steps back on his left leg while protecting himself with a right *jodan uke* (fig. 5-83). The attacker moves immediately forward again, punching with a left *chudan zuki* (fig. 5-84), while the student on the left steps back and defends with a left *chudan uke*. The third attack follows quickly on the end of the second, with the student on the right dropping into a low stance *shiko dachi* before delivering a right *gedan zuki*. This is countered with a backward step, also into *shiko dachi*, followed by a right *gedan barai* (fig. 5-85).

From here, students either step backward away from each other, returning to the starting position (refer to fig. 5-82), or continue with another three attacks, or they can reverse the roles as mentioned before.

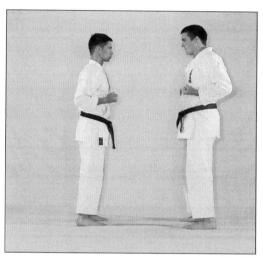

Figure 5-82

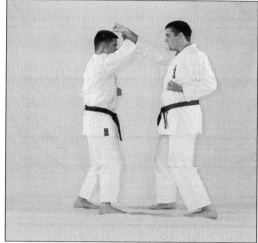

Figure 5-83

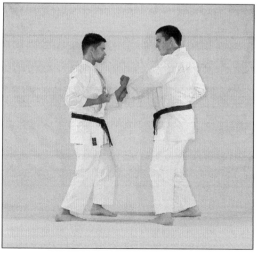

Figure 5-84

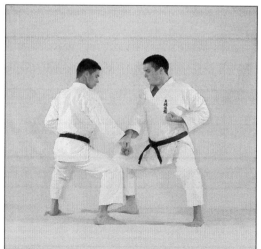

Figure 5-85

Number Two:

From the starting position (fig. 5-86), the attacker moves in with the same three attacks as the first exercise. In this drill only the defense changes. Now the defender drops into *nekoashi dachi* and protects himself with the use of a high block with the wrist, *jodan ko uke* (fig. 5-87). The second attack is deflected by moving off the line of attack, again in *nekoashi dachi*, and the block is made using the back of the hand, *chudan ura uke* (fig. 5-88). While the third attack is swept to one side with an open-handed *gedan barai*, the left hand shields the head (fig. 5-89).

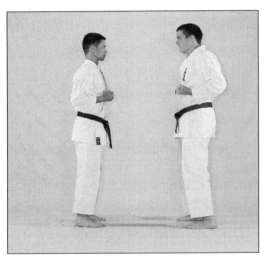

Figure 5-86

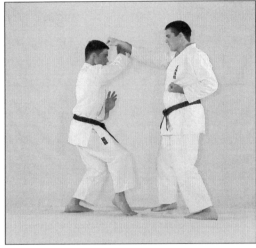

Figure 5-87

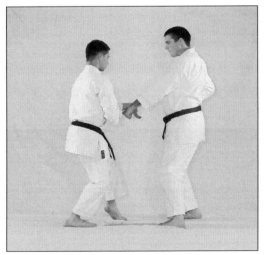

Figure 5-88

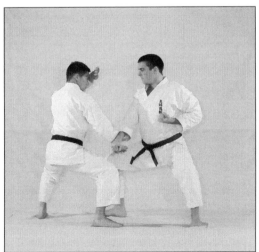

Figure 5-89

Number Three:

Drills number three and four involve a different pattern of stepping, similar to each other but different from the first two drills and the final drill, Number Five. From the starting position (fig. 5-90), the attacker steps in as before and the defender moves backward, blocking with *jodan uke* (fig. 5-91). From here things change a little. The attacker reverses his *sanchin dachi* stance before launching his second attack, but this is parried away by the defender who steps forward and blocks with *chudan uke* (fig. 5-92). The attacker then steps forward once more, this time into *shiko dachi*, and throws his third punch. The defender steps backward, blocking with *gedan barai* (fig. 5-93).

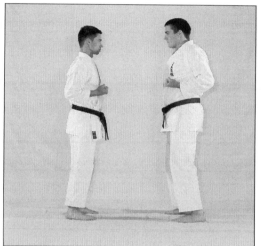

Figure 5-90

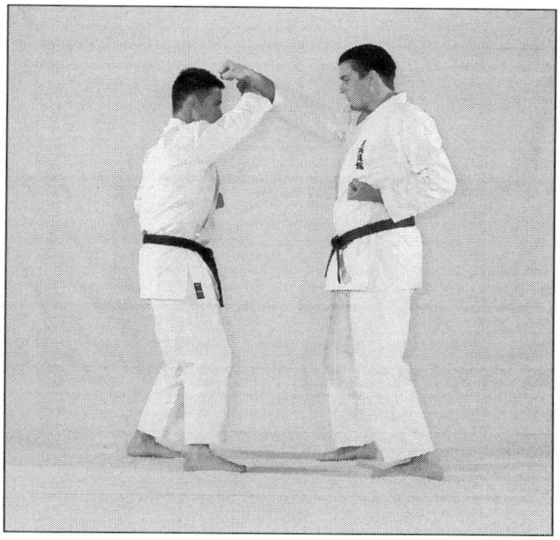

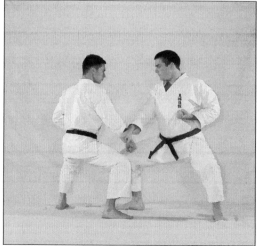

Figure 5-91

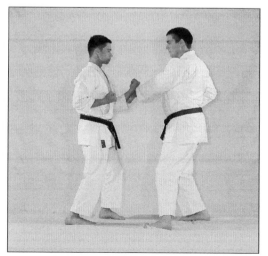

Figure 5-92

Figure 5-93

Number Four:

This drill uses the same blocks as drill Number Two, with the same footwork as drill Number Three. Beginning from the same ready position as before (fig. 5-94), after the first punch has been thrown (fig. 5-95), the attacker once again switches stance and punches again, only this time to the body. As before, the defender steps forward to fill the gap left by the attacker's change of stance and suppresses the mid-level punch before it has a chance to develop (fig. 5-96). From here, the attacker once again steps forward, dropping into a low stance and throws his third punch. The defender mirrors his attacker's movement and steps backward before defending with an open-handed *gedan barai* (fig. 5-97).

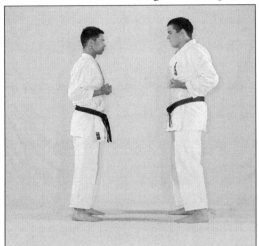

Figure 5-94

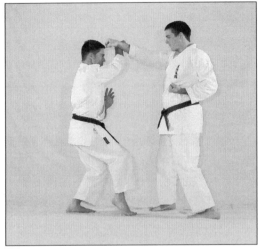

Figure 5-95

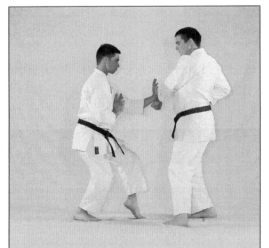

Figure 5-96

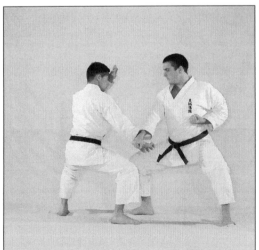

Figure 5-97

Number Five:

The final drill is the same as drill Number One, but with an added exchange of techniques placed on the end. From the position seen in figure 5-98, the attacker moves forward through the three punches found in drill Number One (figs. 5-99, 5-100), while the defender moves backward blocking as before. At this point (fig. 5-101),

(continued on next page)

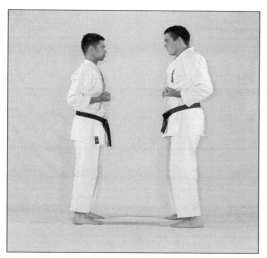

Figure 5-98

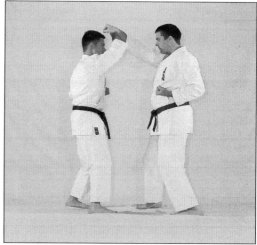

Figure 5-99

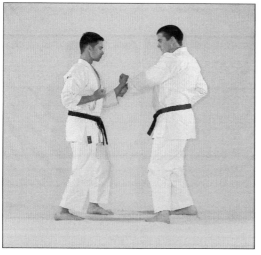

Figure 5-100

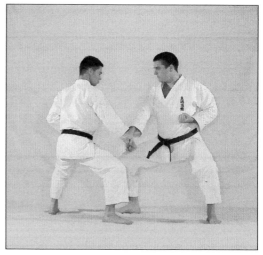

Figure 5-101

the defender goes on the offensive by throwing a left punch to his partner's body (fig. 5-102), which is blocked and countered with a punch from the attacker (fig. 5-103). Here, the defender parries the punch inward, toward his own left hand, which is waiting to grasp the attacker's wrist (fig. 5-104) before delivering the decisive blow, a back-fist strike to the face: *jodan uraken uchi* (fig. 5-105).

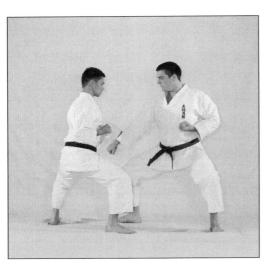

Figure 5-102

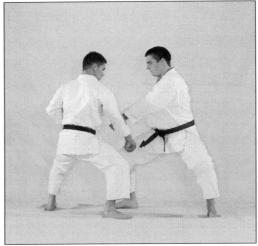

Figure 5-103

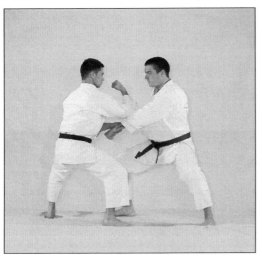

Figure 5-104

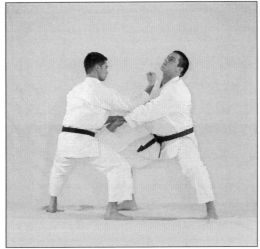

Figure 5-105

6 THE FUTURE FOR KARATE

From Whence We Came: Okinawa

At a little over 26 degrees north of the equator, Okinawa enjoys a subtropical climate, and for much of the year its inhabitants live under clear blue skies. However, during the early summer months, typhoons sweep in off the Pacific Ocean bringing with them strong winds and huge seas often resulting in damage to property, and sometimes loss of life. The older wooden houses, still found in small pockets of undeveloped Okinawa, are characterized by their heavy tiled roofs, which anchor the buildings to the ground when the winds become strong enough to knock people off their feet. Okinawa island (*jima*) lies roughly midway along the *Nansei* archipelago, and is by far the largest of the forty-eight inhabited islands that run in a chain of one hundred and sixty islands stretching from the southern tip of Kyushu (considered part of mainland Japan) all the way to the northern tip of Taiwan. With an overall population of approximately one and a quarter million people, the largest city and the prefecture's capital is Naha, a city that is home to more than three hundred and sixteen thousand people. Densely populated in the south, the island of Okinawa reveals more of its natural beauty as you travel north. Once you get past the sprawling American military bases and the satellite towns that dominate the lower one third of the island, a quieter and gentler way of life is revealed. Although famous these days as the home of karate, the Okinawan culture is rich in its diversity; today its music, textiles, language, ceramics, and architecture, all unique to the ancient kingdom of Ryukyu, still lie waiting to be discovered and experienced by those lucky enough to travel there. Since my first visit to Okinawa, in February 1984, I have returned many times to learn karate from my teachers and to soak up the atmosphere and culture this unique society has to offer. Okinawa may be a political and economic part of Japan these days, but the people and their history tell a very different story from that of Yamoto.[59] I believe the study and practice of karate loses much of its value if you remove it from the cultural environment it evolved in; and while it would be a mistake for foreigners like me to pretend to be Okinawan, it is nevertheless important to develop a level of empathy for the culture. For those who do not yet have a personal experience of Okinawa, I want to introduce here a few of the cultural icons. Becoming familiar with them will help you place karate in its correct historical and cultural milieu. Although the Ryukyu Kingdom[60] has long since slipped into history, this southernmost modern prefecture of Japan continues to stand apart from the rest of the country; separated by the remnants of a different language and culture, its people still remain imbued with a powerful sense of being *Uchinanchu*.

Music

You only have to listen to the music of Okinawa for the briefest of moments to notice the difference between it and the music of Japan; and even though the drum plays a pivotal role in the sound of the island, and other instruments too, like the *sanba* (similar to a Spanish castanet, but with three pieces of wood instead of two), it is the *sanshin* (a three stringed banjo-like instrument) with its instantly recognizable *twang* that best captures the spirit of the ancient Ryukyu Kingdom. With its slow and melodic strumming, often accompanied by an even more solemn vocal delivery from the player, the music can evoke all kinds of images.

From the oppressive heat and humidity of summer to the cooling winds blowing gently in off the East China Sea, the sanshin can portray each with equal subtlety and intensity. Love songs and songs to work by in the fields or on the tiny fishing boats are all sung with the sanshin provid-

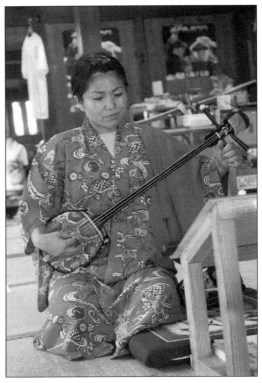

The Okinawan sanshin.

ing a jaunty rhythm by which the islander's dreams and toil are celebrated. The instrument is said by legend to have been invented by Akainko, a musician who lived long ago. Sheltering from the rain one day, he began to notice the sound of the water dripping from the roof. He set about making the very first sanshin (san—three, shin—string) soon afterward and began traveling from village to village giving impromptu performances. His music became so popular among the people that even the royal court began to hear of it, and from that point on the sanshin began to be played for the king himself. As wonderful as this story sounds, the reality is somewhat less romantic. Historians believe the sanshin came to Okinawa from China as a slightly bigger instrument called a *sanxian*; the Okinawans then adapted it into the smaller sanshin we see today. Not to be confused with the Japanese *shamisen*, which the Okinawan instrument predates, the strings of the sanshin are picked, using a plectrum, or *bachi*, which is traditionally made from the horn of a water buffalo.

Drumming too is a major part of the traditional music of Okinawa, and during the summer months huge gatherings called *eisa* are held in various locations. Eisa are said to date back at least four hundred years and to have evolved from Buddhist inspired dances performed by young people during the Bon Festival, a time each summer when the spirits of the dead return to the earth to visit their families. These days there are around a dozen eisa held each year in various locations from Tomigusuku in the south to Nago in the north. With literally hundreds of drummers and dancers taking part, eisa make for a spectacular sight, as well as an incredible sound, and are an important part of the Okinawan culture. The movements of the mass drummers often resemble the *embusen* of karate kata, and the stances they adopt leave you in no doubt that many of the Okinawan traditional dances seen at such celebrations and karate share a common heritage. It is this heritage that I strive to tap into while practicing my karate; for to do otherwise, I believe, would produce something else other than the *feeling* for karate I am trying to find. I struggle each day to make karate my own, while maintaining elements of the culture from which it came. Okinawan music, like all other music, can evoke feelings and emotions that you may otherwise never tap into. It provides the soundtrack to a society that gave birth to the art of karate, an art I have spent the greater part of my life studying. In the early morning, when my personal training is over, I often sit quietly and listen to CDs of the sanshin, allowing its rhythms to wash gently over me as I recall moments of happiness and struggle during my visits to Okinawa. I once heard an archaeologist explain the difference between artifacts that were brought to him by someone else and objects he discovered himself.

> "The first," he said, "was nothing more than an interesting find, something that could tell me little other than what was in front of me. Whereas, when I discover something in the ground for myself, I not only learned about the object itself but the circumstances under which it was used. I can pinpoint its age and sometimes even how it was made. I can even get an understanding of when it had been discarded. From the location of the find, I can often work out the climate at the time the object was in use, and therefore what the location looked like when the object was made and being used by its original owners. By understanding the object in relation to its surroundings my knowledge of it becomes clearer and my appreciation of it much deeper."

As I listened to him speak, it dawned on me that the same was true of karate. If you remove it from its cultural context, you are left with an interesting set of movements that tell you little of their original use. You are left with a set of fighting techniques that say nothing of karate's value to either the individual or society as a whole and provide little or no practical method of protecting yourself from the sometimes harsh realities of life. Karate, once removed from the culture from which it came, becomes something entirely different. Some may think the difference an improvement: I would always disagree.

Textiles

In the time of the Ryukyu Kingdom, Okinawa was a major trading nation within Southeast Asia. This led to the village harbors and city ports of the island thriving, as goods and produce of all kinds came and went, from Japan in the north and Indonesia in the south, to China in the west. And in between these locations, many other countries also traded with Ryukyu, thus exporting not only merchandise but ideas too. This cross-pollination of cultural materials and ideas in Okinawa gave rise to new traditions and reinforced older ones. The wearing of certain clothing not only signified wealth and status within Ryukyu society, but could also pinpoint where the wearer came from. The government, seeking to gain some measure of control over the population, strictly enforced distinct patterns and embroidery on clothing known as *goyofu*. Only people from a particular village were permitted to wear *kimono* with that village's pattern. Not all clothing was subject to such restrictions however; *bashofu*, for example, is a fabric made from the fibers of the banana tree. It is said to take forty banana trees to make one roll of bashofu material, producing a lightweight and smooth garment that could be worn easily in the stifling heat of the Okinawan summer. So popular was it in former times that members of all ranks in the community wore clothing of this kind, from the ordinary worker in the fields to the ruling classes, and everyone in between.

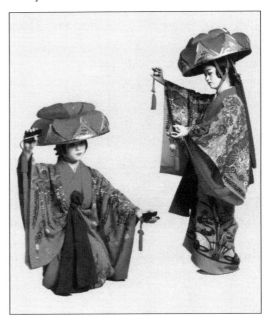

In the royal capital, Shuri, textiles were referred to as *shuri ori* and were woven mostly by the female members of the ruling classes. Made from silk, the silkworms were tended and the yarn produced locally, before the ladies of the court wove it into wonderfully delicate designs of the highest quality. Shuri ori fell into several styles, *shuri hana ori, shuri, hanakura ori, rotan ori, tsumugi,* and *tejima,* each of which displays incredible skill and great beauty. Another Ryukyu fashion is *bingata*, which is the most popular and widespread tradition of textile dyeing in Okinawa. Notable for its use of primary colors, it was at one time reserved for royalty; however, these days it is seen everywhere and its striking designs can be found on everything from postcards to wrapping paper. Along with the sound of the sanshin, bingata forms a unique backdrop to daily life on Okinawa even to-

Traditional Ryukyu dancers, dressed in bingata style kimono.

day. Produced by the use of intricate stencils and the application of brightly colored dyes made from the local indigo plant and the *fukugi* tree, these dyes are also combined with dyes from around the Southeast Asia region to produce a fantastic array of colors. Traditional designs range from flowers to birds, mountains, dragons, and water. The skills needed to produce bingata take time to learn; they also take great patience too, traits not dissimilar to the learning of karate.

Language

In the past I have mistakenly called the Okinawan language *Hogen;* however, I now understand it would be more correctly referred to as Uchinaguchi; another term sometimes used is *Shimakutuba*, meaning the language of the island. The word Hogen implies, in a derogatory way, the language is merely a dialect (*Hogen-fuda*) of Japanese, and this reflects the argument going on among linguists and in other academic circles these days. Is Uchinaguchi a distinct language, or merely a form of Japanese that was somehow separated from its mother tongue long ago and became established on the islands far to the south? With a clearly recorded history as an independent country going back to the twelfth century and the time of King Shunten, Ryukyu remained that way until the Japanese invasion of 1609. Even then, the ruling *Satsuma* samurai clan, once they had established their authority, controlled the population from the sidelines, allowing society to continue on a day-to-day level in much the same way as before. But it was an uneasy peace that lasted for two hundred and seventy years until 1879, when the Ryukyu Islands were officially made a part of Japan. For the next sixty-six years, up to the end of the Second World War when America annexed the island, Japan did what it could to erase the Okinawan culture and replace it with its own. They did this by means of humiliating children who spoke in their native tongue at school and inflicting upon the population a sense of inferiority for those who did not speak Japanese. This was by no means an uncommon method of assimilating one culture into another. All across North America and Canada, authorities were doing the same thing with the 'First Nation' tribes. And in Australia, too, the colonial government of the day was doing its best to stamp out the Aboriginal culture that had existed for at least fifty-thousand years prior to British occupation by forcibly removing children from their families and giving them away to European families and Christian institutions. Choki Motobu, one of Okinawa's more notable karateka, suffered badly from discrimination during his time living in Japan, mainly due to his shockingly poor command of Japanese. Moreover, until Gichin Funakoshi had established himself as a karate teacher, even though he was considered well educated for the day, the only work he could find in Japan was as janitor in a Ryukyuan men's hostel.

In Japan today people use *Nihongo* or *Kokugo*, literally meaning 'the country's language'; therefore, by definition, any deviations from the standard norm must be a dialect and not an individual language. As I have already mentioned, it is an argument that has been going on among academics for many years and I see no end in sight just yet. None of this would matter much, at least not to me, if it were not for the reality that a nation's spirit is best described in its own words, so, take away the language and you start to dismantle the sense of nationhood that binds people together. Americans might call it patriotism, the British perhaps the Dunkirk Spirit,[61] but whatever you call it, a nation stands close to extinction once it loses the ability to pass on its history to the next generation in its own language. Unfortunately, Uchinaguchi is no longer widely used, and is spoken mostly by the old and within a few organizations like the Okinawa Ken Uchinaguchi Kai that have formed especially to preserve it. In December 2008, this organization launched a quarterly newspaper called the *Shimakutuba Shinbun*, which covers Okinawan cultural events and publishes poems as well as articles about Okinawan music and language.

Ceramics

It is said that among the skills brought to Okinawa by the 'thirty-six families' from China who settled in Kume village in 1392 was the art of the potter. These days you have to look a little farther from the coast to find the center of Okinawa's ceramic tradition. Just a few kilometers away from Kume, heading northeast, is the district known as Tsuboya with its restored streetscape aptly named *Yachimun-cho*, or 'Pottery Street'. Here it is possible to find an example of every kind of Okinawan pottery, from the huge jars used in landscaping to tiny figurines made especially as souvenirs (*omiyagi*) for the many thousands of tourists who visit the area each year in search of something uniquely Okinawan. Although heavily influenced by Chinese and other Southeast Asian countries, the ceramics of Okinawa maintain a particular appearance all their own. Prevalent among the items made are the *shisha,* the guardian lion dogs found at the entrance to

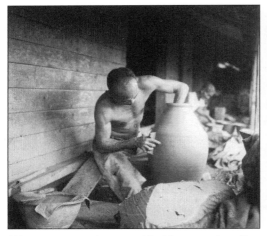

Okinawan pottery has a world-wide reputation all its own.

Okinawan Shisa—guardians against evil.

almost every home and public building across the island. Some of these stand almost as tall as a man, while others are made in miniature to fit on a handy shelf; their facial expressions are fierce and their eyes glare menacingly to scare away any unwanted or evil spirits that may try to gain entry. Alone or in pairs, the shisha are an icon of Okinawan life and although you can find them on sale in every tourist outlet on the island, the handmade guardians found in Tsuboya stand out as something special.

Noted for its plain orange clay finish, as well as the rich glazes sometimes used to embellish a simple cup or vase, the rustic simplicity of the potter's art can be witnessed as a still living part of the Ryukyuan culture. Many of the potteries in Tsuboya today are open to the public, where you can not only buy your own individual piece of Okinawan culture, but also watch the pottery masters at work. Many potters are sixth and seventh generation masters, some even more than that. The skills they possess have been passed down through the ages from one generation to the next until the present day. In a world awash with the mass-produced items people surround themselves with on a daily basis, it is refreshing to find there still exists an opportunity to witness the individual craftsman at work and, as a bonus, be able to take home a little of the results of his skill. Watching a potter at work, as he turns the heavy wheel with his feet and molds the clay into the required shape with deft movements of his hands, it is easy to relate the 'feeling' he has for his art with the feeling a karate master has for his. It seems that regardless of which art is pursued, it is never fully mastered by mere knowledge of technique alone; there is always something else at work, and this becomes evident when you look closely at a person who has absorbed his art and brings it to life at will.

Architecture

Unfortunately it is becoming more and more difficult to find examples of the older, more traditional Okinawan architecture these days. While monuments like the Shuri Palace (*Shuri-jo*) stand out and attract many thousands of visitors each year, the buildings you see today are no more than a few decades old. Shuri-jo was rebuilt over a number of years during the 1980s and opened to the public in November 1992. In fact, I attended the karate and kobudo demonstration that took place on the palace grounds at the time and relished the opportunity to see some of the island's best budoka in action. Although such examples as Shuri-jo give an idea of how Okinawa looked in days gone by, that is all they can do. Within the sprawling metropolis that is present-day Naha, few authentic examples of traditional architecture remain. A number of times I have witnessed bulldozers move into an area and within a few days erase a whole block of old wooden houses, only to have a car park occupy the same spot where the traditional

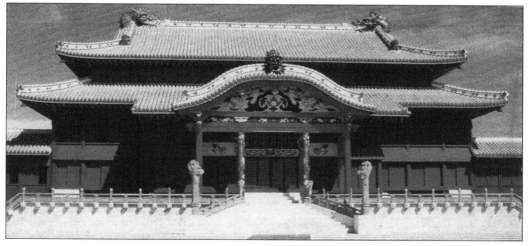

Shuri-jo, the royal palace of the kings of Ryukyu.

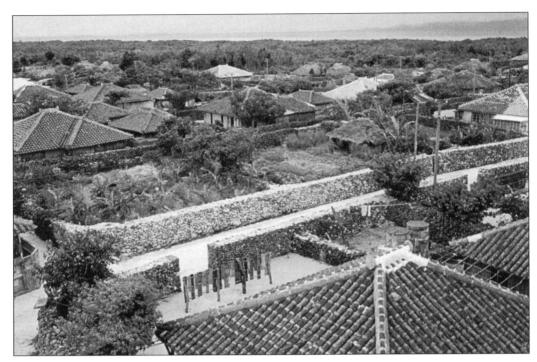

A traditional Okinawan village.

homes once stood. While some would call this progress, the speed at which it occurs always seems a little obscene to me. Today only small pockets of wooden houses with their heavy tiled roofs can be found, although for how much longer I'm not sure, for they are being replaced at an alarming rate by the bland concrete boxes that make Naha look just like any other Japanese city, but then, maybe that's the point.

Whether on a grand scale like Shuri-jo, or the more intimate level of the average home, the architecture of old Okinawa left you in no doubt where you were. The lush vegetation and pitched roofs of the houses gave the island an environment all its own. Those families who could not afford to put tiles on their houses would make a roof of thatch from the reeds found across the island and in this way secure their often basic shelter from the elements. Actually, the roofs of Okinawan buildings, to my mind, provide not only shelter, but also afford even the most mundane of structures an elegance that belies the building's use. Long, gently sloping tile roofs that turn up slightly at the edges provide patterns that enhance their simple sophistication and offer a sense of refinement to the eye.

Cuisine

I once asked a Japanese friend of mine, who had flown down from the mainland to Okinawa to meet me, if she was enjoying her visit to this part of Japan. Her reply surprised me at the time, as she confessed it was like visiting a different country. The food in particular was very different from the type of dishes she ate on a daily basis with her family in Osaka. Now, while it has to be said that each country can boast a regional cuisine, this is not the case here. Because of the Ryukyu kingdom's status as an independent nation prior to the 1609 invasion by Japan, Okinawan food is a reflection of its trading links with China, and many other Southeast Asian countries with which the kingdom did business for hundreds of years. Perhaps the most obvious aspect of Okinawan cooking are the many dishes that do not include rice, and the inclusion of vegetables that are in common use nowhere else in Japan; *goya* is maybe the best example of this. Looking like a large cucumber with a bad case of acne, its knobby green surface gives a good indication of the 'less than smooth' taste to follow. However, blended into a juice and served cold after training, it offers a surprisingly refreshing amount of relief; and many Okinawan dishes use goya in much the same way as Western dishes might use celery.

The *nabera*, a type of pumpkin, and the humble sweet potato also make up a large portion of the vegetables consumed by Okinawans. I have fond memories of waving down the neighborhood sweet potato vendors as they drove around the back streets of Naha in their tiny trucks. On the back, an open fire burning in a metal brazier kept the sweet potatoes hot and ready to be eaten. One hundred yen was a cheap way to keep the nutrition going toward the end of many of my training trips, when funds were running low. Pork too plays a big role in Okinawan food, and it is said that everything from the hoof to the snout is eaten. As well as lean and tender cuts of pork, Okinawans also consume large amounts of the fat too, and some dishes arrive at the table with bubbles of it shining on the surface, something I personally am not a great fan of. Still, when you are training hard every day you tend to get hungry, and when you are hungry it is surprising what you begin to find attractive in the way of food. One day my teacher, Eiichi Miyazato, took my friend and me to a restaurant famous for its noodles, *soba*. I remember his telling us quite clearly, as we left the car and walked across the car park, that this was the best place in the whole of Okinawa for pork. I love pork, it is my favorite meat, and so I was really looking forward to the lunch to come. The waitress took our order, which Miyazato sensei had taken care of, and we settled back with a cold drink to await our meal. Not too long afterward, the waitress appeared again with a tray of food and promptly placed before my friend and me, our lunch. There on the table in front of us were the biggest bowls (like small buckets) of noodles either of us had ever seen in our lives; and sticking out from each bowl were three huge pig's feet! Miyazato sensei had done it again; he had in one clever move solved our hunger problem and at the same time provided us with the challenge to try something new. While providing sustenance he had also managed to remove us both from our comfort zone. He of course faced a far less daunting challenge as he tucked into a rather modest bowl of buckwheat noodles, but it was one of those occasions where I began to understand that when we remove karate from the culture in which it emerged, we really do end up with something entirely different.

Although not strictly a part of Okinawan cuisine, I cannot mention what people eat on the island without taking at least a sideways glance at what they drink also. Of course,

Okinawans drink a large variety of beverages ranging from tea to fruit juices to alcohol, all of which have their place in the overall diet of the population. However, in a final nod of recognition to the uniqueness of Okinawan cuisine I should mention the local rice wine, *awamori*. Strictly speaking, it is more a liquor than a wine and predates the *sake*, rice wine, found in Japan. With a history stretching back over five hundred years from the time of the Ryukyu kingdom, awamori was introduced to Okinawa as a result of the vast trading empire they had established at the time. Long-grain rice from Southeast Asia is used in conjunction with a special mold and the two are allowed to ferment. This produces a liquid that is then distilled into awamori. Noted among the locals not only for its high alcohol content but for its health giving properties too, awamori is often the drink of choice at parties or in the local pub-restaurants (*izakaya*) once a few beers have been consumed and the singing starts to get underway in earnest.

The Nature of Karate, Why We Train

Trying to grasp why individuals practice karate is impossible, you begin for your own reasons, and you continue for your own reasons too. But let me make something very clear here. If all you are doing is learning to kick and punch, to hurt people in a va-

riety of sadistic and highly dangerous ways, then I see little point in karate training at all, for such knowledge and abilities can be found quicker by pursuing other methods. Besides, I know of no karate dojo anywhere in the world where consistent and systematic serious injury is tolerated. Even in dojo where the instruction is considered the toughest, no one leaves training at the end of the night in a body bag. Although karate exploits the medium of conflict to train its followers, the core message of karate is to

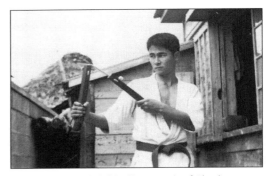

A very young Sokuichi Gibu sensei, of Shorin ryu.

stop violence, or, if a fight should break out, to bring the fight to an end as quickly and decisively as possible. When dealing with a training partner, or even one of the many training tools I use on a daily basis, I am constantly reminded of the necessity to control myself first in order to control my partner or the tool. The correlation is clear: the less control you have over yourself, the less control you are able to bring to bear on your training partner, or the tool you're working with. A poor sense of timing, distancing, balance, or an indecisive mind only contributes to your own downfall. If these things are not in place, if they are not working for you, then they are working against you. Every action and response becomes an effort, and very quickly you find yourself resorting to brute strength to compensate for your lack of control. But look, if all you needed to do karate well was brute strength, then only a handful of extremely fit young men would be able to use it. The rest of us, the over thirty-fives, the vast majority of women, and in fact anyone who was not built like the Hulk, might as well forget karate. If ever proof were needed to show that karate is not based solely on body size and muscle power alone, you need look no further than the physique of the average Okinawan. A cursory glance is all that is needed to understand why such a devastating martial art could never have originated on the island if physical size had been a deciding factor in the genesis of karate. Okinawan men, although often quite broad shouldered and stocky, are small, around five feet to five feet six inches (155 cm–170 cm) in height. Nevertheless, they have a strength that belies their size, and a good Okinawan karateka can punch so far above his weight as to make you seriously wonder how the generation of such power is possible.

That karate when practiced as it was intended, as a method of self-protection, continues to draw people to it even in societies where the need for physical self-protection seems unlikely, Japan being an obvious example, speaks to the broader nature of karate and why people practice it. As I have previously pointed out, there are clear and distinct ways to approach your training in order to get the benefits you are searching for. Having a sound and realistic understanding of why you train in karate removes many of the obstacles encountered by those with a less certain sense of direction. To be on the path and to know why you are being asked to take the steps you are taking can make all the difference. You may not understand your teacher's reasoning at the time he asks you to take a step forward, but if you are training under a teacher, not an instructor, then you can be confident that such a request will lead to progress. For me, fighting has never been an issue; what I am searching for in karate is a way of disciplining myself not to fight because if I don't fight, then I never lose. When I began training, I needed to look at the world in a different way and change my aggressive reaction to the things going on around me. For me, karate provided that discipline and gave me something to push against and struggle with while my nature grew less destructive, and I learned to look beyond the here and now, the then and there, and to glance beyond the obvious. Although I have learned many valuable lessons from all my teachers, it was from Eiichi Miyazato that I learned the most profound examples of how to practice karate. Here are just a few instances of the way he taught me.

When I first began training at the Jundokan dojo, in 1992, I was in Okinawa with my closest friend, Richard Barrett. He had already been a student of Miyazato sensei for some time and spent six months living at the dojo back in the mid-1980s. Through Richard's introduction I was accepted by Miyazato sensei into his dojo, the Jundokan, and whenever I visit the island have trained there ever since. I was warned that Miyazato sensei could be a bit gruff and short-tempered, so I was quite nervous on my first visit. However, I never found Miyazato sensei to be irascible at all. True, he didn't suffer fools gladly, nor did he have much tolerance for people who displayed a lack of good manners, and he was an absolute stickler when it came to punctuality. But none of these things made me feel uneasy; actually they did the opposite. If Miyazato sensei said to be at the dojo for a certain time, you had to be there before, not on time, and certainly not a moment later. On that first visit to the Jundokan dojo I was going to be training twice each day, six days a week for three weeks, a schedule that left little time to do much else except eat and sleep.

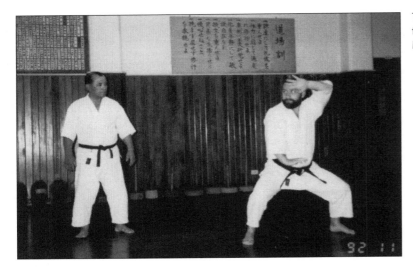

The author under the watchful eye of Miyazato sensei.

Richard was no stranger to the ways of the Jundokan, but for me so much was new. Until that point, I had always lined up when the senior called "Shugo!" and spent the next couple of hours doing as I was told. Karate training had always been structured and the students were led by the commands of the sensei. It was they who set the pace and dictated the type and quantity of training I did. But it wasn't like that at the Jundokan; here I was expected to provide my own momentum and enthusiasm, and every training session was a class of one. I learned to get changed and find an appropriate spot in the dojo in which to train. The harder I pushed myself the more seniors were likely to come over and help me with advice and technical details. The students who did not push themselves were simply left alone, a situation that lasted for as long as the students failed to engage themselves seriously with their training or left the dojo altogether. The Jundokan in those days was open six days a week, from ten o'clock in the morning through to ten o'clock at night, Monday to Saturday. Students were free to come and go as their personal schedule allowed, and it was not at all uncommon for students to train for a couple of hours in the late afternoon, leave for a while to get something to eat, and then return to the dojo until nine or ten o'clock at night.

During that first visit to the Jundokan, Miyazato sensei found many ways to gauge my nature, and cleaning the Jundokan shower room after the school children had used it was only the beginning. One Sunday evening he arranged to have dinner at the apartment my friend Richard and I were sharing. Miyazato sensei duly arrived at the allotted time along with a small group of students, and we set about preparing the vegetables and meat for the meal, *shabu shabu,* a boiling broth into which thinly cut strips of meat are dipped before being taken out and dipped again in a sesame seed sauce and eaten. As the meal progressed Miyazato sensei, who was sitting next to me, took a raw egg and cracked it into a class, *"Tabe, tabe!"* (Eat, eat!), he said, a wry smile forming on his face as he spoke. I looked at the glass and then at Miyazato sensei; he looked at the glass and then back at me. I knew what was going on and so with one big swallow, I downed the raw egg in a single gulp. *"Oishii desu!"* (Delicious!) I said, and then continued eating. Although he said nothing, I could see Miyazato sensei was a little surprised at my reaction to his 'request'. In truth, drinking a raw egg is not something I would do voluntarily, but this was different, this was a test. At the time I thought of my dad and how as a boxer in his youth, he would drink raw eggs as often as he could get them in the belief that they made him stronger. On this occasion I was grateful for my father's example and quietly pleased that my teacher saw no sign of hesitation in my willingness to accept his challenge.

A few years later, in 1996, during one of my regular visits to Okinawa, I was training in the dojo one afternoon when Miyazato sensei appeared and motioned for me to come to the front of the dojo. There he proceeded to examine my every move, kata after kata, until I had completed all thirteen practiced and preserved by the Jundokan dojo. He was being somewhat overly critical, I thought, even for him, or so it felt at the time. Still, I had done my best and in the end that is all anyone can do … right? I remember feeling exhausted and a little confused as I focused on catching my breath and bringing my heart rate down. Miyazato sensei was not one to spend a great deal of time drilling his students. His way was to give students something to work on and then leave them to it, to let them discover the 'feeling' of something for themselves through their own investigation and study. So there I was, standing in the dojo having a one-on-one lesson that had so far gone on for well over half an hour. Strange, then, how it took a while before I noticed Miyazato sensei had gone. He had simply walked off without saying a word and returned to his small office. I stood looking at myself in one of the mirrors for a moment, trying to work out what had just happened. I was also keeping an eye out for his return and kept a careful watch for him coming out of his office at the far end of the dojo. Tetsunosuke Yasuda sensei, one of the Jundokan seniors, was smiling, which only added to my sense of unease and confusion. So I began to stretch. It's what you do in the dojo when you are not sure what to do and yet you are too tired to keep training. One thing you never do in the dojo is stand around doing nothing: so I began to stretch. After a while, Miyazato sensei emerged from his office and called me over, Yasuda sensei came too. As I approached, he extended his right hand, so I instinctively extended mine, and we shook hands. He then unfolded a piece of paper he was holding in his left hand and began to read from it; Yasuda sensei translated. I was surprised to find I had just been promoted to godan (5th *dan*). Miyazato sensei then asked that photographs be taken. As soon as this was done, he bowed; and pointing to the center of the dojo, he looked at me and spoke just one word: "Training!"

I put my certificate with my clothes in the changing room and returned to the dojo to practice. My head was swirling with what had just happened. I had just been promoted to fifth dan; that was master level. Wow! I was a karate master. Just then, Miyazato sensei reappeared and once again called me over. What now … sixth dan, maybe? No. Typically, my teacher was doing what he always did; he was teaching me a lesson.

He asked me to follow him and together we stepped off the dojo floor and put on our shoes before stepping through the front door. Once outside he pointed to a small bucket containing a cloth and large sponge, standing next to a low faucet (tap) over a rather well-kept drain. He pointed to his car standing in front of us. "Can you help please?" he said. "Yes sensei, anything!" was my reply. "Can you clean my car? I have an important meeting this evening and I want to make a good impression when I arrive." And with that he walked back into the dojo, sliding the door closed behind him as he went. I set about filling the bucket and making a start by hosing down the car. Just then, the dojo door slid open and Miyazato sensei popped his head out. "Please do a good job," he said, before sliding the door shut and leaving me to it. All the way through that chore, I could not help smiling to myself. Here I was, 'the big karate master', and what was I doing? I was washing my teacher's car while the junior students were in the dojo practicing their karate. If ever I harbored any serious thoughts of my new rank being important, that lesson well and truly rid me of them. I fin-

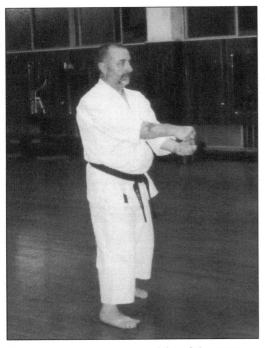

The author training at the Jundokan dojo, 2008.

ished the job, still smiling, and returned to the dojo to practice. That night after training Yasuda sensei took me out for dinner at a Chinese restaurant, where he spoke about being humble even when you have achieved great things.

Why you train in karate dictates how you train. If you are seeking attention, then you will behave overtly and no doubt gain the celebrity you seek. Celebrity, however, often brings more negativity into your life than anything positive, so caution is the key here. The old saying about being careful what you wish for because you just might get it proclaims a wisdom many to-day ignore. It's not wishing or the relent-less hard work it takes to bring your wish to fruition that is the problem; it is what you wish for. Celebrity without substance is like karate without humility: neither enhances the human condition. Still, you walk your own path and in doing so take responsibility for both the good and the bad that you encounter. As I understand karate, and life, you are free to chart your own course and sail as close to the wind as you like; that said you should not complain if your actions leave you high and dry or crash you upon the rocks of failure and adversity. With freedom comes responsibility, a concept not everyone training in karate is willing to live with, it would seem. Traditional karate training, undertaken with sincerity, will not develop your character, but it will reveal it. Once you know who you are and what you are capable of, you can chart your own course and take your life in whichever direction you want it to go.

Modern Trends: Reality-based Martial Arts

The rise in recent years of so-called 'reality' based martial arts reminds me of other great scams committed against the general public, like bottled water, and who can forget the panic that gripped the world in the 1990s over the Y2K dilemma that was supposedly going to see aeroplanes fall from the sky and shut down every computer on the entire planet. Today there are two main streams of 'reality' based martial arts being taught to the public, those based on tactics used by various police and military institutions around the world, and the sporting 'reality' engaged in by young men who have something to prove to themselves and others. While the military approach to self-protection sounds compelling, I fear the mindset of those teaching it to the public is little different to that of the average karate instructor who sets up shop in the local scout hut and solicits for business in the usual way. Military 'Close-Quarter-Combat' is a tool with a precise purpose, to kill! I'm not sure what good that skill is in most people's everyday life. Still, the dream of having the largest knife, the biggest gun, or the most deadly fighting techniques, should you be confronted, remains a powerful draw card to those who live their lives in fear of violence.

While I have nothing but admiration for those folks who train hard in any martial art, and for those who enter the various cage-fighting tournaments around the world, I have to say what they do is no more real in terms of fighting than the kind of training I have done in the past in various karate dojo in Okinawa and elsewhere. If you want to get into a really 'real' fight, you should join the police, prison service, or the military. In any of these situations you will come across plenty of people who will happily kill you: that's real fighting! All the other stuff, in rings, in cages, in dojo, in *kwoon*, and in *dojang* around the world, that's all sport. Okay, I admit, some of this sport is brutal, and a lot closer to reality than others, and it takes no small amount of courage to enter into these *fights*, but it's still sport, and as such has rules and safety measures in place to avoid serious injury. Walk into the local Hell's Angels clubhouse and give the sergeant-at-arms a big kiss; then you will have a real fight on your hands. Sorry, but as tough and as demanding as these 'reality based' and martial sports are, they are no more real than any other rule-bound, combat-based sport.

So, is there anything else you can do to engage in a real fight, short of searching for a Hell's Angel to cuddle or joining the armed forces? Well yes there is. You can turn the fight away from others and look inward toward the negative aspects of your own character. Once you take your gaze off others and start to focus on your 'self', you will find an opponent who is not so easily defeated, an adversary who will take real commitment to control, let alone vanquish. Too much eh? Yes, I thought so. It is a common enough reaction when faced with the prospect of engaging in a 'real' fight. People usually back off and start looking for excuses or find ways to avoid this particular confrontation. If your life is not fulfilling then how do you go about changing it? If you do not have contentment, how are you going to find it? If you do not have control of your own future, then how can you regain that control? If fighting for such things in your life is not 'real' then I don't know what is. Regardless of which martial art you train in, the important thing to remember is this: it's not what you do that adds value to your life, but how you do it. Fighting others is not easy, but such battles pale into insignificance compared to the brawl you engage in when you take on your own ego: that is about as 'real' a fight as it gets.

What you see now in terms of fighting sports is nothing new, the ancient Romans did it, and the ancient Greeks did it too. In actual fact, they really did fight for real. Gladiators entering the arena could only guarantee coming home for dinner if they killed their opponent; now that's a real fight. And the fighters of the first Olympic games who took part in the *pankration*[62] tournaments knew their opponent was out to inflict life-threatening damage if they could: also real. What you see on TV today is a highly developed version of the oldest male dominated activity in the world: fighting. It appeals to the cave man in those whose aggression has yet to be domesticated. After all, there are few creatures walking the planet today more gullible and headstrong than the average human male between the ages of sixteen and twenty-five. Fueled by testosterone and raging hormones, and guided through their formative years by a brain not yet fully developed, adolescent boys are easily turned toward their natural tendency to fight. If young men have even the slightest inclination toward pugilism, the seemingly 'new' and exciting approach of cage fighting in the martial arts hits the nail squarely on the head. Those of you who have been around the block a few times have witnessed other such realities in the martial arts before. I sometimes wonder how many ex-*ninja* there are walking around out there today, each one a highly trained assassin, expert in 'Black Ops' and covert surveillance techniques, and masters of the one-touch death grip. In spite of all the hype surrounding *Ninjitsu* in the 1980s, I always figured I was safe.

Any training in the martial arts, if entered into seriously with a sincere desire to engage the 'self', will make your fight real. But just as real as the training is the desire of a few individuals who claim anything and everything if it will help them part you from your hard-earned cash. There is nothing new about the modern trend in martial sports; the packaging and promotion may have changed and will no doubt change again in the future, but the product is the same. For, at the end of the day, the only thing being bought and sold are dreams. Aggression is a natural part of being a male; it is in our genes, but we do not have to fight each other, we can choose another path. In my opinion aggression is not the problem here; the problem lies in identifying where to aim your aggression and identifying exactly who or what you should be fighting against. You can choose to fight another person, you can choose to fight the 'system', or you can choose to fight your own negativity and the things about your character that lead to your unhappiness. While the first two options will undoubtedly create more problems than they solve, the third approach will direct you toward contentment. But it's not an easy path to walk; on the contrary, fighting your own ego offers far less 'instant gratification' than any other alternative, and yet its rewards are intensely meaningful and lasting.

We Stand Alone Surrounded by Many

When you embark upon the path of karate you do so on your own. Although others surround you on all sides, you nevertheless stand alone in your efforts to make progress. While others may inspire you, and still others seem to be the source of all your problems, your situation will not change so long as you remain unable to rely upon your own sense of self. When you strive to understand fully the concept of balance and how it might best be applied in your daily life, you make the inexorable move from being exclusively a student who is dependent on your teacher's generosity, toward the role of being a teacher yourself, where you extend the gift of guidance to others. You discover the rewards inherent in giving more than taking and in doing so come to understand the nature of your tradition. All this is wrapped in the continual ritual of training and contained in the simple act of going to the dojo and applying yourself, body and mind, to the study of your art. The difficulty found in simplicity is often a cause of dismay in those new to, or unfamiliar with, karate training. Still, with sincere effort and the pas-

sage of time, the difficulty subsides and the mystery of your martial art begins to fade; as Jon Franklin once said, "Simplicity, carried to an extreme, becomes elegance." It's a quote that often comes to mind when I observe senior karateka on Okinawa going about their daily lives.

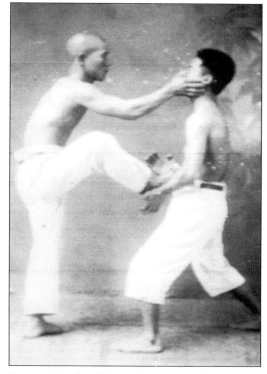

I have already mentioned my teacher, Eiichi Miyazato, and the advice I heard him issue many times to foreign students who asked him questions: "Just do it!" At first, I wondered if his response meant he was perhaps fed up with being asked questions, and for a time, I had some sympathy for those disgruntled visitors who left the Jundokan believing they had met a cantankerous old man. In time, however, I came to understand the profound simplicity of my sensei's method of instruction. Not for him, the overly-long explanations or the jaw-dropping demonstrations of fighting prowess that some karate teachers like to feed their followers. What Miyazato sensei

Karate at its simplistic and destructive best.

did was set you on a course of self-discovery. He simply pointed his students in the right direction and let them make their own way, step-by-step, day-by-day. Every once in a while he stopped by to see how things were going and to offer advice when he felt it was needed; if not, he would simply leave you to get on with it. Now, this method of teaching may seem beyond the ability of many karate students today, and quite frankly, that's because it is! Miyazato sensei's approach to teaching was not for everyone, but I feel he was the most sincere, simple, and direct of all my teachers; and I now employ this method myself when I teach yudansha level students. If teaching is only a matter of showing what is possible and learning is making it possible for yourself, then the responsibility for learning falls squarely in the lap of the student and is beyond the dominion of any teacher. As you continue to train throughout your life, you need to be aware that your successes and your failures are yours and yours alone. Others may have contributed to them both, but you own them; they are yours. The good news is that both success and failure are great teachers, and how you react when you experience either provides the lesson, as well as a clear indication of how you are progressing as a karateka, and a human being.

Miyazato sensei came to me in the dojo one afternoon and asked, "Are you still here?" I didn't get his meaning straight away. I mean, obviously I was still there; who else was he talking to? But he did things like this; he planted seeds and watched to see what grew. I often thought too much into his words and at times imagined all sorts of meanings in what he said to me. I should have known better, he didn't play games, he was a direct kind of person who left you in no doubt where you stood, and I liked that, so why did I sometimes fail to appreciate what I already knew? Looking back, I think I had yet to stop over-engineering my karate; and so every now and then I would find myself fretting over the simplest of comments that came my way. Miyazato sensei was not actually asking me if I was still in his dojo. He could see that, but he was asking me to re-examine what I was doing there. He was asking me to confirm that I was fully engaged in my pursuit of karate and my own self-improvement, or was I simply in the building doing a bit of training. I don't think he was being judgmental but was acting like a mirror and inviting me to ponder what I saw. When my thinking was over, what action would I take? Lessons like this cannot be given to large groups of karateka, for there is a level of intimacy and trust in play here that is lost if you are learning karate in a large group simply doing as you are told by the man at the front of the class.

Since entering a dojo for the first time, in 1974, I have witnessed massive changes in the way karate is practiced, the kind of people who practice it, and even the way the general public thinks about it. I am sometimes asked by curious readers of my books and magazine articles how many students I have, or how many 'clubs' I run. Implicit in the question is the assumption I have many students and teach karate far and wide. When I explain my situation, the most common reaction is one of surprise. Due to reading my work over the years, many have built a particular image of me in their minds, but the reality of how I live and the way I teach karate often comes as a big shock. I am reminded when something like this happens of the need to remain levelheaded. For insomuch as you bestow celebrity upon others, you diminish your own sense of self in equal measure. In my work for martial arts magazines, I have met, over the years, many truly amazing martial artists from many different backgrounds and cultures. A lot have been somewhat less spectacular as people than the image I had of them prior to our meeting. To say I have been left a little bit disappointed at times is an indication of two things: the reality of the person when I met him and my own expectations. I now understand that expectations are unwise. Besides, it is exactly this kind of thinking, of projecting your own imaginings onto others that leaves the door open to all kinds of negative experiences, experiences that you must, as they are of your own making, accept full responsibility for. There is an old story that illustrates the dangers you face when you do not follow your nature and put yourself under the control of others; it goes like this:

> A tortoise stood on the riverbank trying to get across, but the river was in flood and to swim across would mean certain death. No matter, he was a patient tortoise and decided to let the water level drop. He was in no hurry, he had everything he needed and all the time in the world; and he knew his journey would continue once the current slowed down a little. After all, it wasn't like he couldn't swim; it was just that his journey would take a little longer if he waited.
>
> From the middle of the river a huge crocodile emerged and slowly made its way toward the tortoise. The tortoise grew nervous and backed off a little.
>
> "Hey tortoise, do you need any help?"
>
> "No thank you. I'm making my own way just fine thanks."
>
> "Jump on my back and I'll get you across."
>
> "That's okay, I'll just wait for a while. Besides, you will only eat me if I accept your offer."
>
> "No I won't … I promise!"
>
> The tortoise thought for a while; he had his doubts, but then he began to wonder how long he might be stuck waiting for the river to calm down. So eventually, against his better judgment, the tortoise decided to trust the crocodile and accept his offer of help. He jumped on the crocodile's back and off they went into the middle of the river. As soon as they reached the deep water, the crocodile rolled over, tipping the hapless tortoise into the raging torrent. The last thing the tortoise said was, "I knew you would eat me!"
>
> On the riverbank, a bird sitting in a tree had been watching the events unfold; he asked the crocodile, "Why did you eat that tortoise, even though you promised not to?"
>
> "I couldn't help it," said the crocodile. "It's my nature!"

Although many variations of this story are told in many different cultures, the moral of the story can be appreciated on a number of different levels. First of all, you behave according to your nature. If you insist on denying your nature you will never learn to change it, but if you understand the nature of others you can protect yourself. If you go against your better judgment, you must accept the consequences. When people say they are doing you a favor to make your life easier, perhaps it's best to remind yourself that life, or karate, was never meant to be 'easy'. When you have all you require for the journey, there is no need to accept an easy option. In all your dealings with others remember, patience is a virtue and actions speak louder than words. And finally … stay away from crocodiles: they will always eat you!

Okay, so the chance of meeting a real live crocodile in the dojo is extremely rare, but I have seen many a slippery reptile posing as a sensei over the years, and I have seen many a tortoise-like student only too willing to accept his promises too. When you bestow 'celebrity' on the people who teach you, you are allowing them to take control of your thinking. You listen to their words even when they are at odds with their actions, and you give both of these things more value than they deserve; not to put too fine a point on it, you abandon your own opinions in favor of theirs. Why do you think advertisers use celebrities to sell their products? If you have ever bought something solely on the endorsement of a celebrity, then you have fallen for the same deception the tortoise fell for. Thankfully, your decision to buy the home gym equipment now gathering dust in the bedroom hasn't resulted in as high a price for you as the tortoise had to pay.

I once asked a very famous Shotokan karateka in England why he had never been to Japan to train. He said he felt he had everything he wanted from karate right there in England. He was a national and international sporting champion at both kata and kumite and frequently appeared on the cover of karate magazines. He and I were both nidan (2nd *dan*) level at the time, and in complete contrast to him, I had dreamt of training in Japan for as long as I had been training in karate. At the time his attitude toward training in Japan came as a big surprise. This young man's level of karate ability was simply astonishing; he had fought and won against the best in the world, including the Japanese, so why did he not want to train there? The truth is I don't know, nor am I about to speculate. I do know this however; when you travel to Japan you often find the most difficult aspect of the trip lies outside the dojo. Karate training in Japan is no more different or difficult than training in a well-run dojo anywhere else in the world; the difference lies in the emotions you have to deal with when you are out there alone with no one but yourself to rely on. As demanding as the training might be, it is usually the most familiar part of the experience; the emotional challenges appear when you are outside the dojo trying to live, and they can often prove severe. What most visitors to Japan struggle with is their immediate illiteracy; they can't read, they can't write; they can't even ask a question. As strange as it might sound to those who have never practiced their karate in Japan, becoming the 'foreigner' is often the hardest part of the entire trip. Learning to navigate such obstacles on your own requires a certain strength of character and teaches you a lot about your true nature and the kind of person you really are. If you practice Japanese karate, this is the value of going to Japan! If you do not have the heart to step out of your comfort zone and put yourself out there, on your own, then perhaps you should ask yourself, "Are you still here?"

Regardless of who your instructor is, which club or dojo you train at, which association you may be affiliated with, or what type of karate training you think you are involved in, it is important to remember why you started and why you continue: why you are still here! Karate is a solo journey, albeit made in the company of others sometimes; but you do not 'belong' to anybody or anything, not unless you allow it. I learned long ago that people treat you the way you allow them to. Fall into line and become a subservient automaton and you will end up wherever others want to put you. This is not karate. A traditional karate teacher will not insist on your unquestioning obedience or loyalty. Instead, he will make available to you an education that provides an opportunity to comprehend your own nature as well as the nature of others. Having acquired such an education, you decide either to go or stay, training with your teacher, according to your nature. Okay, so, perhaps finding a teacher able to provide such an education is easier said than done; but then, being a sincere student is not so easy either. Appreciating karate is much easier said than done too; like many things in life, it is always easier to talk than get off your butt and do something. Thought followed by action is the nature of karate.

Celebrity instructors are not sensei; and you can tell this by the way they cultivate their fans. Traditional sensei are often not particularly friendly toward their students, whom they often keep at arm's length. Why do they do this? They do it because familiarity breeds contempt. These sensei may not be a student's best friend, but they are great examples, not only of the physical aspects of karate but as individuals who have found a way to live a well-balanced life, and in doing so freed themselves from many of the concerns that cause problems for others. Regardless of what some people try to do with it, traditional karate is not a spectator sport, it is not a career path, nor is it some kind of intellectual, semi-scientific pastime. It is a civilian method of self-protection, the learning of which will change your outlook on life. It produces individuals who are capable of dealing with the negativity that inevitably comes with living. But wait. If you think you can get such skills by passing promotion tests and going to seminars, think again! All karate asks of you is honest effort on a regular basis. That's it! When I come to think about it, that is all Miyazato sensei was asking of me too. My body was in the dojo and my limbs were moving in accordance with the kata I was doing, but was 'I' there, in the moment, bringing my karate to life; or was I just in the dojo doing a bit of training? My sensei wasn't asking me if I was still in his dojo in a physical sense, but if I was still completely present in mind, body, and spirit. This idea of doing karate with your whole body is encapsulated in the term, 'Shin Gi Tai', a literal translation of which is 'mind, technique, and body', but more broadly it points to the unity of the physical and the cerebral acting as one through the medium of your spirit. The application of spontaneous movement born from the unity of mind, body, and spirit is, for me at least, something worth working for. If you ever get it, you will be invincible! You do not need to know the science behind karate techniques or what mathematical formula can be best used to articulate it to others; what you need is the self-discipline to put yourself in the dojo often and to be fully engaged in your pursuit of karate when you are there. Am I still here? I never left … how about you?

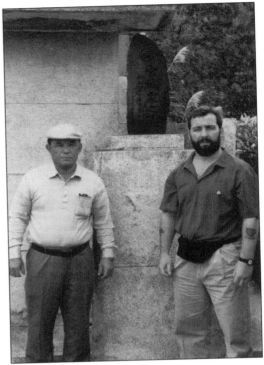

Eiichi Miyazato and author at the tomb of Chojun Miyagi sensei.

STORIES OF THREE GREAT MEN

There is an aspect of training on Okinawa of which I am particularly fond, the story telling. It can happen at any time but most often it occurs after training, when the sweating is over for the day and everyone retires to a local izakaya, where food and a few cold beers help ease the body's aches and pains, relieve the tiredness, and deepen the bonds between student and teacher. At such times as this, Okinawa's rich oral history surrounding karate and kobudo begins to flow from one generation to the next, and stories of former bushi emerge from the past to enrich the present and inspire the future. I am conscious of the fact that an opportunity to sit around a table with various Okinawan masters is beyond the reach of many, and so before this book comes to an end I would like to share a few budo stories with you. To do so I have plucked from the past three men who have, each in his own way, contributed greatly to the art. They all lived and came to prominence as bushi at different times in Okinawan history and represent the three main streams of Okinawan karate, namely, Tomari te, Naha te, and Shuri te. But remember, these stories are just that: stories! Although they are told about real people and 'sometimes' real events, they are not to be taken as hard-core facts. The purpose the stories serve is inspirational, to help motivate you to do better when you're next in the dojo, or as you move through life. Like the parables found in Christianity and the lessons found in the study of Zen, the veracity of many karate stories do not always stand close inspection, but as I said, that's not the point: the tales are told for reasons other than the transmission of facts.

Another function of these stories in the learning of Okinawan karate is to give depth and history to the activity you are engaged in, to show what you are pursuing today was pursued by others long ago, and that the challenges you are currently facing were also faced by budoka decades before you were even born. Learning that others have stood where you stand now, and that they found ways to move forward, to improve, and to go beyond the seemingly overwhelming problems in front of them, can afford immense support when times are tough. Appreciating that you walk the budo path alone while remembering you walk in the shadow of others who have traveled that way before offers hope. Listening to stories from karate's past has a way of making your way ahead seem less impossible, although only a fool would think the stories made the path any less difficult. If your predecessors had to make sacrifices to make progress, it would be a mistake to believe you won't have to also. The stories are there to point you toward the attributes you need to make these sacrifices. Bringing forth courage, humility, honesty, charity, and integrity when you need them will be no easy task. But the pursuit of budo karate is the pursuit of all of these attributes and more, so take heed, listen to the tales of those who have gone before you, and learn. Learn that the way of karate is about more than kicking and punching, more than trophies and titles, and more than fame and fortune. If you come to understand this through your efforts on the dojo floor and the stories you hear from your teachers and seniors, then you will understand why such stories need to be told and retold to each generation of karateka that comes along. If we who teach karate today fail to do this, then we become responsible for the loss of something precious.

Kosaku Matsumora (1829–1898): The Ethical Master of Tomari te

Perhaps best remembered today for disarming a sword-wielding samurai with nothing more than a wet towel, the life of Tomari's Kosaku Matsumora reads like a novel. Born in 1829, he was the eldest son of Koten Matsumora, an indirect descendent of the first Okinawan King through his connection to the Yuji clan. His childhood name was Taru-kane; but he was also known by the Chinese name, Yuikan. Small in stature, even for an Okinawan, he nevertheless grew into a strong young man with broad shoulders and a chest that was said to be as big as a bull's; contemporary accounts often describe Matsumora's physical appearance as impressive. How fortunate then, that his moral education was as comprehensive as the tutoring he received in the martial arts. As a child he studied the Chinese classics as well as Confucianism. This seems to have been the educational standard of the day for children coming from families with 'connections'. Although his father's link to the Yuji clan no doubt brought with it a certain measure of prestige among his Tomari vil-

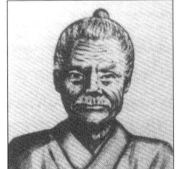

Kosaku Matsumora

lage peers, it was of no great use in financial terms. Kosaku was going to have to make his own way in the world, at a time when the social upheaval unfolding within the King-dom of Ryukyu was steadily moving toward its inevitable conclusion. Japan, which had invaded Ryukyu in 1609, was changing from a feudal system into a constitutional based nation, and Okinawa, as the center of the Ryukyu King-dom, would be required by its masters to comply.

Tomari village, like other locations around Okinawa, had for many years operated a level of jurisdictional con-trol over its inhabitants. While it acted as the official port for the royal capital, Shuri, it also maintained a certain level of fiscal independence. Tomari was not unique in this, as each village had its own 'communal property' in the form of small plots of land and, to some extent or other, its own store of funds with which it paid for activities the village elders felt were benefi-cial to the community. These days we might think of this arrangement as being similar to paying local or state taxes to take care of local needs, and consider these as being separate from government taxes. In Tomari village, the communal wealth was known as *Neewagumuchi* (knee-wa-goo-moo-chee) and it was to play a significant role in the life of Matsumora in the years to come. But more about that later; for now, let's go back to the middle years of the nineteenth century, to a time when the young Tarukane was taking his first tentative steps toward becoming a master of his homeland's fighting arts. His early childhood instruction in the fighting arts of ti—the word 'karate' was still unknown at this time—began under the guidance of Giko Uku (1800–1850) who, for three years, taught his young student the foundation kata of the Tomari system: naihanchi. Although still known by this in present-day schools of Okinawan karate, the kata are also widely known by their Japanese name: tekki, shodan, nidan, and sandan, respectively. As well as kata, Matsumora was taught how to use the hips to generate power and various training methods to build strength in his legs and torso. After three years his instruction came under the direction of another of Tomari's great bushi, Kishin Teruya (1804–1864). Over the following years the young Matsumora grew in both stature and ability. Teruya had taught him the kata passai and wanshu, the latter said to have been Teruya's favorite training drill. The martial arts at that time were a closely guarded secret. Students were accepted only if they had a good character and were thought unlikely to bring dishonor to either their teacher or their village. To this end the training was conducted privately, either in the early hours of the morning or late at night. The locations where training took place were also kept secret from prying eyes, and so deserted beaches, wooded glades, and even graveyards were regularly pressed into service as venues for the passing on of knowledge. Sometimes the most dedicated student would train at the site of his teacher's family tomb, but such sites were reserved for only the most devoted of students, and to receive an invitation like this was a sign of the master's trust in his student. Matsumora received such an invitation from Teruya, and it was here that he was introduced to the hidden combat strategies found in the kata his teacher had been teaching him. Today this kind of information is known as 'bunkai', and among traditional schools of Okinawan karate it is considered just as important as kata training in thin air, if not more so. In common with many of the family tombs of that time, the Teruya tomb was an imposing structure and an expensive one too. Gravesites in the Ryukyu Kingdom followed the fashion in China, and large 'turtle-back' graves (*kameko baka*) dotted the island. During the American invasion of Okinawa, in April 1945, many of these historic monuments were destroyed. The Japanese military had commandeered scores of them and integrated the tombs into their defensive battle lines. After the war, the demand for land by the occupying American military saw more ancient graves destroyed, annexed, or moved to locations with no association to the family whose ancestors were being unceremoniously shifted around the island. The Teruya family tomb was built in 1774, at the cost of over three hundred thousand dollars (U.S.) in today's currency. It represented not only a massive investment by the Teruya family but also a measure of the level of respect in which the Okinawans held their ancestors. To be invited to practice his karate at the family gravesite was no small thing, and the solemnity of the gesture was not lost on Matsumora. In Shoshin Nagamine's excellent book, *Tales of Okinawa's Great Masters*, translated by Patrick McCarthy, Nagamine has this to say about Matsumora's invitation:

In the eyes of an Okinawan, nothing was as important as the character or personality of a potential deshi [disciple] of karate. There was, and to some extent still is, an unwritten law that karate should never be taught to anyone who is rude, arrogant, or disrespectful, and that also held true for brothers and children of the master's family. The reason master Teruya taught Matsumora at the family tomb was not only because he was so talented, but largely because he was a modest and genuine person, a man who understood that the essence of karate was *shingitai* and deeply embraced its principles. To master Teruya, Matsumora was the perfect deshi. Hence, it was at the family tomb in front of Teruya's ancestors, that master and deshi sincerely exchanged vows. For Matsumora, this honor reinforced his commitment, well being, and enthusiasm to continue his training even harder than before.

Nagamine's book goes on to tell many inspiring tales about Matsumora and other great budoka from Okinawa's past, and I would strongly recommend this book to anyone interested in the history of karate. Matsumora lived at a time of great social upheaval in Okinawa. The Satsuma clan from southern Japan had administered the Ryukyu Islands since they invaded in 1609, and from that time the Ryukyuan king was, in reality, no more than a puppet of the ruling bakufu, the military government back in Japan. For centuries there existed an uneasy treaty between the native Uchinanchu population and their Japanese overlords. Abuse was fairly common in certain quarters and was on display almost daily in the way the Japanese of samurai rank viewed the locals. Matsumora, now a young man and a well-respected bushi in his own right, often wondered what would happen if he had to face a samurai. To that end he began experimenting with ways to deal with a sword. Te, or toudi, was essentially a bare hand fighting art and even though certain weapons in the form of horseshoes, walking sticks, and some farming tools, were in common use among the fighting men of Okinawa, bushi had long since been banned from carrying swords. To level the odds a little, Matsumora devised a way of turning something as ordinary as a towel, into a weapon. He began by wetting a towel to give it a little weight, and placed a few stones in it before giving it a few twists to keep the stones

in place; then, he had a student attack him with a wooden sword (*bokken*). With this kind of training Matsumora is said to have devised a way to avoid the sword with the use of tai sabaki, or body shifting, and used the towel, with the stones in it, to strike the swordsman's hands, arms, and head. After some time training this way, he was able to disarm his student even when the attacks were fast and furious. Because of this, he grew confident in his ability with

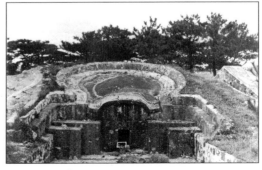

A 'turtle-back' tomb, this one bears witness to the ravages of war.

his new-found weapon. As fate would have it, his training was about to come in handy. In an incident that changed the course of his life and saw him lose a finger to the blade of a samurai's sword, Matsumora's training and confidence was put to the test one day as he walked close by the Takashi Bridge.

From a distance he heard the sound of shouting coming from a large and angry crowd. As he drew closer, he began to take in what was happening, his eyes falling on the samurai, sword raised high as if ready to strike, standing over a local who was cowering on the ground. The samurai was screaming abuse at the man and from the look of things, he was just about to dispatch the local to meet his ancestors; Matsumora had seen enough and pushed his way through the crowd, coming to a halt between the samurai and his intended victim. This act alone demonstrated the uncommon courage of the young bushi from Tomari, for he was determined to stop the samurai from having his way. With the two men now facing each other, the level of tension in the air was palpable and the crowd moved a little farther back as they anticipated the combat that was about to get underway. Matsumora removed the concealed towel he had become accustomed to carrying and stood his ground. Without warning the samurai took a swing at the young bushi, but Matsumora was able to avoid the deadly blade by means of tai sabaki and countered with a lightning fast flick of the towel which wrapped itself around the blade. This move was followed instantly by Matsumora pulling the sword from its owner's hands and tossing it to the ground; in doing so the razor sharp blade sliced through one of Matsumora's fingers, and both sword and finger flew through the air in a spray of blood. The whole encounter was over in flash. Matsumora knew his disarming of the samurai was not the end of the matter; indeed, it was only the start of his problems. Thinking quickly, he picked up his finger and the sword from the ground and ran from the scene as quickly as he could, throwing both finger and weapon in the Azato River as he made his getaway. The samurai did not give chase; he was now facing a crisis of his own. To lose his sword in a fight was a massive loss of face for the samurai, but to have lost it to an unarmed Okinawan was, frankly, unimaginable. He left the area as quickly as he could. With his sword lost, his symbol of authority was gone and his pride was in tatters. Later, if he could find Matsumora, he would have his revenge. The locals were elated by the encounter they had just witnessed and word soon spread around the area about the bushi from Tomari who had defeated one of their oppressors so decisively. Having suffered a humiliating defeat, Matsumora knew the authorities would be discreet in their pursuit, but pursue him they would. He wouldn't be hard to identify either, not with a freshly severed finger on one hand; besides, Matsumora's face would have been etched deeply into the samurai's memory. He wasn't about to forget the face of the Okinawan who had shamed him in a hurry. That same night Matsumora packed a few belongings and headed north to Nago at the base of the Motobu peninsula, and there he remained for the next ten years. He lived in the forest outside the village, during which he continued to train himself in the martial arts, as well as maintain his strength by regular use of kigu undo training with the chiishi, makiwara, and various other tools. Finding work as a rent (debt) collector for a wealthy local landowner, Matsumora was able to act as mediator and smoothed the way for those in debt to repay what they owed without enduring painful levels of hardship. His ability to sort things out gained Matsumora a reputation for being fair and good-hearted, and he became a well-liked figure in Nago.

As much as life was good in Nago, Matsumora longed to return home to Tomari. A decade had passed since he last walked its streets; the time was right to return, and so this he did: quietly. His reputation however was sufficient to alert the locals to his return and soon he was the talk of the village. There were still many who remembered his combat with the samurai official and how he lost his finger. And his status as a bushi had not been diminished by his long absence. A challenge match was arranged between Matsumora

and a young bushi from Kaneko by the name of Toguchi, a young man with a growing reputation. The oral account of their meeting, handed down over generations, states that Matsumora defeated his younger opponent without a single blow being thrown from either party. It is said that the look in Matsumora's eyes and his physical presence alone was enough to make Toguchi concede defeat.

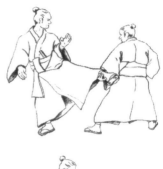

Until 1879, when the Ryukyu Kingdom formally ended, each village raised its own community chest in the form of money, property, and land. Some villages were more successful than others and Tomari residents were considered quite well provided for in this respect as their nest egg, the Neewagumuchi, was quite substantial. Once the kingdom was abolished, and the king, Shotai, abdicated and he and his family forced to relocate to To-kyo, Japanese officials began the systematic plunder of the kingdom's wealth in the name of the new National Government. As part of that process each village and town throughout the Ryukyus was visited and local assets seized. When officials arrived in Tomari they were met with firm resistance; if they wanted the Neewagumuchi they were going to have to fight for it. The officials met with village elders and made their demands, as they had done in other communities, but instead of compliance they met with stern-faced villagers who refused to hand over their property. As the afternoon passed the argu-ments back and forth grew more acrimonious on both sides and the ever-growing crowd of young men outside the Uku residence, where the meeting was taking place, began to worry the Meiji Government Officials. Many of the young men were armed with *bo* (staff) and *sai* (iron

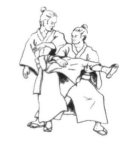

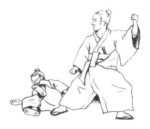

Although Tomari te is no longer a 'stand alone' tradition in its own right, many of its fighting strategies, like the one seen here, are still found in the kata of most Shuri te schools of karate.

truncheon) and knew how to use them. Not only that, but they made it clear they were prepared to use them too! The Japanese officials, appreciating their position, made a tactical withdrawal. Noting that the situation had not been resolved and would therefore have to go to a second meeting at some time in the future, the second meeting took place a few weeks later at the Tamanaha residence; only this time, the funds held in the Neewagumuchi had been placed in a strongbox and positioned in the middle of the room where the meeting was to take place. The Japanese officials must have been somewhat surprised to see it sitting there in the middle of the floor, but this was going to be the least of their surprises that day. In a tone the officials were unused to, the village elders made their feelings clear. They could take the Neewagumuchi if they wished, but they would have to run the gauntlet of bushi led, as before, by Matsumora if they did. From outside the home taunts of "Go ahead, remove it if you think you can" came from the men who were gathered in the courtyard. It became clear to the Japanese officials that the citizens of Tomari were not about to give up their community wealth without a serious

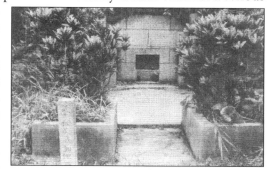

Tomb of Kosaku Matsumora. The stone pillar reads "Bushi Matsumora Kosaku."

confrontation. They departed empty handed and did not return again; Matsumora's show of strength had worked, and the Neewagumuchi remained intact and working as it was intended until 1974, when the assets were used to establish the Senkaku Kenshokai, an organization set up for the welfare of Tomari village.

When Kosaku Matsumora died in November 1898, he was seventy years old. His life had been shaped by the ancient traditions of his homeland, Ryukyu, and the birth pains of its transition from the old ways to the new. He left behind a body of thought and practice that can still be found in Okinawan karate today. Although Tomari te as an organized school in its own right no longer exists, much of its techniques survive in the kata practiced by students of the various Shuri te schools. The kata, *rohai, wankan, chinto, wanshu*, and Tomari *passai*, are often seen in demonstrations, signifying their continued practice in the dojo. Matsumora taught many students who went on to become karate masters in their own right, and of these Kodatsu Iha was the most

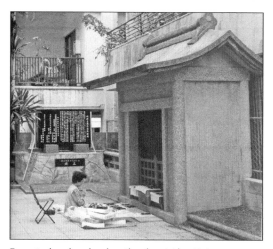

Even today, locals give thanks at the Matsumora monument in Tomari.

enthusiastic propagator of his sensei's teachings after Matsumora died. In May 1983, a monument to Matsumora was erected in Arayashiki Park in Tomari. In part, the tablet reads, "…The name of Kensei (Fist Saint) Matsumora Kosaku, a man of honor and justice, will live on forever."

Kanryo Higaonna (1853–1915): The Fist Saint of Naha te

Born on March 10, 1853, into a family descended from lower rank officials (*keiomachi*), Kanryo Higashionna (pronounced Higaonna in Japanese) was one of eight children whose father, Kanyo, made his living as a merchant. As the owner of three small boats known as *yanabarusen*, Kanyo bought goods in Naha and sailed to the north of Okinawa selling his wares in coastal villages and to the people living on the islands of Oshima, Kudakajima, and Ihejima, among others. When the goods were sold he bought firewood and upon his return home sold it in Naha. From the age of ten Kanryo, whose childhood name was Moshi, accompanied his father on many voyages and as such was acquainted early in life with hard work and even danger. Perhaps it was the hardships he faced and overcame as a youth that led to him becoming one of Okinawa's most famous bushi. For in those formative years of his transition from child to adulthood the foundations of his character were laid. Years later he went on to produce a method of karate training that lives to this day in the hearts and minds of many millions of people around the world: Naha te. In the history of Okinawa, and Japan in general, 1853 was a deci-

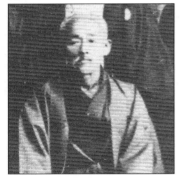

Kanryo Higaonna

sive year. Just two months after Moshi was born, his father awoke to see three strange-looking ships at anchor in Naha harbor. On board were over two hundred American sailors and marines led by Commodore Matthew C. Perry of the United States Navy. It was an extraordinary sight indeed greeting the local population that spring morning. Large black ships the likes of which few if any had seen before sat motionless in the harbor, belching thick smoke from the single tall funnel that stood erect amid the web of rigging. The Americans had arrived in vessels that were leaving the old world of sail behind; a blend of wind and steam power had pushed them across the Pacific Ocean. This was not exactly a display of gunboat diplomacy, but it was a show of force. For the Okinawan people and the secret art of toudi (karate), things would never again be the same.

In January 1867, thirteen years after the Americans first arrived, Moshi took part in a ceremony to mark his entry into manhood. The *katagashira* ritual involved tying his hair into a topknot, where it was held in place by a large pin known as a *kanzashi*. He would no longer answer to his childhood nickname, Moshi, and from that time used the name we know him by today: Kanryo. Sadly, the same year he became a man he was also left fatherless. Life on the waterfront of Naha was rough and tough and far removed from life in the more sedate hillside town of Shuri, the royal capital. Amid the commercial hustle and bustle of Nishimura village, men like Kanyo Higaonna worked hard to make a living. With a wife and eight children to provide for his situation was tough, but by no means unique. Often the friction caused by too many men chasing too few opportunities led to fights, a lot of which developed into more than just fistfights. Kanyo was killed in one such altercation, tragically stabbed to death, an event that left the family devastated.

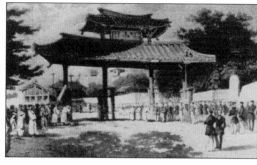

Commodore Perry and officials gather at the Shurei mon and prepare to meet the king. Shurei mon, the gateway to the royal palace, proclaims Ryukyu as the 'Land of Propriety'.

According to some legends, the death of his father caused Kanryo to swear revenge, and to this end he sought instruction from the famous bushi of nearby Kume village. That he managed to become a student of Seisho Arakaki is testimony to his ability to overcome the challenges of life. As a member of the lower classes and a non-resident of Kume village, he would have found it extremely difficult to gain acceptance, and yet, he did. He was around sixteen or seventeen years old when he began to practice karate; the exact date is unclear. Seisho Arakaki worked as a translator of Chinese and in this capacity had traveled to China on several occasions on behalf of the Ryukyu government. Although he had trained in the fighting arts since he was a young man growing up in Kume village, Seisho Arakaki is thought to have received instruction in China also. As well as his mastery of the empty hand arts, he was known for his abilities with the sai and the bo.

Exactly how Higaonna managed to find himself in China is also open to debate. By all accounts this is where he wanted to be so he could learn the fighting arts that were legendary in the eyes of the Okinawans. But travel to China was restricted at this time and obtaining the right documentation was no easy task. I'll leave it to the historians to discover how this was done; what I can say for sure is that Kanryo Higaonna arrived in the Chinese city of Fuzhou as a young man in his early twenties, and after an uncertain beginning found work in a small family factory producing items crafted from bamboo. His employer later became his teacher (*sifu*) and by all accounts the relationship between student

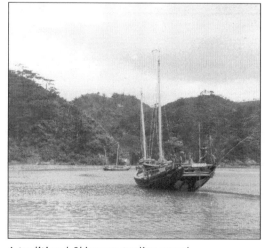

A traditional Okinawan trading vessel.

and teacher became a strong one. Soon many people began to hear about the young man from Ryukyu with a talent for the martial arts. Higaonna became known in Fuzhou as *Ryuchu no To'onna* (Higashionna of Ryukyu). Upon his return to Okinawa some years later, and after many difficult lessons from his teacher Xie Zhong Xian (also known as Ryu Ryu Ko), Higaonna was a changed man and no longer held a desire to seek revenge or indeed harm anybody. Instead, he settled down in Nishimura village and continued to sail his yanabarusen north, trading goods and buying firewood. He kept his fighting abilities to himself and did not accept students.

The Chinese city of Fuzhou, where Higaonna lived, had been a center of both commerce and the martial arts since early times, and many masters lived within its boundaries. One day two groups of students from the same style, but different kwoon, began to argue about who had the best technique. With neither group willing to concede defeat, the argument became heated by the passion of the young men on both sides. Both factions insisted their technique was the original and therefore the best and most correct.

Because the argument occurred in a public place, the sifu of both groups soon heard about it and between them decided to put their students to the test by holding a contest. On the day of the gathering, students from each kwoon took their turn to demonstrate a kata. Remember, even though they were from different kwoon the style was the same; therefore, the kata they did should have been the same also. According to the story, Kanryo Higaonna was the last student to display his kata and chose to perform sanchin. As he was Okinawan and not Chinese his performance came under even more scrutiny than the others, but his long hours of training became obvious. After the contest was over the sifu from the other school announced that students of Ryu Ryu Ko had the better technique. It is said it was because of this incident Higaonna's fame as a martial artist began to grow in Fuzhou.

Even before Higaonna left Fuzhou to return to Okinawa, his notoriety was beginning to precede him. Another story from his days in China tells of his attempt to engage in *Kaki Damashi*. This custom had long been a part of Chinese and Okinawan martial arts and refers to the testing of one's fighting skills by engaging in street fights. Flowing through the city of Fuzhou is the Min River and one of the many ways people crossed it was by the Manju Bridge. On either side of the bridge stood two guardian statues in the shape of lions, and people who wanted to challenge others would sit on the back of one of these statues. There they waited for anyone who was willing to fight them to make himself known. One night Kanryo Higaonna went to the bridge and climbed onto the back of a lion. It is said in the story that such was Higaonna's reputation as a martial artist that no one was willing to accept his challenge. The fierce look in his eyes alone was said to have been enough to change the mind of any would-be challenger, and all those who came close enough to see his glare simply carried on walking.

On his return home to Okinawa he lived close to the sea, at Naha-ku, Nishishinmachi 2-chome, in a type of house known as a *nagaya.** Higaonna kept his fighting skills

---

* Nagaya were single-story dwellings divided into several compartments and were home to the poorer members of Okinawan society.

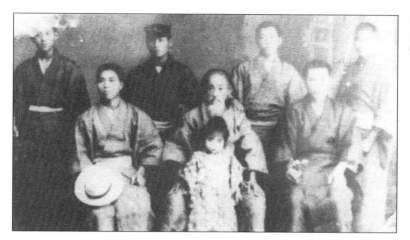

Kanryo Higaonna (center). The child is his granddaughter.

a closely guarded secret, preferring to work on his boat, and he was persuaded to accept students only after many appeals. Around the year 1889, he began to teach a few individuals on a private basis. One of these students was known to be Choki Yoshimura, the second son of the man who had helped him gain permission to travel to China years earlier. A little over a decade later, in the early years of the twentieth century, a small group of students was training regularly with Higaonna. Instruction took place at the Higaonna home and it was said that the severity of the lessons was the main reason he had so few students, for only a small number were able to endure the harshness of the training. (Author's note: While I'm sure the training was 'intense' for the students in many ways, I personally don't believe the training was 'severe', at least not in the way I think of severity. If you look at the age of some of his students they would have been mere boys at the time; I'm not sure how severe the training could have been under these circumstances. Still, the value of these stories, as I have already indicated, lies not in their historical accuracy, but in their ability to inspire successive generations.) Included among Higaonna's students, training around this time, were Juhatsu Kyoda, Chojun Miyagi, Kenwa Mabuni, and Seko Higa.

In September of 1905, at the invitation of the school principal, Junichi Kabayama, Kanryo Higaonna began teaching karate twice a week at the Naha Commercial High School. In those days (1905–1913), the school was a two-story building known as the *Nanyo-kan* and stood in the Kumoji district of Naha. Earlier, in 1901, karate was introduced into the public school system as a way of keeping the art alive, while at the same time it provided the youth of Okinawa with a wonderful method of physical and mental discipline. Because of this, many young people got a taste of what karate training was like. Although it has to be said, the type of instruction given in the public school system bore little resemblance to the type of training going on in the private dojo of the sensei at that time. Stories of karate training from so long ago still fire the imagination of today's karate enthusiasts. But we should not forget that before the introduction of karate into the public school system, it was not so easy to find a sensei. Everyone in the

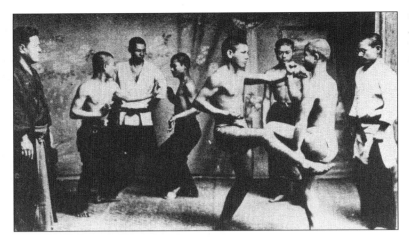

Chojun Miyagi (left) and Juhatsu Kyoda (right) watch over younger students training.

neighborhood knew who they were, of course, and the fame and reputation of some sensei, especially from the Shuri, Naha, and Tomari areas, stretched the length and breadth of Okinawa and throughout the Ryukyus. However, knowing who these men were and gaining access to their instruction were two very different matters. Unlike today, students at this time had to gain their sensei's trust and prove themselves to be of good character. Quite often they would have to be introduced by someone who was already known to the sensei. Many stories still survive to illustrate the importance of this in the history of karate. Here are a few concerning Kanryo Higaonna.

One day a man by the name of Zencho Tokeshi asked Kanryo Higaonna for instruction, but his reputation as a street fighter had preceded him and so he was refused. This angered Tokeshi who returned several times to press home his request, but each time he was met with the same answer. This annoyed Tokeshi to the point where one day he lay in ambush, his attack coming while Higaonna was using the toilet. As was common back then toilets were placed away from the main living area of the home. Higaonna's was next to his pigpen and close to the stack of firewood he sold to make his living. Tokeshi picked his moment carefully, when Higaonna was preoccupied, and let fly with a large piece of wood from the stack. The missile missed its intended target but proved the point that such a character was not ready to learn karate.

A second story involved a student who was already training with Higaonna. Fresh drinking water on Okinawa has always been vital to the harmony and wellbeing of the people, and local springs were treated with the utmost respect. Not every neighborhood had a spring however, and so a few enterprising boat owners made their living by collecting, transporting, and selling fresh water to people who had no other means of collecting it for themselves. Several small boats would leave the port at Naha each day and sail up river to Utenda, a place east of the city that could be reached easily by boat. Here they would fill their barrels with the fresh spring water before returning downstream to Naha. Everyone knew that drinking water was a precious commodity; without it people simply could not live. So one day, when Kanryo Higaonna found one of his students had been

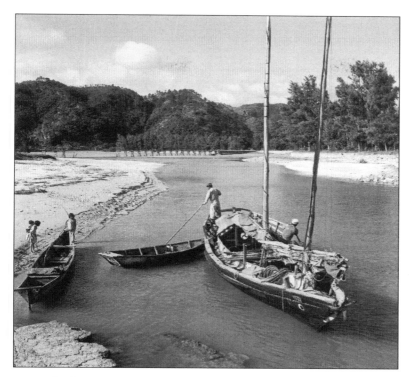

On boats similar to this one, Okinawans carried fresh water to Naha.

using fresh spring water to bathe in, he found the student's lack of consideration and good judgment intolerable, and telling him so, refused to teach him further.

Although not from the upper classes of Okinawan society, unable to read or write, and with little or no formal education, Higaonna nevertheless displayed the warm hearted and hard working characteristics so typical of the Okinawan people. Intelligent and with experience of life gained from his years living abroad, he settled down and married a woman called Makado, from the island of Iheyajima. At the time of their marriage Makado was already pregnant with another man's child, and later gave birth to a boy on May 15, 1882; together they named him Kan. Kanryo Higaonna adopted the boy as his own and bestowed upon him the role of chonan: the son who bears the responsibility of carrying on the family line. Many of today's karateka owe a debt of gratitude to Kanryo Higaonna, for without him, men such as Chojun Miyagi and Kenwa Mabuni would not have received the training they did and perhaps not gone on in later years to establish two of the four main schools of karate in the world today: Goju ryu and Shito ryu. Another famous student of Higaonna, Juhatsu Kyoda, established the Tou'on ryu school of karate. Although not as widespread or as popular as the two previously mentioned schools, it is nevertheless an important piece of Okinawa's karate heritage and can be considered a tangible treasure of Ryukyu. In fact, many of those who learned karate from Higaonna went on to achieve success in life. Whereas Chojun Miyagi and Kenwa Mabuni devoted their lives to teaching karate, Juhatsu Kyoda became a schoolteacher and retired many years later as a headmaster (principal). Other students achieved success in calligraphy, music, medicine, and commerce. Knowing this we can gain some insight into the true value of training in the martial arts of Okinawa.

In October 1915, Higaonna fell ill and his health deteriorated quickly over the following weeks to the point where his death was imminent. In spite of the medical attention provided by doctors and the care given to him by his student Chojun Miyagi, Kanryo Higaonna passed away at the relatively young age of sixty-two (sixty-three by Okinawan reckoning) on December 23. His funeral was held at his home in Nishishin-machi 2-chome. Apart from his years in China, he had lived his entire life in the same area, how amazing therefore that his influence has managed to spread to every corner of the globe where karate is now practiced. Following the Okinawan custom, his bones were laid to rest in Tsujibara cemetery; however this site was an-

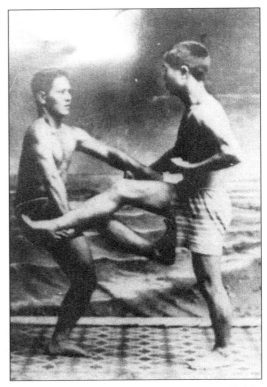

Students of Kanryo Higaonna: Chojun Miyagi (left) and Juhatsu Kyoda (right).

nexed by the American military after WWII and the Higaonna family grave was then moved to Ukishima Dori. It remained at that location (behind the Ukishima hotel in Naha) for a while before finally being relocated to Ontake cemetery in Shuri, where it remains to this day.

Throughout his life Higaonna was known by many names. In China he was known as Ryuchu no To'onna, for his fighting prowess. On his return to Okinawa he was referred to as Ashi no Higashionna[*] because of the speed of his kicks. He was also referred to as bushi even though he was not educated in the formal sense; yet he was knowledgeable of the world beyond Okinawa. Later in life, he was often called Tanmai, a term of respect and affection reserved for older people. Now, in death, he is frequently referred to as Kensei (Fist Saint). Perhaps the most significant name budoka can have attached to their name is 'sensei'. I believe Kanryo Higashionna was that, and more.

_____

[*]   Ashi, in this case, means 'legs'.

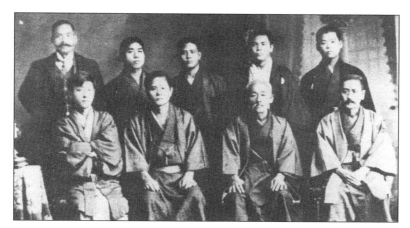

In this photograph of Kanryo Higaonna, a young Chojun Miyagi is seen standing in the back row, center.

Gichin Funakoshi (1868–1957): The Gentle Teacher of Shuri te

Perhaps it was always Funakoshi's destiny to shed light on a part of Okinawan culture that had for centuries remained hidden from the gaze of the general population. He shone like a bright star in a dark sky and pointed the way forward for the many millions around the world who would take up the challenge of learning Okinawa's 'Way of the Empty Hand'.

Whether this is true or not there can be no denying the impact this gentle man has made on the world of karate and why these days the name Gichin Funakoshi is known wherever the art is practiced. He was not born into a family that practiced karate, although his father, Gisu, was known to have possessed some skill in *bojutsu* (techniques using a six-foot staff) and was a minor official from the privileged shizoku class. But Gisu was also, according to Gichin himself, responsible for the decline in the family's financial status due to his fondness for alcohol. Born in Yamakawa-cho in the Ryukyu capital of Shuri in 1868, Gichin Funakoshi's childhood was often difficult. Being born prematurely and into a family that had fallen on hard times meant he spent much of his childhood with his maternal grandparents. Having survived the first few years of life, he began his formal education and made friends at school with the eldest son of the famed karate master, Yasutsune Azato,* and through this friendship was

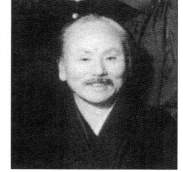

Gichin Funakoshi

introduced to karate, the art that would alter the course of his life forever. Funakoshi was only eleven or twelve years old at the time and by all accounts found karate training very difficult at first, but he managed to continue throughout his teenage years and eventually made the practice of karate his life-long challenge. Karate in Okinawa at that

---

* Yasutsune Azato belonged to the Tonochi class of shizoku families. Tonochi were hereditary chiefs of towns and villages throughout Okinawa, and the village of Azato (present day Asato) was the family seat of Funakoshi sensei's teacher.

time was practiced secretly, and even though the masters were well known to the general public, the people who trained under them were not. Even among those who practiced karate, the identity of their fellow students was a closely guarded secret, so well kept in fact that often close neighbors who were training with the same master knew nothing of the other. Indeed, for many years Funakoshi believed he was the only student of his teacher. Much of his training was conducted either late at night or in the early hours of the morning, and in his autobiography, *Karate-do: My Way of Life,* [*] he relates some of the problems resulting from his training schedule, many of which called into question his reputation as a citizen of good standing:

> I made my stealthy way in the dead of night, carrying a dim lantern when there was no moon, to the house of Master Azato. When, night after night, I would steal home just before daybreak, the neighbors took to conjecturing among themselves as to where I went and what I was doing. Some decided that the only possible answer to this curious enigma was a brothel. (page 5)

Of course, the truth of Funakoshi's night-time ventures could not have been further from the imaginings of his neighbors, for even as they slept peacefully in their beds, he was undergoing the most rigorous training imaginable under the watchful eye of his teacher. He continues in his memoirs:

> Night after night, often in the backyard of the Azato house as the master looked on, I would practice a kata (formal exercise) time and time again week after week, sometimes month after month, until I had mastered it to my teacher's satisfaction. (page 6)

Not all his early training was conducted in secret however. A visitor to Okinawa, the Japanese writer, Yukio Togawa,[†] made the following observation during one of the many storms that hit the island each year:

> The sky above was black, and out of it came a howling wind that laid waste to whatever stood in its path. Huge branches were torn like twigs from great trees, and dust and pebbles flew through the air, stinging a man's face. Okinawa is known as the island of typhoons and the ferocity of its tropical storms defies description. To withstand the onslaught of the winds that devastate the island regularly every year during the storm season, the houses stand low and are built as sturdy as possible; they are surrounded by high stone walls, and the slate tiles on the roofs are secured by mortar. But the winds are so tremendous (sometimes attaining a velocity of one hundred miles per hour) that despite all precautions the houses shiver and tremble. During one particular typhoon that I remember, all the people of Shuri huddled together within

---

* Funakoshi's autobiography was first published in English in 1975, by Kodansha International, Tokyo.
† Yukio Togawa, "Training for Life: Against a Typhoon," in *Karate-do: My Way of Life*. In his humble manner, Funakoshi used an article written about him by Mr. Togawa, a prize-winning author and friend of his family.

their homes, praying for the typhoon to pass without wreaking any great damage. No, I was wrong when I said that all the people of Shuri huddled at home: there was one young man, up on the roof of his home in Yamakawa-cho, who was determinedly battling the typhoon.

Mr. Togawa goes on:

Anyone observing this solitary figure would surely have concluded that he had lost his wits. Wearing only a loincloth, he stood on the slippery tiles of the roof and held in both hands, as though to protect him from the howling wind, a tatami mat. He must have fallen off the roof to the ground time and again, for his nearly naked body was smeared all over with mud. The young man seemed to be about twenty years old, or perhaps even younger. He was of small stature, hardly more than five feet tall, but his shoulders were huge and his biceps bulged. His hair was dressed like that of a sumo wrestler, with a topknot and a small silver pin, indicating that he belonged to the shizoku. But all this was of little importance. What matters is the expression on his face: wide eyes glittering with a strange light, a wide brow, copper red skin. Clenching his teeth as the wind tore into him, he gave off an aura of tremendous power. One might have said he was one of the guardian Deva kings. Now the young man on the roof assumed a low posture, holding the straw mat aloft against the raging wind. The stance he took was most impressive, for he stood as if astride a horse. Indeed, anyone who knew karate could have seen that the youth was taking the horse-riding stance, the most stable of all karate stances, and that he was making use of the howling wind to refine his technique and to further strengthen his body and mind. The wind struck the mat and the youth with full force, but he stood his ground and did not flinch. (pages 45, 46)

Stories like this one about Funakoshi and similar stories relating to other bushi abound in the annals of Okinawa's long karate history. In a time before sports science and modern gym workouts, karate practitioners used the things they found around them and the forces of nature to improve their abilities. Opportunities for Gichin Funakoshi to stand on roofs were however coming to an end, and so too was the topknot he wore as a mark of his family's status. In the year 1888, at the age of just twenty-one, and having gained a position as an assistant teacher at a primary school, the question of his topknot became an issue that threatened to alter the course of his entire life. For if he insisted on keeping it, his career as a schoolteacher would have ended before it had even begun. Keen to move toward a more modern world the young educator was ready to do away with the symbol of his social standing, but his family had other ideas. On the day he visited his parents to inform them of his new position, dressed in the official teacher's uniform,* his parents took an altogether different view of the matter. His father could

---

* In the early years of the twentieth century, junior schoolteachers wore a uniform similar to the high school uniform worn by present day students, consisting of dark trousers and a dark jacket that buttoned up to a high neck collar. The brass buttons bore the governmental cherry-blossom design that was standard at the time.

hardly believe what his son had done and, clearly upset, cried angrily, "What have you done to yourself? You … the son of a samurai!" His mother was even more upset and refused point blank to talk to him. Even before he had had a chance to explain himself to her she left the house by the back door and fled to her parent's house. Like it or not, Funakoshi had turned a corner and there was no going back.

There is a common misconception that the karate of Gichin Funakoshi was, and is today, called Shotokan. Unfortunately, this misunderstanding was established many decades ago and has now become a fact in the minds of many. Nevertheless, it is a simple misunderstanding, and one that can easily be put right. The name, Shotokan, was given to the dojo built in the Toshima ward of Zoshigaya in Tokyo, and opened in the spring of 1936. A year earlier a committee had been formed to coordinate the collection of funds to build the mainland's first dojo dedicated solely to karate. Karate had been taught in mainland Japan for over a decade before this time, but always in borrowed or rented premises.[*]

Never before had a dojo been built specifically for the study of karate; upon completion the committee also chose a name for the dojo, calling it the Shotokan. To Funakoshi's surprise the committee had chosen the pen name he had used when signing the Chinese poems he wrote as a young man. In his autobiography, he explains why he used that name during the years of his youth:

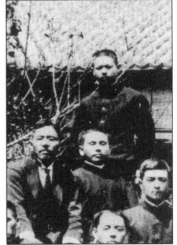

> The word 'shoto' in Japanese means literally 'pine waves' and so has no great arcane significance, but I would like to tell you why I selected it …
>
> My native castle town of Shuri is surrounded by hills with forests of Ryukyu pines and subtropical vegetation, among them Mount Torao, which belonged to Baron Ie Chosuke. The word torao means 'tiger tail' and was particularly appropriate because the mountain was very narrow and so heavily wooded that it actually resembled a tiger's tail when seen from afar.

Gichin Funakoshi (center) wearing the uniform of a junior school teacher.

> When I had time, I used to walk along Mount Torao, sometimes at night when the moon was full or when the sky was so clear that one stood under a canopy of stars. At such times, if there also happened to be a bit of a wind, one could hear the rustle of the pines and feel the deep, impenetrable mystery that lies at the root of all life. To me the murmur was a kind of celestial music.
>
> Poets all over the world have sung their songs about the brooding mystery that lies within woods and forests, and I was attracted to the bewitching

---

[*] Kanbun Uechi established his first karate dojo in Japan in 1925; however, training was held in secret and restricted to Okinawans only. In 1932 Uechi moved his dojo to the Tebira district of Wakayama and opened up the training to the general public. This took place a full two years before Funakoshi began teaching karate to the Japanese in 1934 at the Okinawan men's hostel where he lived, and four years before the 'Shotokan' dojo was built.

solitude of which they are a symbol. Perhaps my love of nature was intensified because I was an only son and a frail child, but I think it would be an exaggeration for me to term myself a 'loner'. Nevertheless, after a fierce practice session of karate, I liked nothing better than to go off and stroll in solitude. Then, when I was in my twenties and working as a schoolteacher in Naha, I would frequently go to a long narrow island in the bay that boasted a splendid natural park called Okunoyama, with glorious pine trees and a large lotus pond. The only building on the island was a Zen temple. Here too I used to come frequently to walk alone among the trees. By that time I had been practicing karate for some years, and as I became more familiar with the art I became more conscious of its spiritual nature. To enjoy my solitude while listening to the wind whistling through the pines was, it seemed to me, an excellent way to achieve the peace of mind that karate demands. And since this had been part of my life from earliest childhood, I decided there was no better name than Shoto with which to sign the poems I wrote. (pages 85, 86)

From this story we discover the reality of the name; it was his dojo's name and not the name of the art that was being practiced there. Funakoshi's karate lineage was impressive and 'cast a straight shadow', a saying used in Japan to indicate a direct line of succession. For his main teacher had been Azato Yasutsune who in turn had been a disciple of bushi Matsumura Sokon of Shuri, who himself had been a student of the Chinese military attaché, Iwah. I believe such a pedigree was of more value to Funakoshi than being known as the originator of a particular 'style' of karate. Indeed, during his lifetime he made his feelings on that subject very clear. Along with many of his predecessors and contemporaries, he did not like the idea of karate being packaged into 'styles' and saw only rivalry and enmity coming from such a move.

On March 6, 1921, Funakoshi, along with others, demonstrated his karate and kobudo skills before the Japanese Crown Prince who stopped over in Okinawa on his way to Europe. A year later, in the spring of 1922, Gichin Funakoshi sailed from Naha as the head of a delegation that was to demonstrate Okinawan karate at the first National Athletic Exhibition in Tokyo. As the president of the Okinawan Association for the Spirit of the Martial Arts, he was invited by the Okinawan Educational Affairs Office to take part in the display. The demonstration took place in May at the Kishi Gymnasium in the Ochanomizu district of Tokyo and was by all accounts received with great approval. As well as the physical display of karate, Funakoshi gave a lecture and erected an exhibit featuring photographs and drawings of karate in action and a number of scrolls detailing the history of karate on Okinawa. The audience was a mix of academics from various universities, military officers, and men with professional backgrounds—lawyers, doctors, and the like; as such, Funakoshi was deliberately introducing karate to Japanese society at a particular level in order to ensure it was not viewed as a brutal or barbaric form of fighting. For the next three decades, he remained in Japan, spreading the word by teaching and demonstrating karate whenever and wherever he was invited. Because of this his life was not an easy one, and we can look back now and appreciate the many sacrifices he endured in order to fulfill the promise he made in one of his many beautiful poems. This elegy, found in John Stevens' book *Three Budo Masters,* page 67, was written shortly after Funakoshi made the decision not to return home to Okinawa, but instead, to remain in Tokyo and do what he could to oversee the dissemination of karate in Japan:

> The superlative techniques of the South Seas, this is karate!
> What a pity to see the true transmission threatened.
> Who will take the challenge to restore karate to its full glory?
> With a steadfast heart, facing the azure sky, I make that solemn pledge.

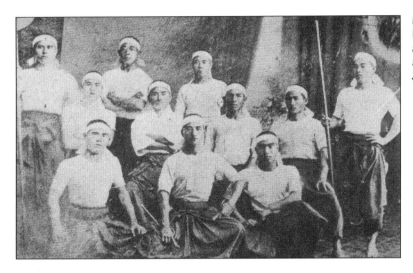

March 6, 1921, Funakoshi (center) with arms folded. Taken after a demonstration for the Japanese Crown Prince.

Of course, Funakoshi was not alone in his concern for the introduction of *authentic* karate into Japan. Concerns, I might add, that were not altogether unjustified, for by the time he arrived in Tokyo there were already a small number of Japanese claiming to know karate well enough to teach it, a situation he points to in the second line of his poem. Other notable Okinawans also left their island home to teach karate to the Japanese. Kanbun Uechi, Gochoku Chitose, Choki Motobu, Juhatsu Kyoda, and Kenwa Mabuni are among the best known of Okinawa's masters to teach in Japan, although there were many others too. Nevertheless, it can be said that it was Gichin Funakoshi who made the most impact and therefore led the way. History records his life-long efforts and the astonishing proliferation of karate that came as a result. Today, it is said that approximately forty-million people practice karate in almost every country in the world. You can't help but wonder what kind of poem Funakoshi sensei might write about karate if he were alive today.

On Friday, April 20, 2007, eighty-five years after Funakoshi left his island home and fifty years after he passed away, a monument was erected to the memory of this

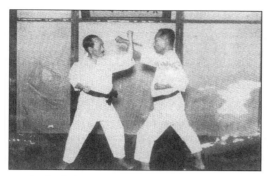

Funakoshi (left) engaged in ippon kumite training.

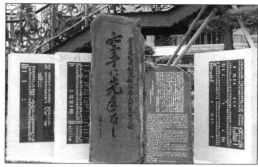

The Funakoshi monument in Okinawa. The kanji reads: "Karate ni sente nashi," which means "No first attack in karate."

remarkable man. Situated close to the Okinawan Budokan Hall, on reclaimed land that was once part of the harbor in the town of Naha, a large stone monument dedicated to Funakoshi sensei now stands. It is close to the location of the long narrow island where he had once walked among the trees and listened to the sea breeze blowing through the pines. Since its unveiling, the monument has become a place of pilgrimage for karateka, and these days people come from all over the world, to visit the monument to show their gratitude and offer their thanks. They come also to celebrate the life and times of the humble schoolteacher from Shuri, who oversaw the development of karate and watched it grow from a provincial martial art into an activity that was practiced throughout Japan. Karate today is enjoyed as a sport, practiced as a way of staying healthy, and for some, as a form of budo. Regardless of which way karate is pursued it remains a force for good in the world, and for that reason alone we should all embrace it. Gichin Funakoshi was a pioneer and a great example to us all of how a humble manner and strong spirit can overcome all obstacles in life. He passed away on the Japanese mainland on the twenty-sixth day of April 1957 at the age of 88, leaving behind a legacy of thought and practice that continues to this day.

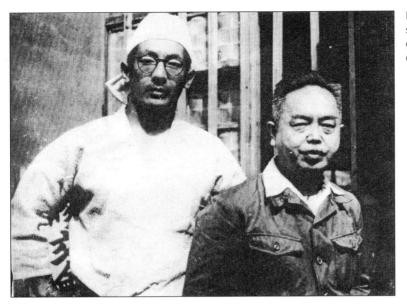

Kenwa Mabuni with his student, Chojiro Tani, outside Mabuni's Osaka dojo, ca. 1948.

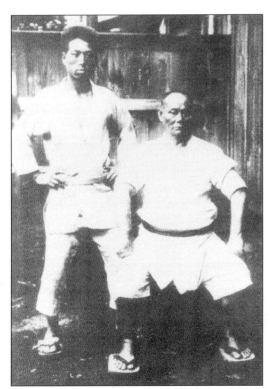

Choki Motobu and his student, Miyashiro.

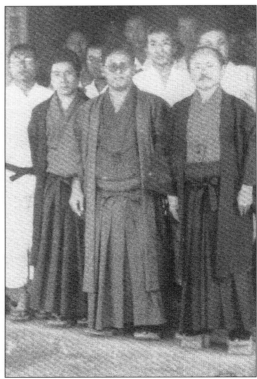

Chojun Miyagi (center) and Gichin Funakoshi (right) meeting in Japan.

8 IN CONCLUSION

The pursuit of progress is often arrogant because it fails to take into account lessons from the past and the extent to which our present understanding is built upon them. Tradition, on the other hand, is often paralyzed by rigidity of thought and action; in such cases, the tradition dies a slow and painful death. The key to personal growth lies in understanding balance.

—the Author

The aim of this book has been to point you toward the hidden depths of appreciation and the tangible benefits that come with the study of Okinawa's indigenous fighting arts. But be aware that it barely scratches the surface of what awaits those who take the plunge into the world of traditional Okinawan karate training. I make no claim to be the best or the only person teaching karate; in fact, I am happy to proclaim my limitations as both a student and a teacher of the art. There are sensei living throughout the world today with far more experience than I have and are far more able in their teaching methods too. But if the content of this book has captured your imagination or inspired you in any way, then I would urge you to seek out individuals who are teaching budo through the Okinawan fighting arts. They are people who by their very nature actively avoid the glare of publicity and celebrity, so finding them won't be easy, and neither will your attempts to gain access to their dojo. You will have to be patient, use your intelligence, and approach with humility. You may have to travel a great distance from your home, but that alone should not discourage you, for nothing of any value in life is gained without sacrifice in one form or another. Once you gain access to a traditional dojo, you will discover that was the easy part; the most difficult challenge budo has to offer is revealed in the continuous training, day after day, year after year. Karate is not limited to budo; it can also be engaged through the medium of keeping fit, and sport. If you're looking for a different kind of challenge to that offered by budo, then fix your sights in another direction and consider joining a karate club. They are far more common and have much to recommend to those who would like to know something of karate, yet don't want what budo has to offer. Please remember, though, the choices you make in life dictate

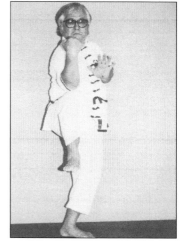

Ko Uehara sensei, ca. 1989, prefers to train in a Chinese shirt.

the experiences you have; you won't find budo where budo can't be found. So make your choice between a karate dojo and a karate club, and then immerse yourself wholeheartedly in your new-found pursuit.

If you are determined to discover a dojo, find a sensei, and face the challenges of training in karate in the traditional Okinawan way, then the following advice will help. First, approach the sensei with humility and patience, not with a list of requirements and requests. Next, don't expect the sensei to want to teach you just because you want him to teach you. Even before you approach a dojo, educate yourself as much as you can in the history of the martial art being taught there; but don't speak as if you comprehend the training. Remember, at this point you have only a little knowledge of the tradition; you don't have an understanding of it. Of the two, knowledge is inexpensive, you can get it from a book, but understanding is a lot more costly. You will pay for your understanding over a long period of time with the currency of experience; for in budo, experience is the only recognized method of payment for understanding. Should you be lucky enough to gain entry to a dojo, leave your expectations at the door, as they will be of no use to you now; and besides, you are there to learn from your experiences, not behave as if you have already had them. Remember what the late Okinawan karate master Shoshin Nagamine had to say about a dojo:

> The dojo is a special place where guts are fostered and superior human natures are bred through the ecstasy of sweating in hard work. The dojo is a sacred place where the human spirit is polished. Purify your mind and cultivate the power of perseverance by strengthening your body and overcoming the difficulties that arise during training.[63]

Karate, at least in Okinawa, was never intended to be a sport, nor was it intended to provide individuals with an income. Since its earliest days, karate has been a civilian method of self-protection, undertaken by young men who felt a need for such training. Although not exclusive to any one section of Okinawan society, prospective karate students were vetted for signs of negative character traits, and even though some individuals slipped through the net, by and large, the system worked to keep the knowledge of karate, and kobudo, free from those who might use that knowledge mindlessly. Arguments are regularly put forth these days that karate would have died out long ago had it not taken the sporting and commercial route, and the reason there are tens of millions of karateka around the world today is due to the appeal of sport and the ingenuity of the commercial entrepreneur. I have to concede, at least a little. This argument is not without some merit for I also believe karate, if it had continued to be passed from one generation to the next in the traditional manner, would certainly not have the millions of followers it has today. That said, I lament the current situation, with its shift away from the dojo and from teachers and students taking personal responsibility for their karate. I'm disappointed that many karate teachers accept students based on their ability to pay rather than their character. I'm saddened that many karate teachers no longer understand why they teach the things they teach, other than they have been told to teach that way by the leader of the organization they are affiliated with. And I despair the lack of guidance coming from many of those who have assumed the mantle of leader. All of these "changes" in the way karate is passed on from teacher to student these days have come about as a result of meddling with something that wasn't broken in the first place. The transmission methods employed for generations prior to the turn of the twentieth century worked just fine! True, there were a lot less people training in karate back then, but was that a bad thing? I don't think so. I believe those who were teaching and training in karate prior to its emergence from the shadows of secrecy understood the karate they were training in and could back up their understanding with action, not in the sporting arena, but on the streets where it was designed to be used. I would also refute the notion that karate would have died out by now had it not been for a small number of enterprising Japanese who repackaged karate in their own nationalistic image before selling it to the rest of the world. My sensei, the late Eiichi Miyazato, would still have trained with his teacher, Chojun Miyagi, and I would still have eventually found my way to Miyazato sensei's dojo in Okinawa, albeit perhaps by a different path to the one that did eventually lead me to his door. The same holds true for many other karateka around the world today who continue to practice and pass on the karate they have learned in the time-honored way from their sensei. Without recourse to gimmicks or commercialism, many karateka have discovered teachers of great merit who have been able to guide them. Unlike the millions of people who declare their involvement with karate, traditional karateka are counted in far smaller numbers. Budo training is an extraordinarily confronting activity, and something so confronting will never be popular.

I don't believe traditional karate training is attractive to the majority, it never has been in Okinawan society, and I see nothing in Western societies that makes me think otherwise. The 'idea' of mastering karate techniques is appealing, but that's something different altogether. Not many people want to deal with their own negativity on a regular basis and struggle with the ensuing confrontation. Budo places you squarely in the cross hairs of your own shortcomings, and then steps back to see what happens next. It does this, not once or twice, but constantly. It's a tough place to stand on a regular basis, but this is the essence of budo training—going to the dojo and standing in the full glare of your own inadequacy. When you think about karate training like this it doesn't sound too inviting, but this is exactly my point; it's not and was never meant to be. Karate only becomes "attractive" to a mass audience when you factor in prizes and promotions, a phenomenon not lost on those who make their living on the dream others have of mastering a martial art. Dealing with the extremes of your own nature and restoring a sense of balance in your character is not something others can do for you; you must tackle that job alone. However, when your training begins, you will need the guidance of others who have made more progress than you; such people are called 'sensei'. They will point you in the right direction and encourage you to find your own way forward, and will stop you from becoming lost in the façade of karate, thus missing out on the profound rewards budo training has to offer. Okinawan karateka of old did not broadcast their study of karate; they kept it to themselves. It wasn't so much a big secret as it was something they considered personal, something they were doing for themselves. Even today in Okinawa quite a few people adhere to this practice. A good friend and *sempai* of mine at the Jundokan dojo still hasn't told his colleagues at work or most of his extended family that he trains in karate. When you consider he has been going to the dojo for well over forty years, it puts into perspective the humility of the man's character. Outside of karate circles, few of the people I interact with on a daily basis know I practice karate, and only my immediate neighbors know of the dojo that stands discreetly at the rear of my home. Compare this behavior with someone who continuously posts himself on YouTube, Twitter, or Facebook. The psychology involved when you embark on the expansion of your mind through the development of your body stems from the cultivation of your spirit. Understanding this important point—that everything begins in your mind—is vital to understanding how your true nature is revealed through the practice of karate. This is the essence of Shin Gi Tai in action. Let us suffer no ambivalence here. Until the physical techniques of karate flow from your body free of conscious thought through the medium of your spirit, you cannot say you 'know' karate; nor can you say karate has become a natural part of who you are. Until you can move through life with good manners and live a balanced lifestyle, you cannot say you live well.

Karate needs to return to dojo-based training, away from the national and multinational organizations that have failed and continue to fail the art so badly. Karate students, once again, need to connect to the type of transmission that serves karate best: the personal relationship between teacher and student. For karate (not commerce) to thrive and maintain any relevance at all in the modern world, I strongly believe the responsibility for progress must once again rest squarely on the shoulders of the individual karateka. Training has to step back from the mass activity the majority of karateka are involved in today and return to the dojo floor. Chojun Miyagi said the ultimate aim of karate was

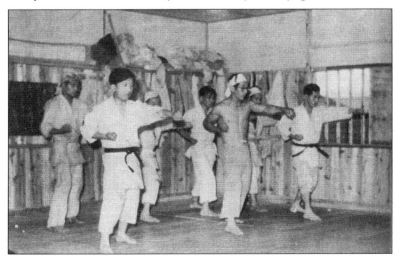

Japanese students training at the Mabuni dojo in Osaka. Chojiro Tani is in the front row (center).

to develop a balanced nature, to become gentle from a position of strength, and to live a modest life by being confident in your humble approach to the world around you. I must admit I find his teachings are by no means easy to follow. I constantly struggle with the shortfalls in my character and the perceived injustices I see around me on a daily basis. It has taken some time to realize I cannot change the world; I can only change me. So this is who I work on: me! I work on the way I react to and interact with the events and the people I come into contact with each day. What little progress I make I cherish, while my frequent failures give me plenty to continue working on. By taking this approach to my karate training I have come to understand the Okinawan adage: "One lifetime is not enough." Just as I work on me, you should work on you.

When it comes to pointing you in the right direction, in a physical sense, I would like nothing more than to provide you with a roadmap to the nearest traditional sensei and his dojo. But the truth is, even if I knew where such people were, telling you their location would only shorten your odds of being accepted as a student. If you take anything away from this book, I hope you take away the idea that you have to develop your own karate and your own life. You have to stop depending so much on the drip-fed information provided by others, start thinking for yourself, and begin learning from your own experiences. I want to encourage you to stand on your own two feet and take responsibility for your failures and your successes, and grow and mature into a capable and accomplished human being: a person who is respected by his community for his humility, not ridiculed for being timid; admired for being principled, not despised for being arrogant; and well-liked for being fair, not derided for being naïve. I'm not quite there myself. I still have some way to go, but I believe the study and practice of karate is bringing me closer to having the kind of character I have just described. All I have to do is maintain the resolve to continue one step at a time, one day at a time. Many others have done this before me, and many others are doing it today. I draw encouragement from this and remind myself often that if others can find it within themselves to pursue traditional karate then so can I; and if I can, you can too!

Although the study of karate is not 'the' answer to all the problems in the world, if studied with conviction under the guidance of a traditional teacher, it can help provide the solution to many of the problems in 'your' world. The word karate literally means 'empty hand', and yet the technique first studied by karateka is, ironically enough, a punch. As the student matures, his hands open and from then on the possibilities are endless. Prominent among these possibilities is the option not to fight at all but to follow instead the fundamental principle of budo, that is, to stop violence; this is the ultimate aim of karate. Although karateka take as their primary source of inspiration the Okinawan masters of long ago, I hope I have shown that 'truth' can come from many sources and is not confined to one culture or one philosophy alone. To go deeply into your martial art you will be required to go deeply into your own character, and to do that, you will have to become a seeker of truth. Not the 'mystical' kind of truth that places you at the center of the universe, but the plain and simple kind: the honest truth that exposes your true nature. I want to end this book with a quote from a great teacher and fighter, a man who faced hostility almost all his life and learned to triumph over it by means that were thought impossible at the time. He was a teacher whose greatest battle toppled an entire empire, a man whose methods are still written about in books today. He was a fighter who understood the principles of conflict well and how to use gentleness to overcome brute strength. During his lifetime his millions of followers gave him the name, 'Mahatma' meaning 'Great Soul', but we know him today as Ghandi. In a turn of phrase that captures the very essence of karate, Mahatma Ghandi once said: "You can't shake hands with a clenched fist."

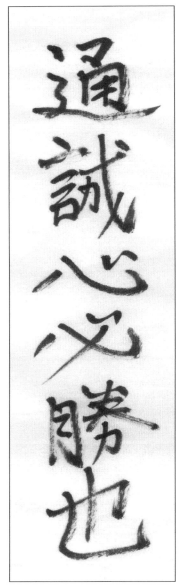

"Victory comes from a sincere heart"

Notes

Chapter One

1. Profiles of many of these individuals can be found in Tetsuhiro Hokama's book, *100 Masters of Okinawan Karate* and Masahiro Nakamoto's book, *Okinawa Kobudo.*

2. An English translation of the March 23, 1934, document was published in 1993 by the International Ryukyu Karate Research Society (IRKRS). The second document is the January 28, 1936 speech given by Chojun Miyagi following a demonstration of karate in Sakai Suji, Osaka; it can be found on page 81 of Morio Higaonna's book *The History of Karate.* In each of these documents, the information being presented is essentially the same.

3. Shoshin Nagamine (1907–1997) was the founder of the *Matsubayashi* school of *Shorin ryu karate.* The co-creator of the *gekisai kata,* along with Chojun Miyagi, *gekisai dai ichi* reflects the karate of Shuri, whereas *gekisai dai ni* leans more toward the karate of Naha. I met Nagamine sensei a couple of times in 1992 and spoke with him at length about karate.

4. Chuan fa is another term for Chinese martial arts otherwise known as *kung fu* or *wushu.*

   The Eight Precepts of Chuan fa are

   1. The human mind is one with heaven and earth
   2. Blood circulates the body with the movement of the sun and moon
   3. Inhaling is gentle, exhaling is strong
   4. Adjust to changing circumstances
   5. The hands should move without conscious thought
   6. Distance and bearing will dictate the outcome
   7. See beyond the obvious
   8. Expect the unexpected

5. Sun-Tzu (ca. 500–400 B.C.) was a Chinese military commander best known as the author of *The Art of War.*

6. Many stories of Okinawan masters being the worse for alcohol have been passed down through the ages in the rich oral tradition of karate on the island. Almost all the great teachers of the past have one or more tales attached to their name, highlighting their ability to defend themselves from ruffians and thieves, even when they were intoxicated. Kanryo Higaonna (Higashionna) is no different in this regard. As a youth living in China he took part in street fights to test his fighting skills and later, upon his return to Okinawa, it is known he frequented the Tsuji district of Naha, an area of the city well known, even today, for its seedy drinking establishments and brothels. On page 27 of his book, *The History of Karate,* Morio Higaonna relates a story of a drunken Kanryo Higaonna making his way home from Tsuji and how he defended himself from a surprise attack by a much larger antagonist. The veracity of the story is not in doubt, at least not by me; but like many of the stories you hear in Okinawa, there is a common and often familiar ring to it.

Chapter Two

7. Beginning in 1603, and lasting two hundred and sixty-five years until 1868, Japan was ruled by one family: the Tokugawa. This reign began when the country was unified under one military warlord, Ieyasu Tokugawa, following his success at the battle of *Sekigahara* in 1600. In 1603, Ieyasu was proclaimed *Shogun,* a title first granted by the Emperor to Yoritomo Minamoto toward the end of the twelfth century. Meaning "commander-in-chief for the suppression of barbarians," it was a title used by the person holding the real power in Japan, for the emperor had long since lost it. Successive Shogun ran Japan as they saw fit, which usually meant by military force. Ieyasu, however, came up with a system to keep the country's warlords under control. Part of each year the warlords, or *daimyo,* were expected to live in the capital where Ieyasu could keep an eye on them. For the remaining months, when they were free to return to

their domain, they were obliged to leave their families behind in the capital. It was a system that worked well, and the Tokugawa *Shogunate* faced few serious challenges to its rule.

8. In F. J. Norman's excellent little book *The Fighting Men of Japan*, he talks of his encounter with a former samurai. The book is a memoir of Norman's time living in Japan during the 1880s, and in part, he covers his interest in Japanese fencing and wrestling. One of the first, if not 'the' first Westerner to study kendo, Norman began training in 1888. This is what he had to say about one of the men he met at the dojo:

> Among the many swordsmen who used to put in their daily attendance at the Takanawa fencing room–dojo–was one who very early attracted my attention. He was an elderly man, and in some respects a finer swordsman than Umezawa, who introduced me to him one day as his sensei or teacher. Onoda was his name, and though he was exceedingly tall for a Japanese he was quite the best built one I have come across. For a long time I could gather nothing more about him than that he did not like foreigners, and that it would be just as well if I did not thrust my acquaintance-ship upon him. Later on, I learned he was, or had been, the hereditary fencing master to the late Shogun or "generalissimo" of Japan.

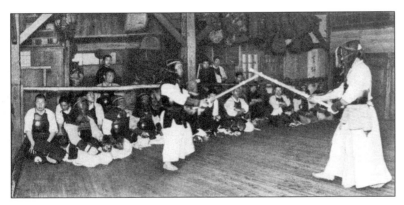

Former samurai turn to teaching martial arts and ken-jutsu.

9. The term "salary men" is used to describe men who work long hours for their company, take few holidays, and can be found napping on trains and buses in every major city in Japan.

10. The Shotokan Karate International Federation (SKIF) was established in 1978 by Hirokazu Kanazawa.

11. Like most translations from Japanese to English it is difficult, if not impossible, to find an exact meaning that bridges the gap between the two languages. I have always found it more useful to think of the meaning of what I am trying to say, rather than get bogged down in the technicalities of syntax. Onagaishimasu, or a variation of it, is used in many different situations. It suggests a feeling of friendliness and good intentions toward someone in your future dealings with him. In karate it is used when bowing prior to training with a partner, or sometimes when you arrive at the dojo and make your initial bow to the shomen. Sometimes translated as "Please help me," broadly speaking it means something more like, "I hope we can work well together and achieve good things."

12. For the most part, it was the Japanese who spread karate around the world, hence the link between karate and the Japanese language. Nevertheless, there remain many Okinawan words and phrases connected to karate that are not found in standard Japanese; muchimi, for example, is a word used to describe a heavy almost magnetic feeling with either the ground or an opponent. The difference between Nihongo (Japanese) and Uchinaguchi (Okinawan) is clear and undeniable. The word Hogen points to Uchinaguchi being nothing more than a regional dialect of Japanese and is considered a derogatory term by many older Okinawans; they have a saying, "*Umarijimanu kutuba washine kuninwashinyun*": "Forget the language of your island and you will also forget your country."

13. *Kana* are phonetic symbols used to write words not covered by kanji. There are two types of kana: hiragana, used to write the inflectional endings to kanji, and katakana, which are used to write foreign words. Although hiragana and katakana make the same sounds, they are different in appearance, hiragana being more soft and rounded and katakana being sharp and angular.

14. Keinosuke Enoeda (1935–2003). The book, *Keinosuke Enoeda: Tiger of Shotokan Karate,* detailing the life of this exceptional exponent of Shotokan karate, was written by Rod Butler in 2004 and published by Karate-London in London, England.

15. For several years I was a member of the English branch of the Shukokai World Karate Union, and for two years, 1976 and 1977, represented England in various kata and kumite tournaments around Britain and in Europe.

16. Hirokazu Kanazawa, born 1931–. I have had the pleasure of training under Kanazawa sensei a number of times in various locations around the world. He has visited my home and my dojo, on more than one occasion, and I learned much from listening to his conversation. Two excellent chronologies of Kanazawa sensei's life exist in English: his autobiography, *Karate—My Life,* and Dr. Clive Layton's biography, *Kanazawa, 10th dan: Recollections of a Living Karate Legend, the Early Years (1931–1964).*

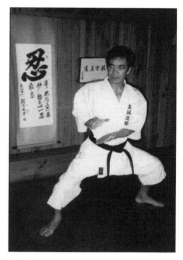

Hirokazu Kanazawa practicing seiyunchin kata in the author's dojo.

17. For a number of years in the 1990s, I wrote a monthly column called "Sugao" for *Traditional Karate* magazine in England. Sugao is a Japanese term used to describe a face without makeup, in other words, your true face. Back then there was no such thing as a blog; even so, each month I wrote my thoughts and ideas, and surprisingly, to me at least, attracted a fairly large following.

18. The *Bubishi,* an in-depth treatise on military arts and sciences, is a Chinese martial arts book written in 1621. In the eighteenth, nineteenth, and into the twentieth century, it held almost biblical status among Okinawa's karate teachers.

19. The battle at Sekigahara on the Nakasendo, the middle mountain road in central Japan's Mino province, in the year 1600, came about as a result of Ieyasu Tokugawa's enemies' attempts to draw him out of Osaka in order to kill him. But they had underestimated Ieyasu's ability to gather intelligence about their plans; and secondly, they overestimated their ability to stop the Tokugawa army moving west from their capital of Edo (modern day Tokyo), capturing the castles along the Nakasendo and to the south, the Tokaido or eastern sea road. Both these major arteries were important to maintaining control over central Japan. A campaign lasting months ensued as castles fell or were besieged out of contention, as two great armies fought for supremacy. With their plans in tatters and the possibility of defeat becoming more and more real, a frantic effort to stop the Tokugawa army reaching its objective at Sawayama had to be made. A plan was hatched to meet them head-on in a narrow wooded valley along the Nakasendo: a place known as Sekigahara.

20. In the closing months of 1614 a garrison of over 113,000 samurai and *ronin* (samurai who for whatever reason had no master; they often acted as mercenaries, fighting for whichever side would pay them) led by Hideyori Toyotomi had entrenched themselves in Osaka castle and were besieged by a Tokugawa army consisting of over 194,000 men. Throughout that winter there were many skirmishes as supply routes to the castle were fought over, taken and retaken. As the summer of 1615 approached, the momentum of the campaign grew, with the battle at Tennoji being the last major confrontation. It ended with thousands of Tokugawa troops swarming into the castle grounds and with their artillery, smashed the castle keep until it began to burn. Having lost the siege which had raged on and off for almost a year, Toyotomi committed *seppuku,* (the less vulgar name for the act of ritual suicide more commonly known as *hara-kiri*).

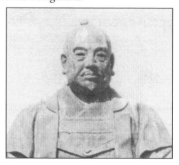

Shogun Ieyasu Tokugawa, the undisputed ruler of Japan.

21. The Shimabara rebellion came about as a result of the cruelty of the ruling daimyo, Shigeharu Matsukura, whose habit it was, among other things, to punish the peasantry by dressing them in straw clothing before setting them on fire. In September 1637, an uprising broke out, with some estimates putting the number of people involved at more than half the 45,000 population of the Shimabara peninsular. Even with the help of a Dutch ship brought in from Nagasaki to bombard the fortress of Hara Castle, where the rebels were besieged, it took six months for the blockade to succeed. The castle was finally stormed by Tokugawa troops and a mass slaughter of its occupants ensued. After this, there would be no more serious opposition to the rule of the Tokugawa.

22. From some time in 1710 to September 1716, Tashiro Tsuramoto began to visit the reclusive Mitsushigi Yamamoto, and during that time he recorded many of their conversations. This was an age when samurai had little to do with regard to war and were instead being encouraged to better themselves through the study of art and poetry. Tsuramoto had recently been removed from his position as a scribe when he began to visit Yamamoto; perhaps he felt he could connect to a bygone age through his conversations with the older man.

23. Often referred to as the "Rape of Nanking," the invasion of the city by the Japanese imperial army which occurred on December 9, 1937, covers a six-week period where the Japanese systematically murdered, raped, and plundered their way through the city, leaving behind an estimated 300,000 dead or wounded, and committing between 20 and 80 thousand acts of rape. Brushed aside by successive Japanese governments and prime ministers since the end of the war as "overly exaggerated propaganda," there seemed to be a change of heart in Japan in 1995 when Prime Minister Tomiichi Murayama and Emperor Akahito both expressed sorrow and regret in "statements of mourning." True to form, however, at the last moment, the "written apology" promised to China failed to materialize and was instead replaced by a verbal comment expressing Japanese regret for any tragedy that "might" have taken place. In 2007 a hundred or so members of the ruling Liberal Democratic Party (LDP) declared the whole Nanking massacre a lie, a fabrication made up by the Chinese to embarrass Japan. They cited the "fact" that no evidence exists to prove anything happened. Perhaps they should have read the despatches and reports written at the time by men like Harold Timperley and John Rabe, or spent time viewing the truly shocking images captured by John Magee.

24. Chomo Hanashiro (1869–1945) was born in Yamakawa village, Shuri. On his gravestone, the inscription reads in part, "Here lie the remains of Hanashiro Chomo, the first mayor of Mawashi village, who revealed the name of karate to the world for the first time in 1905."

25. The Tang dynasty in China lasted almost three hundred years, from A.D. 618 to A.D. 907.

26. Donn Draeger was born in Milwaukee, Wisconsin, in 1922. As an officer in the U.S. Marine Corps, he spent a great part of his life living in Asia. He achieved teaching licenses and senior ranking in several schools of Japanese budo, and was a Western pioneer as far as the Asian martial arts are concerned, achieving many firsts for a Westerner and breaking the ground for those who would follow years later. A prolific writer, he authored some twenty books and contributed to many martial arts periodicals worldwide. Like a true warrior, he returned home to die, passing away in his home town of Milwaukee in October 1982.

27. The word *Shoto* was the pen name used by Funakoshi to sign his poetry. It is a word that, for him, brought to mind the soft evening breezes blowing in from the sea that whispered through the pine trees of his native island home: Okinawa. The word *kan* simply means hall or building. When his supporters raised enough money to establish a dojo, they gave it the name, Shotokan, "Shoto's building." Over time, the name became synonymous with the sort of karate training going on there and was adopted as the name for the style of karate as well as the dojo.

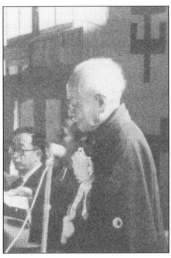

Gichin Funakoshi worked tirelessly to propagate karate in Japan.

28. Kanken Toyama (1888–1966). Born in Shuri, he is said to have taken up training in the martial arts as a young boy. As was the way in Okinawa back then, Toyama learned his skills from a variety of teachers. He learned *bojitsu* from Oshiro and *saijitsu* from Tana and Chosho Chibana. His karate came from a number of sources: Anko Itosu, Kentsu Yabu, and Kuwae Ryosei, who was the senior student of Sokon Matsumura, from the Shuri te tradition. As well, he trained for a while in Naha te with Kanryo Higaonna. In 1932, he moved to Tokyo and soon afterward opened his own dojo, which he called Shudokan.

29. The Dai Nippon Butokukai–The Great Japan Martial Virtue Society–was founded in 1895 and established in Kyoto by the Japanese Ministry of Education, under the patronage of the Meiji emperor.

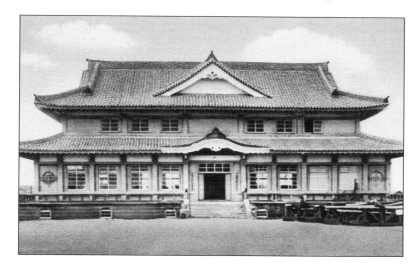

The Okinawan Butoku Den training hall before the war.

30. A *shinkokai* is an organization or group set up to promote a particular activity, in this case: karate.

31. Kumite, or sparring, can be practiced in a number of ways: *ippon* kumite–one attack sparring, *renzoku* kumite–consecutive attack sparring, and *jiyu* kumite, where the students are free to attack at will.

32. Chojun Miyagi traveled to Hawaii in the spring of 1934, arriving on May third. Celebrating his forty-sixth birthday on the voyage across the Pacific, he remained on the islands for several months, teaching selected groups of enthusiasts and lecturing to large audiences.

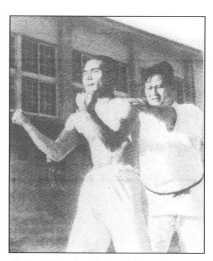

Chojun Miyagi assisting his student, Kotara Kohama, with shimi during sanchin training, ca. 1941.

Chapter Three

33. Mark Bishop is an Englishman who lived in Okinawa for fifteen years during the 1970s and 80s; he is best known for authoring the landmark volume, *Okinawan Karate: Teachers, Styles and Secret Techniques*, (1989, A & C Black Publishing, London). His lesser-known work, *Zen Kobudo: Mysteries of Okinawan Weaponry and Te*, (1996, Tuttle Publishing, Vermont), is also a great resource for serious students of Okinawan martial arts culture.

34. A school of karate founded by Kanbun Uechi (1877–1948). As a 19-year-old teenager, Kanbun Uechi left Okinawa and traveled to China to avoid conscription into the Japanese army. He lived in China for several years and during that

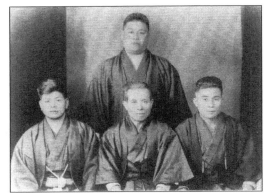

Kanbun Uechi (center) with students in Wakayama, Japan, ca. 1937.

time he studied *Pangainoon*, a school of Chinese combat taught by Chou Tsu Ho (1874–1926) who was also known as Shushiwa. Upon his return to Okinawa, he taught Pangainoon ryu to a small number of people both in Okinawa and on the Japanese mainland. After Kanbun died, the type of combat he taught was renamed Uechi ryu: Uechi's school.

35. Morio Higaonna (1938–) was my first Okinawan teacher when I abandoned Japanese karate training in favor of the Okinawan approach in 1984. His first experience of karate was watching his father training at home. His formal training began when he entered the garden dojo of Chojun Miyagi. Miyagi had already passed away by this time and the training was led by Eiichi Miyazato. Shortly after Higaonna became a student, training moved from the Miyagi family home to the Jundokan, a purposely-built dojo in nearby Azato. Although the number of Okinawans training under Morio Higaonna has always been small, as a result of his large following outside of Okinawa, he is arguably the best known Okinawan karate teacher in the world today.

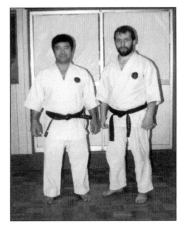

The author in Tokyo, 1986, with Morio Higaonna sensei.

Kenwa Mabuni with Doshisha University karate club. Chojiro Tani is fifth from right, back row. (See note 36, next page.)

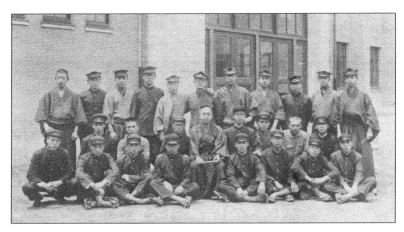

36. Founded by the Okinawan Kenwa Mabuni (1889–1952). He began karate training under Anko Itosu in 1903, and five years later, in 1908, became a student of Kanryo Higaonna. A graduate of the Okinawa Fishery School, he worked as a police officer and taught karate in Shuri for thirteen years from 1916–1929. He then moved to Osaka in Japan and established a dojo there. The first name he gave his karate was Hanko ryu, meaning 'half-hard'; but later he settled on the name Shito ryu to pay honor to his two main teachers.

37. Karma is the law of cause and effect. You reap what you sow, you get what you give, what goes around comes around, do now—pay later. Karma is the belief that everything you do, past, present, and future, is connected.

38. In April 1985, Kathy and I married. To this day, she remains the foundation upon which my life is built.

39. Keiji Tomiyama (1950–) is a graduate of Doshisha University. Having tried Western boxing in high school, his introduction to karate came when he entered the University in 1968 and began training under the direction of Chojiro Tani, head of the Tani-ha Shito ryu and founder of the Shukokai karate organization. After graduating in 1972, he moved to Paris to assist Yasuhiro Suzuki who was then the chief instructor for the Shukokai in Europe. He later moved to Brussels before settling in England where he still lives today. I owe much to Tomiyama sensei, and credit his example, both as a karateka and human being, for turning me away from the negativity I carried within me during my time as his student. He opened many doors and dared me to step through them.

40. Inner-city Manchester has never been one of the world's most affluent places to live. The district of Charlton-on-Medlock, where I grew up, has appeared in classical English literature over the years, but only to depict the kind of hell the English working class lived in during the years following the industrial revolution. Even as late as the 1950s and 60s when I was growing up there, living in a neighborhood where drunken brawls were commonplace and prostitutes plied their trade on the pavement and in houses close by, goes some way to painting the picture of my surroundings as a child. That said, growing up in a slum is in many ways advantageous, as the only way from there is up!

41. *Enigma 2: The Cross of Change*, 1993, Virgin Schallplatten GmbH, UK, ref: CDVIR 20. If you come across this CD, make sure you play it loudly … but please, check with your neighbors first.

42. I have fond memories of sitting in a sauna with Higaonna sensei swapping stories about the various scars on our bodies. He was genuinely impressed by the bullet hole in my right leg until I confessed it wasn't really a bullet hole at all, just a large round scar left by an accident with a broken bottle when I was eight years old. When I showed him the scar on my stomach left by a real stabbing, he just flat out refused to believe me. I think there's a moral in all this somewhere.

43. *Izakaya* are my favorite places to eat when I am in Okinawa. They are small, family run eateries, which offer heart-warming food and thirst-quenching cold beer in a lively atmosphere. They are the places where the locals go to eat.

44. "They Really Are That Old: A Validation Study of Centenarian Prevalence in Okinawa," by D. C. Willcox, B. J. Willcox, Q. He, N. C. Wang, and M. Suzuki, in the *Journal of Gerontology: Biological Sciences,* 2008, v. 63A (4): pp. 338-349.

45. Charles (Joe) Swift is a native New Yorker who has lived in Japan since 1994. He has translated several historically important texts on karate and kobudo and continues to research and write about the classical martial arts of Okinawa. Moving from Osaka to Tokyo in 2001, Swift opened a branch dojo of the Mushinkan where he acts as the chief instructor. Skilled in both karate and the use of Okinawan weaponry, his research has proven to be of invaluable assistance to budoka wishing to learn more about the traditional fighting ways of Okinawa.

46. A native of Los Angeles, California, John Sells began training in karate as a child. He has been published widely both in America and abroad and holds senior ranks in both karate and Okinawan kobudo. He also holds the title of *Hanshi*, awarded to him in Japan by Kenzo Mabuni, son of Shito ryu's founder, Kenwa Mabuni.

47. I have known Graham for almost twenty years, and yet know almost nothing about his life. A native of England's North East, his early years in martial arts began with Shotokan karate and Western boxing. Quick to see that the institutionalization of karate was not for him, he separated himself from the organizations running karate in England and has remained staunchly independent ever since. A prolific writer

on and researcher of not only karate, but jujitsu and Western wrestling too, Graham's articles continue to be published and used as a scholarly reference by researchers. His generosity and assistance with my own research has been gratefully received on many occasions.

48. Terry O'Neill is a legendary figure in English karate. As well as being an accomplished karateka, he is also an accomplished actor, appearing in many English television dramas, as well as Hollywood feature films such as *Entrapment, Dragonheart*, and the *Conan* movies. Having worked previously on a karate magazine, he began publishing a very modest periodical himself in 1972, called *Fighting Arts*. Over the next two and a half decades it grew into arguably the world's most popular martial arts publication with a circulation of over twenty thousand copies each issue. Although suffering a few setbacks and undergoing a change of name, the magazine was always known for its high production quality, as well as the depth of its interviews and articles and stunning photography. The magazine ran for twenty-four years until its eventual demise in late 1996 after a production run of 93 issues.

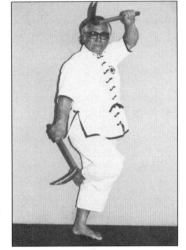

49. Seiko Kina (1911–1994) was a carpenter by trade who in his later years opened a small confectionary shop and café at the back of Heiwa Dori market in central Naha, Okinawa. His dojo, the Junkokan, was above the shop and I visited it a number of times during my first visit to Okinawa in 1984. A student of Chojun Miyagi, and later, Seko Higa, Kina taught at the Higa dojo for a number of years during the 1950s and into the 1960s. He later became an advisor to Morio Higaonna when the latter established his own world-wide karate organization, the IOGKF.

50. "Do-gi" is a term used for the uniform worn by karateka when training. Also known as a "keiko-gi," or simply a "gi," it is a relatively recent addition to karate training, gaining prominence only after karate became established in mainland Japan and the push was on to make the Okinawans conform to Japanese standards. Even so, the wearing of a do-gi did not become universal in Okinawa until as late as the 1960s, and even today there are some senior teachers who don't wear it, Ko Uehara being just one name that comes to mind.

Ko Uehara, ca. 1989, demonstrating an 'on-guard' posture with a pair of kama (sickle).

51. *Tai sabaki*—body shifting; *suri ashi*—sliding the legs, by pushing and then pulling quickly from one place to another; *chakuchi*—replacing one foot with the other while your body remains in the same place.

52. The shakuhachi is a Japanese wooden flute made from the root of a tree. It takes great skill to be able to select an appropriate root and produce an instrument that can deliver the haunting tone the shakuhachi is famous for.

53. The makiwara, or as the Okinawans call it, *machiwara*, is the one training tool that seems to have been adopted by the Japanese when karate was first introduced to them by Okinawans in the early years of the twentieth century. Traditionally a stout post set in the ground with a small target of straw wrapped around the top, it is used to train the entire body for the rigors of impact.

54. In the sense that no matter how proficient you may become there is always something more you can do to improve. Nothing stays the same, so adapting to change is endless. Implicit in understanding the concept of mu—nothingness—is the realization that it relates to everything.

55. In 1995, the Okinawan government published their *Okinawa Karate "Kobudo" Graph*. In it, the editor noted there were over 40 million practitioners of karate and kobudo in the world at that time.

Chapter Four

56. In his book, *The Essence of Okinawan Karate*, (1976), on page 104, Shoshin Nagamine writes: "The two fukyugata practiced today were composed by (me) Shoshin Nagamine, the originator of Matsubayashi ryu karate, and Chojun Miyagi, the originator of Goju ryu karate, because the kata of the Shuri and Naha schools had been too difficult for beginners. In 1940, two of the compositions were authorized to be the formal basic kata by the special committee of Okinawa karate-do organized and summoned by Gen Hayagawa, then Governor of Okinawan Prefecture." Nagamine also demonstrates the kata on page 109.

Chapter Five

57. According to Morio Higaonna in his book, *The History of Karate,* pages 99-100, Chojun Miyagi did not re-establish his dojo immediately after the war ended.

58. Three of Chojun Miyagi's children perished during the Second World War: his son, Jun, and two of his daughters, Tsuneko and Shigeko.

Chapter Six

59. An ancient name for Japan.

60. The Ryukyu Kingdom was established in the mid-fifteenth century when the Three Kingdoms (*San-zen*) era came to an end in 1429, and King Sho Hashi ruled the whole of Okinawa Island. Over time, the kingdom grew to encompass the other island in the archipelago and stretched from the Japanese island of Kyushu in the north to Taiwan in the south. It was taken over in 1609 by the Japanese Satsuma clan and became a Prefecture of Japan in September 1872. In 1945 the American and allied invasion saw Okinawa fall under American control until it was handed back to Japan in 1972.

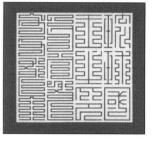

The Royal Seal of the old Ryukyu Kingdom.

61. A term used in Britain to describe the kind of resolve and determination needed to see something through to the end. In 1940 the British Expeditionary Force, which had been dispatched to Europe to challenge Hitler's Germany to withdraw from Poland, found itself in desperate retreat. The German forces were far superior in both number and firepower and soon had the British and French armies in full retreat and pinned down in the harbor and surrounding beaches at Dunkirk in northern France. Desperate to save as many troops as possible, British Naval Command launched 'Operation Dynamo' in May 1940. A call went out across Britain for volunteers to sail to France to rescue as many as they could from Dunkirk. Hundreds of boats, some no bigger than family pleasure craft, set sail in an armada the likes of which the world had never seen before; and for nine days and nights, ferried the bulk of the Expeditionary Force and combatants from the French army, back to Britain. Although many died on the beaches and in the rescue attempt, it was a defining moment for the British in the early days of the Second World War. It was a moment that saw the entire nation pull together to achieve a seemingly impossible outcome.

62. This was a brutal form of boxing where contestants fought, usually naked, with only leather straps around their fists. The aim was to literally beat your opponent into submission; the fight lasted for as long as it took for one or the other to achieve the required outcome.

63. In his book, *The Essence of Okinawan Karate-Do,* Shoshin Nagamine writes this in his list of dojo ethics, page 49.

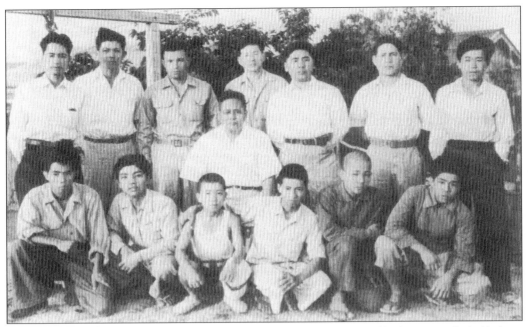

Chojun Miyagi with post-war students, back row starting third from left, Eiichi Miyazato, Meitoku Yagi, Seikichi Toguchi, Eiko Miyazato, Seikichi Kinjo.

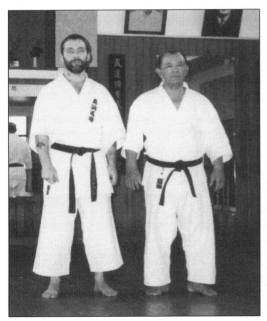

The author with his teacher, Eiichi Miyazato sensei, Okinawa, 1996.

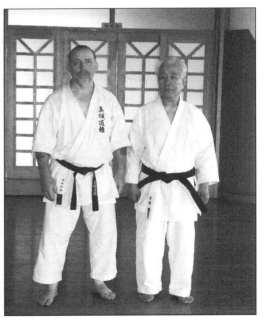

The author with Seikichi Kinjo sensei, Okinawa, 2011.

Glossary

aikido. A Japanese martial art based on the teachings of Morihei Ueshiba.

ashi barai. A leg or foot sweeping technique used to destroy an opponent's balance.

ataraxia. A word used by the Greek philosopher, Pyrrho of Elis, to describe "inner peace."

awamori. An alcoholic drink popular in Okinawa made from distilled rice (different from sake).

bachi. A large plectrum made from buffalo horn and used on Okinawa in the playing of the sanshin.

bakufu. Literally meaning, 'camp office', it was the name given to the military government system, which ruled Japan until the Meiji Revolution in 1868.

bashofu. A type of Okinawan textile made from the fibers of the banana tree.

bassai. See also **passai**. A karate kata with several variations, of which bassai dai and bassai sho are the best known in Japanese karate schools.

bingata. A type of brightly colored print design found throughout the Ryukyu Islands.

bo. A staff of wood approximately six-feet in length, used in the practice of kobudo.

bojutsu. The techniques used to fight using a 'bo'.

bokken. A wooden sword used for training purposes.

Bubishi. See also *Wubeizhi.* Translation: *Account of Military Art and Science,* a Chinese martial arts book written in 1621, which for centuries has been held in great esteem by Okinawa's fighting men.

budo. The 'military way'. A term used these days to describe learning a martial art to help develop a person's character.

budoka. A person who puts into practice the lessons taught by budo teachings.

Budo Mountain. A term used to describe the physical, philosophical, and psychological journey undertaken by budoka.

Bunbu ryo do. A term used to describe the balance of training in the martial arts and achieving scholarship as a way of deepening an appreciation of both.

bunkai. A word used to describe the techniques that make up a kata, but also used to denote the practice of breaking down a kata into workable strategies based on sound fighting principles.

bushi. In Japan this title applies to samurai; in Okinawa it denotes a gentleman who is also highly skilled in the martial arts.

bushido. The way of the warrior.

bussho. Doing something every day, which brings you closer to the place you want to be.

Butokukai. (Dai Nippon Butokukai). A martial arts organization set up in Japan in the nineteenth century to govern the practice of all martial arts throughout the country.

chakuchi. Changing legs, from forward to rear, without changing position in relation to the opponent.

Ch'an. This is the Chinese reading of Zen.

chiishi. Chi—strength, ishi—stone: a tool used in Okinawan karate to promote strength in the arms, wrists, and hands.

chinto. A karate kata practiced in schools originating from Shuri te.

chonan. Usually the eldest son, the boy destined to become the heir to a family business.

chuan fa. A term that more correctly describes Chinese fighting arts than the term 'kung fu'.

chudan kamae. An 'on-guard' posture with at least one arm covering the middle (chest) area of the body.

chudan ura uke. Mid-level block using the back of the hand.

chudan uke. A block which covers the middle (chest) area of the body from attack.

dachi. Stance.

daimyo. A rank within Samurai, a daimyo was the equivalent of a European Baron in medieval times. A Lord who had absolute power of life and death over all who lived within his domain.

dan. Japanese word meaning, 'position'. In karate, it denotes a person's position, 'rank' within the art.

dan-i. The ranking system used in karate and other martial arts to rank its practitioners.

deshi. Student.

do-gi. See also **keikogi, gi,** and **karategi.**The uniform worn during karate training,

dojang. The Korean name for the place where martial arts (Taekwondo, Hapkido, etc.) training takes place; it can be thought of in the same way as the Japanese word, dojo.

dojo. Literally meaning 'the place of the way,' this word was borrowed by early Japanese commercial instructors from the Buddhist tradition where a room (called a dojo) in a monastery is set aside for the students to learn from their master.

doryoku. To make a great effort.

eisa. Mass gatherings of dancers and musicians on Okinawa held during the summer months.

embusen. The 'line' followed during kata practice in Japanese schools of karate.

empi. Old Japanese word for elbow.

empi uchi. Striking with the elbow.

fukugi. A type of tree used in former times throughout the Ryukyu Islands to line roads and mark village boundaries.

fukyugata ni. The name used in the Matsubayashi School of karate for the gekei sai kata found in Goju ryu.

gasshuku. To lodge together, to gather for the practice a martial art without distraction.

gedan barai. A sweeping block covering the lower (stomach–groin) area of the body.

gedan zuki. A punch to the lower part of the body.

gekisai. To smash and destroy: the name given to the two kata devised by Chojun Miyagi and Shoshin Nagamine in 1940.

gekisai dai ichi. The first of two gekisai kata, this one devised by Shoshin Nagamine.

gekisai dai ni. The second of two gekisai kata, this one devised by Chojun Miyagi.

genkan. An area just inside a Japanese home, or dojo, where shoes are removed. To go beyond the genkan wearing shoes is considered extremely bad mannered.

gi. See also **keikogi, do-gi,** and **karategi.** The uniform, based on peasant clothing, worn by karate practitioners while training.

godan. Literally, fifth position: the title given to holders of the fifth dan rank in karate.

go no sen. To block an attack and immediately respond with an attack of your own.

goya. A bitter cucumber-like vegetable found in Okinawa.

goyofu. A fabric design law, which was strictly enforced by the government during the days of the Ryukyu Kingdom.

hachidan. Eighth dan rank.

Hagakure. Translated as *Hidden by Leaves.* A book dealing with the thoughts of a retired samurai.

hanakuri ori. A type of design found in Okinawan textiles.

Hanshi. Teacher by example, a title bestowed upon only very senior budoka.

hara-kiri. See also **seppuku.** A rather vulgar name given to the ritualistic suicide sometimes conducted by samurai.

hikei uke. An open-handed, grasping block.

hiragana. A form of written Japanese, often used to assist with the reading of kanji.

Hogen. A term, meaning dialect, erroneously used to describe Uchinaguchi, the language of Okinawa.

Hogen-fuda. A derogatory term used still to describe Uchinaguchi, the language of Okinawa. In the past, a Hogen-fuda–"dialect-card"–was hung around the neck of any child found speaking his native language in school. It was a belittling experience similar to the wearing of a 'dunce's cap' in the West.

hojo undo. A wide range of supplementary training found throughout Okinawan karate, done in order to better equip a karateka for the rigors of karate itself.

hombu. Headquarters.

hosshin. Making a start.

iaido. The Japanese martial art of drawing a sword, making a cut–or series of cuts–before returning the sword to its scabbard.

ikken hisatsu. One hit–one kill, also used to denote a certain attitude when facing an opponent.

ippon. One.

ippon kumite. One attack–one response sparring practice.

ippon kumite bunkai. One attack–one response sparring where the response is taken directly from a kata.

ippon uke barai. One-step blocking practice.

irimi. Entering–to move in on an attacker in order to take control or avoid being hit.

ishi sashi. A training tool used in Okinawan karate for conditioning the body.

izakaya. A neighborhood restaurant/bar where Okinawans go to unwind at the end of the working day.

jari bako. A container filled with stones or sand, and used in Okinawan karate to condition the fingers.

jikaku. Self-realization, sometimes called 'waking-up'.

jima. Japanese word for island.

jodan ko uke. Upper-level block using the wrist.

jodan shuto uchi. Upper level (head height) strike with the outside edge of the hand.

jodan uke. Upper-level block.

jodan uraken uchi. Upper level (head height) strike with the back of the fist.

jodan zuki. A punch to the neck, head, or face.

joseki. The part of a dojo where senior students train.

judan. Tenth dan rank.

judo. The 'gentle way', a Japanese martial art based on using an opponent's strength against him.

jujutsu. A form of Japanese unarmed combat utilizing strikes, kicks, throws, and joint locks.

junbi undo. Warming up (preparation) exercises.

jutsu. A word used to endorse the practicality of the techniques, rather than their sporting application.

kai un. Developing your own fate.

kakato geri. A kick where the heel is used as the point of impact.

kakemono. A hanging scroll found on a wall in the dojo.

kakie. A form of sparring used in some Okinawan schools of karate, similar to the 'sticky-hands' training found in Chinese martial arts.

kameko baka. Large turtle-back shaped tombs found all across Okinawa.

kamiza. See also **shinzen** and **Shinto** shrine. A small wooden shrine found in some karate dojo.

kanzashi. A type of hairpin worn by Okinawan men to keep their topknot in place.

kangeiko. Mid-winter training.

kanji. The Chinese written characters used in the Japanese language.

kara. Empty, as in a void.

karate. Empty hand.

karatedo. The way of the empty hand.

Karate-do Gaisetsu. A document on karate written and presented by Chojun Miyagi in 1936.

karategi. See also **do-gi**, **keikogi**, and **gi**.

karateka. A person who practices karate.

karma. The law of cause and effect.

kata. Means 'form' in Japanese. A word that is used to describe the correct way to do almost everything.

katagashira. An ancient ceremony on Okinawa for boys passing into manhood, which took place at the age of 14 years old when their hair was gathered into a topknot.

katakana. A form of written Japanese, used to write all foreign (non-Japanese) words.

keikogi. See also **do-gi, gi,** and **karategi.** The uniform worn while practicing karate.

keiomachi. A class of lower-ranking official during the Ryukyu Kingdom era.

kempo. A school of Japanese martial art very similar to karate.

kendo. The 'way of the sword', a martial art/sport using swords made from bamboo.

kenko. An activity undertaken to maintain good health.

kihon. Basic techniques.

kihon ippon. A term used to indicate one-step/one-point sparring.

kigu undo. Training with tools.

ko uke. A blocking technique found in karate using the wrist.

kobudo. Literally translated, means the old martial way. Today the word refers more to the practice of fighting with home-made weapons, as used by Okinawans against the Japanese occupation forces from 1609 onward.

kobudoka. A person who practices with weapons, which originated from Okinawan farming and fishing tools.

kongoken. A heavy, iron, ring used in Okinawan karate to condition the body.

kun. Guidelines, for example: dojo kun.

kung fu. See also **chuan fa.** The term 'kung fu' means to be 'very good' at something, not necessarily fighting.

kumite. A meeting of hands—sparring.

kururunfa. A karate kata found in schools originating from Naha te. It emphasizes holding and trapping, and the use of quick movements to break free from various grips.

kuzushi. To make an opponent unstable by destroying his balance.

kwoon. A Chinese name for a martial arts school, similar in meaning to the word 'dojo'.

kyogi. Sports.

Kyoshi. A title given to senior martial artist, meaning 'expert teacher'.

kyu. A word used for all ranks below that of *dan*.

kyudan. Ninth dan rank.

makiwara (machiwara). A stout post usually set in the ground, around the top of which is placed a target used by karateka to develop the strength of their punch.

mawashi uke. A circular block using both hands.

michi. A road or path, also the name of the kanji usually read as 'do', as in karatedo, judo, etc.

morote uke. A block where one hand is used to assist the other.

muchimi. A word from the Uchinaguchi language meaning sticky, in the magnetic sense, and used to describe the feeling employed to connect with an opponent, or with the ground.

musei jinko. To reveal or impart something to others by being a good example of it yourself.

nabera. A pumpkin-like vegetable found in Okinawan cuisine.

nafuda. A small wooden peg upon which a dojo member's name is written before being hung on the nafudakake.

nafudakake. A board found in traditional dojo showing the names and ranks of the dojo members.

nagaya. Single-story dwellings divided into several compartments that were home to the poorer members of Okinawan society.

naginatado. The way of the halberd, a sword-like blade attached to the end of a long staff.

naifanchin (naihanchi). See also **naihanchin** and **tekki**. The name of Shuri te karate's foundation kata.

nanadan. Seventh dan rank.

Neewagumuchi. The name given to the Community Chest of Tomari village in Okinawa.

nekoashi dachi. Cat stance, a posture where energy is loaded into the rear leg, ready to pounce (cat like) toward or around an opponent.

nidan. Second dan rank.

nigiri gami. Gripping jars, used in Okinawan karate for conditioning the body.

Nihongo. The Japanese language.

Ninjitsu. A type of special training undertaken by spies and mercenaries during Japan's feudal era, the name means the 'techniques of endurance'.

nintai. To endure.

omiyagi. Souvenir.

pankration. A type of full-contact fighting found in the original Olympic games of Ancient Greece.

passai. See also **bassai**. In Okinawan karate, this kata has a number of versions including Oyadamari no passai and Matsumura no passai. Passai is the Okinawan pronunciation of bassai.

reigi saho. Etiquette–good manners.

Renshi. A title awarded to advanced martial artists meaning, 'expert practitioner'.

renshu. Training.

renzoku. A term used to indicate more than one attack.

renzoku kumite. A type of sparring where two or more attacks are instigated in quick succession.

rohai. A karate kata found in schools originating from Tomari te.

rokudan. Sixth dan rank.

ronin. Literally 'wave-man', a term used to describe a masterless samurai.

rotan ori. A type of design found in traditional Okinawan fabrics.

ryu. School, as in tradition.

Ryukyu. The name of the old kingdom, which today forms the Okinawa Prefecture of Japan.

sabaki. A term used in karate to describe methods of moving or shifting from one place to another.

sai. An iron fork-like truncheon used, usually in pairs, in schools of Okinawan kobudo.

saifa. A karate kata found in schools originating from Naha te. It emphasizes powerful strikes with the clenched fist, to smash and break an attacker's bones.

sake. A Japanese alcoholic drink made from distilled rice.

samurai. A class of people in Feudal Japan, meaning, 'those who serve', the samurai class rose to prominence and eventually overthrew the monarchy. The class system was officially abolished during the Meiji Restoration.

sanba. A musical instrument found on Okinawa; similar to Spanish castanets, the Okinawan samba is made up of three small pieces of hard wood that produce a distinctive 'click'.

sanchin. A karate kata said to have originated in the Shoalin temple in China and found today in schools from the Naha te tradition. The name means 'Three Battles'. This kata is a tangible expression of Shin Gi Tai.

sanchin dachi. A defensive stance used in karate.

sandan. Third dan rank.

sandan uke barai. Three step blocking practice.

sanseiru. A karate kata found in schools originating from Naha te. Although the name means 'thirty-three hands', this kata also contains ten attacking moves using the legs.

sanshin. Okinawan three stringed, banjo-like instrument.

sanxian. Chinese three stringed, banjo-like instrument.

seipai. A karate kata found in schools originating from Naha te, meaning 'eighteen hands'. This kata emphasizes open hand techniques.

seisan. A karate kata found in schools originating from Naha te, meaning 'thirteen hands'. It contains tripping techniques as well as arm locks and kicks.

seishin tanren. Forging the spirit through hard training.

seitei gata. A term used in sports karate for the obligatory kata-like displays used in competitions.

seiyunchin. A karate kata found in schools originating from Naha te, meaning to 'control and pull'. This kata emphasizes techniques to escape from various holds, as well as taking an attacker to the ground.

seiza. Sitting in the traditional Japanese (kneeling) fashion.

sempai. Someone who is senior to you.

sen no sen. To capture (anticipate) an opponent's intention to attack and strike first.

sen ren shin. 'Polish the spirit' a maxim reminding us of the purpose of budo training.

sensei. Literally translated, means 'ahead in life'. It is a title used in karate when addressing a teacher.

sento. A public bathhouse.

seppuku. The act of ritual suicide among the samurai class; men disembowelled themselves, while women cut their own throats.

shabu shabu. A delicious stew, cooked at the table, into which thinly-cut slivers of meat are placed and retrieved before eating.

shakuhachi. A type of Japanese flute carved from the carefully selected roots of trees.

shamisen. A three stringed Japanese musical instrument.

Shidoin. A title used in some schools of Japanese martial arts, meaning teacher.

Shihan. A title used in some schools of Japanese martial arts, meaning advanced teacher.

shiko dachi. A low, wide stance used in karate when pulling an opponent to the ground.

Shimakutuba. A term meaning, 'the language of the island' referring to the everyday language of Okinawa.

shimoseki. The area in a dojo where junior students train.

shimoza. Lower wall in a traditional dojo.

Shin Gi Tai (shin gi tai). Literally translated, means Spirit—Technique—Body. A deeper meaning behind this phrase is the striving for unity between the body and the mind, through the cultivation of the spirit.

shinjin. Consciousness; in budo terms, to wake up to the realization there is a better way to live.

shinkokai. A name that can be applied to any practice or promotional group within a martial art without a defined leader.

Shinto shrine. See also **kamiza** and **shinzen**. A small alter found mostly in Japanese dojo, and less so in the dojo of Okinawa.

shinzen. See also **kamiza** and **Shinto shrine**.

shisha. The lion-dog creatures found throughout the Ryukyu Islands on rooftops and outside entrances to ward off evil spirits.

shisochin. A karate kata found in schools originating from Naha te, the name means 'fighting in four directions'. This kata emphasizes twists and turns, arm locks, elbow strikes, and escaping from holds.

shizoku. A title given to families from a mid-level class of officials during the time of the Ryukyu Kingdom.

shodan. Literally translated, means first position. This name is given to the first dan rank in karate.

Sho-go. A series of titles beyond 'rank' used in karate: Renshi, Kyoshi, Hanshi, etc.

shomen. The main/front wall in a dojo.

shoshin. Literally–first mind, used to denote open mindedness, or the mind of a beginner.

shugyo. Austere training, training above and beyond the intensity of regular training.

shu ha ri. The three stages of learning according to Eastern philosophy: to preserve, detach, and transcend the knowledge of those who taught us.

Shuri. The Royal Capital of the old Ryukyu Kingdom.

shuri hana ori. A type of design found in Okinawan textiles.

shuri ori. A type of design found in Okinawan textiles.

sifu. Chinese word for 'teacher'.

soba. Pasta-like noodles.

soji. Cleaning, an activity undertaken by students in every traditional dojo.

Sun-Tzu. (ca. 500–400 B.C.) Chinese general and master of military tactics.

suparinpei. A karate kata found in schools originating in Naha te, meaning 'one hundred and eight hands'. This is the longest kata in the Goju ryu canon. It emphasizes the use of grappling as well as quick evasive movements and the use of open hand techniques against vulnerable areas of the attacker's body.

suri ashi. A type of moving the body around quickly, found in karate.

Tai Chi. The Grand Ultimate Fist, a school of Chinese martial arts.

tai sabaki. Body shifting.

tan. A barbell-like tool used in Okinawan karate to condition the body.

tanden. A point just below the navel considered to be the point of origin for the generation of physical power.

Tassei. Achievement.

Tasshi-shihan. A title used in some Japanese schools of karate; it means, an exceptional master teacher.

tejima. A style of Okinawan textile design origination in Shuri.

tekki. See also **naifanchin, naihanchin.** A karate kata found in schools originating from Shuri te.

tetsu geta. Iron sandals, used in Okinawan karate to condition the body.

ti. An old term given to the martial arts in Okinawa; also, a fighting method which involves applying pressure to disrupt an adversary's central nervous system.

tokunoma. An alcove found in the main wall of an Okinawan dojo.

Tomari passai. A version of the karate kata indigenous to Tomari village.

to te jutsu. An alternative name, in olden times, given to the fighting arts on Okinawa.

tou. A tool used in Okinawan karate to condition the fingers.

toudi (tode). A name used prior to 'karate' for the fighting arts of Okinawan.

tsumugi. A type of Okinawan textile originating from Shuri.

tsu shin gen. Insight.

Uchinaguchi. The language of Okinawa.

Uchinanchu. A native Okinawan.

ude kitae. A tool used for conditioning the body, particularly the arms, through continuous pounding.

ude tanren. Forearm conditioning.

ura zuki. A punch using an upturned fist (palm up) in a jabbing or thrusting action.

wankan. A karate kata found in schools originating from Tomari te.

wanshu. A karate kata found in schools originating from Tomari te.

Wubeizhi. See also *Bubishi.*

yanabarusen. A small wooden trading boat in common use throughout the Ryukyu Kingdom.

yen. The currency of Japan.

yoi. A position of readiness.

yondan. Fourth dan rank.

yudansha. A person who holds a dan rank in Japanese or Okinawan martial arts.

zanshin. Awareness.

zazen. A meditative posture used in some schools of Zen training.

Zen. See also **Ch'an.**

Bibliography

Adams, Brian C. *The Medical Implications of Karate Blows*. 4th reprint. New York: A.S. Barnes and Company, 1976.

Bishop, Mark. *Zen Kobudo: Mysteries of Okinawan Weaponry and Te*. Rutland, Vermont: Tuttle Company Inc., 1996.

———. *Okinawan Karate: Teachers, Styles and Secret Techniques*. 2nd ed. London: A &C Black Publishers Ltd., 1999.

Bittmann, Heiko. *The Teachings of Karatedo*. Kanazawa, Japan: Heiko Bittmann Publishing, 2005.

Butler, Rod. *Keinosuke Enoeda: Tiger of Shotokan Karate*. London: Karate-London Publishing, 2004.

Clarke, Michael. *Hojo Undo: Power Training for Traditional Karate*. Wolfeboro, New Hampshire: YMAA Publication Center, Inc., 2009.

Coelho, Paolo. *The Pilgrimage*. Rio de Janeiro: Editora Rocco Ltd.,1986.

De Mente, Boye Lafayette. *Kata: The Key to Understanding and Dealing with the Japanese*. Boston: Tuttle Publishing, 2003.

Dollar, Alan. *Secrets of Uechi-ryu Karate, and the Mysteries of Okinawa*. Antioch, California: Cherokee Publishing, 1996.

Draeger, Donn. "Karate-do." *Modern Bujitsu and Budo*. Chap. 7, in Vol. 3, *The Martial Arts and Ways of Japan*. New York: Weatherhill Inc., 1974.

Funakoshi, Gichin. *Karate-do: My Way of Life*. Tokyo: Kodansha International Ltd., 1975.

Gow, Ian. *Okinawa 1945: Gateway to Japan*. London: Grub Street Publishing, 1986.

Hadamitzky, Wolfgang, and Mark Spahn. *Kanji & Kana*. Rutland, Vermont: Tuttle Company Inc., 1981.

Haines, Bruce. *Karate's History and Traditions*. Rutland, Vermont: Tuttle Company Inc., 1968.

Higaonna, Morio. *The History of Karate*. Westlake Village, California: Dragon Books, 1996.

Hokama, Tetsuhiro. *100 Masters of Okinawan Karate*. Okinawa: Hokama Publishing, 2005.

———. *Timeline of Karate History*. Okinawa: Hokama Publishing, 2007.

Kanazawa, Hirokazu. *Karate—My Life*. English ed. Trans. by Alex Bennett, Ph.D. Singapore: Kendo World Publications Ltd., 2003.

Layton, Clive. *Conversations with Karate Masters*. Birkenhead, England: Ronin Publishing Ltd., 1988.

———. *Kanazawa, 10th dan: Recollections of a Living Karate Legend, the Early Years (1931– 1964)*. Middlesex, England: Shoto Publishing, 2001.

———. *Training with Funakoshi*. Norfolk, England: Kime Publishing, 1992.

McCarthy, Patrick and Yuriko McCarthy. *Gichin Funakoshi Tanpenshu: Untold Stories*. Aspley, Australia: International Ryukyu Research Society, 2004.

Miller, Rory. *Meditations on Violence; A Comparison of Martial Arts Training & Real World Violence*. Wolfeboro, New Hampshire: YMAA Publication Center, Inc., 2008.

Murphy, Wendy. Tradition and Revolt: Islands of the Rising Sun. London: Cassell Ltd., 1980.

Nagamine, Shoshin. *The Essence of Okinawan Karate-Do*. Rutland, Vermont: Tuttle Company Inc., 1976.

—————. *Tales of Okinawa's Great Masters*. Boston: Tuttle Publishing, 2000.

Nakamoto, Masahiro. *Kobudo: Okinawa Traditional Old Martial Arts*. English ed. Trans. by Miguel da Luz. Okinawa: Bunbukan Publishing, 2008.

Nicol, C. W. *Moving Zen: Karate as a Way to Gentleness*. 1st (paperback) ed. London: P. H. Crompton Ltd., 1975.

Norman, F. J. *The Fighting Men of Japan: Training and Exercises of the Samurai*. New York: Dover Publications, Inc, 2006.

Okinawa Prefecture Board of Education. *Okinawa Karate: Kobudo Graf*. Naha, Okinawa: 1995.

Okinawa Media Planning Co., Ltd. *The Okinawan* (magazine), (2009) vols. 2-6.

Simson, Vyv, and Andrew Jennings. *Dishonored Games: Corruption, Money and Greed at the Olympics*. New York: Shapolsky Publishers, Inc., 1992.

Stevens, John. *Three Budo Masters:* Jigaro Kano (Judo), Gichin Funakoshi (Karate), Morihei   Ueshiba (Aikido). Tokyo: Kodansha, 1995.

Tomiyama, Keiji. *Fundamentals of Karate-do; Essential Elements for Development Through Karate Training at All Levels*. Nottingham, England: S K Enterprises Publishing, 1990.

Turnbull, Stephen. *The Samurai Sourcebook*. London: Arms & Armour Press, 1998.

Yahara, Hiromichi. *The Battle for Okinawa*. New York: John Wiley & Sons, Inc., 1995.

Recommended Reading

At the beginning of each year, I place a list of books on the dojo notice board. These are titles I feel will help the students at the Shinseidokan dojo to grow and develop as karateka. I want to do the same here. If you have found this book valuable then I believe you will find much in the recommended titles in this list. When you train yourself in karate you are obliged to train your whole body; this includes your mind. A well-developed physique without a well-developed brain to control it is of limited use to either you or the community. Reading exercises the brain and improves your intellect. It broadens your appreciation of life and of karate; therefore, reading—studying—as a natural part of your training should not be neglected. Although I feel all the books listed here are worth reading, I have avoided listing them in order of importance: you will be the judge of that. I haven't even listed them in alphabetical order. I have, however, grouped the books into broad categories and, to help you identify the book you are looking for, I have given the ISBN reference where one exists, as well as the title and author. But please note, many of the best books written about Okinawan martial arts that I've discovered have been privately published and no ISBN was assigned to them; so, if you cannot find some of these titles in bookshops, try looking for them on the Internet, or contacting the author directly. The list is by no means exhaustive; I have not read every good book written on karate, nor have I listed what I consider to be the 'best' books. I am merely pointing you toward books I think are worth reading. So please treat this list as suggestive only.

Okinawan Karate

The Essence of Okinawan Karate, by Shoshin Nagamine: ISBN 0-8048 1163-6

Tales of Okinawa's Great Masters, by Shoshin Nagamine: ISBN 0-8048 2089-9

Okinawa's Complete Karate System, by Michael Rosenbaum: ISBN 1-886969-91-4

The Teachings of Karate, by Heiko Bittmann: ISBN 3-9807316-2-6

The History of Karate, by Morio Higaonna: ISBN 0-946062 36 6

Okinawa Kobudo, by Masahiro Nakamoto

Zen Kobudo, by Mark Bishop: ISBN 0-8048-2027-9

Okinawan Karate (Second Edition), by Mark Bishop: ISBN 0-7136-5083-4

The Art of Hojo Undo, by Michael Clarke: ISBN 978-1-59439-136-1

Roaring Silence: A Journey Begins, by Michael Clarke: ISBN 0-9544466-1-5

Karate-do: My Way of Life, by Gichin Funakoshi: ISBN 0-87011-463-8,
    ISBN 0-87011-241-4

Three Budo Masters, by John Stevens: ISBN 4-7700-1852-5

Training with Funakoshi, by Dr. Clive Layton: ISBN 0-9513406-3-8

Secrets of Uechi-ryu Karate, by Alan Dollar: ISBN 0-9651671-1-9

Tanpenshu: Untold Stories of Gichin Funakoshi, by Patrick & Yuriko McCarthy

Karate My Art, by Choki Motobu; Translated by Patrick & Yuriko McCarthy

Timeline of Karate History, by Tetsuhiro Hokama
100 Masters of Okinawan Karate, by Tetsuhiro Hokama
History & Traditions of Okinawan Karate, by Tetsuhiro Hokama: ISBN 0-920129-19-6

Japanese Karate

Fundamentals of Karate-Do, by Keiji Tomiyama: ISBN 1-873764-00-6
The Way of Sanchin Kata, by Kris Wilder: ISBN 978-1-59439-084-5
The Karate Experience: A Way of Life, by Randall G. Hassell: ISBN 0-8048-1348-5
Karate My Life, by Hirokazu Kanazawa: ISBN 4-9901694-2-5
Karate Training: The Samurai Legacy and Modern Practice, by Robin L. Rielly:
    ISBN 0-80481488-0
Moving Zen by C. W. Nicol: ISBN 0-981764-515
Spirit of the Empty Hand, by Stan Schmidt: ISBN 0-911921-00-2
The Budo Karate of Mas Oyama, by Cameron Quinn: ISBN 0-7316 1119 5
The Human Face of Karate, by Tadashi Nakamura: ISBN 4-07-975055-2
One Day—One Lifetime, by Tadashi Nakamura: ISBN 9780804830645
Karate: Technique and Spirit, by Tadashi Nakamura, ISBN: 4-07-974179-0
Periodical: *Shotokan Karate Magazine*

Recommended (DVD) Viewing

Okinawan Karate: Dojo and Masters, vols. 1 and 2. Produced by *Karate Bushido Magazine,*
    Paris, France.
Okinawan Karate: Indomitable. Shorin ryu Shobukan, Uema dojo (Okinawa). Produced by
    Okinawa Eizou Center Co, Ltd, Okinawa.
The Empty Mind—The Spirit and Philosophy of Martial Arts. Produced by Budo Films,
    Miami Beach, Florida, United States.

Online Resources—Blogs

http://www.Okinawakarateblog.blogspot.com
http://www.Gojukenkyukai.blogspot.com
http://www.Karatejutsu.blogspot.com
http://www.Chibanaproject.blogspot.com
http://www.Yamada-san.blogspot.com
http://www.Shinseidokandojo.blogspot.com
http://www.kowakan.com

Websites

http://www.shoryukan.com   Okinawan Shorin-ryu karate (Williamsburg, VA)
http://www.shinkendojo.net   Okinawan Goju-ryu Ryusyokai (England)
http://www.shinjinbukan.com   Okinawan Shorin-ryu karate (New York)
http://www.portaskarate.org   Okinawan Goju-ryu Shobukan (New Jersey)

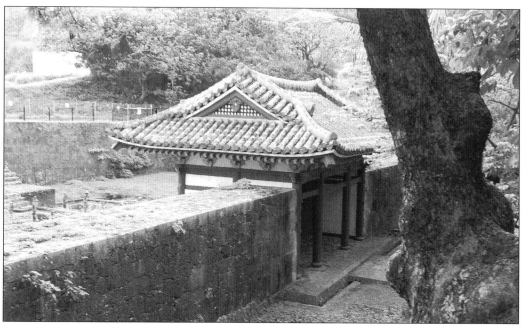

The gate to Enkakuji shrine, part of the royal palace in Shuri, was first built in 1492.

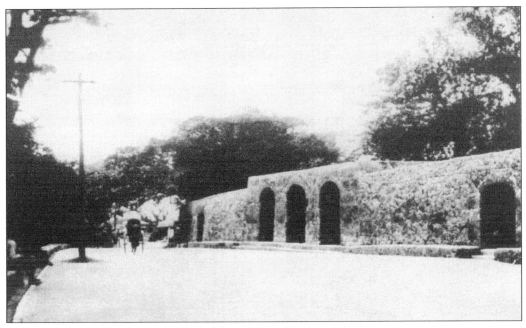

The gates of Sogenji temple as they looked from the outside, ca. 1900.

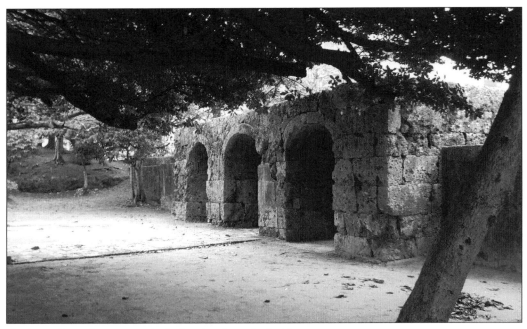

The Sogenji temple gates as the look today, from the inside.

Index

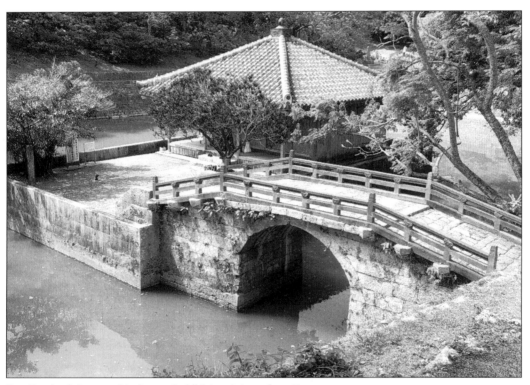
Bezaitendo shrine, used to house Buddhist scriptures from Korea.

About the Author

Michael Clarke was born in Dublin, Ireland, in May 1955, and moved to England with his family at the age of three. He grew up in one of Manchester's less affluent neighborhoods and left school as soon as legally possible, at the age of fifteen. His later teenage years were fraught with violence on the streets, at soccer games, in pubs and bars—in fact, anywhere a crowd gathered and an opportunity to brawl presented itself. It was a lifestyle that saw him arrested and facing a court of law on more occasions than any young man should. His final conviction landed him behind bars, and it was from here he began his slow climb back to propriety and self-respect.

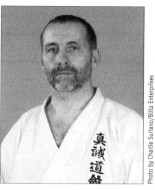

Photo by Charlie Suriano/Blitz Enterprises

Walking into a karate dojo for the first time in January 1974, his mind was slowly opened to the possibilities of another way of life, a life where problems were solved by fighting the belligerence that smoldered within him at the time. He never stopped fighting: he just turned his aggression inward, away from the focus on others, and aimed it squarely at his own character. Today that fight continues. Michael has been practicing karate for more than two-thirds of his life and has traveled the world to do so.

As well as the years of physical training and research into the art of karate, his articles and interviews have been published over the past twenty-five years in magazines from New Zealand to England and America to Japan. As well, he has had four books published, including his previous multi-award winning book, *The Art of Hojo Undo: Power Training for Traditional Karate*. Often confrontational, Michael's writing attracts both support and disapproval in large measure. Nevertheless, he is one of the few internationally recognized karateka writing today who is able to point the way to a more meaningful future by observing lessons learned in the past.

Michael lives quietly in Northern Tasmania with his wife, Kathy. He trains in karate and kobudo by himself each morning in the small dojo standing discreetly at the rear of his home and teaches only those few students who are willing to make the necessary commitment. He continues to visit Okinawa regularly to practice karate with his sempai (seniors) and friends at the Jundokan dojo and to immerse himself ever deeper into kobudo, the ancient weapon arts of Ryukyu.

Also by Michael Clarke . . .

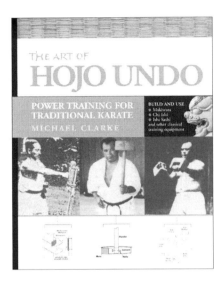

The Art of Hojo Undo

Power Training for Traditional Karate

By Michael Clarke, Kyoshi 7th dan

Adding Power to the Fighting Techniques of Karate

Hojo Undo means 'supplementary training', and using these tools is the key for developing the devastating power of Karate techniques. Without Hojo Undo training, a practitioner cannot reach the profound strength levels required for a lifetime of Karate training.

This book details how to construct and use many training tools, provides accurate mechanical drawings, comprehensive training methods, and an historical context to understand why Hojo Undo was created in 'old' Okinawa.

- Warm-up exercises
- Detailed construction drawings
- Build your own Hojo Undo tools!
- Learn how to use the tools to develop devastating power
- Link your increased power to fighting techniques
- Read what Okinawan Masters say about Hojo Undo training

"With the absence of any work on hojo undo, this book is destined to become an instant success and I am pleased to be able to lend my name to its publication. Mike Clarke's empirical experience and deep knowledge of both Okinawa's fighting arts and the culture in which it evolved make him uniquely qualified to produce a book of this nature." – Patrick McCarthy, Hanshi 8th dan, from his Foreword

222 pages • 360 photos and illustrations
Code: B1361 • ISBN: 978-1-59439-136-1

SKILL LEVEL
Ⓘ Ⓘ Ⓘ

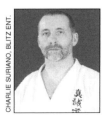

CHARLIE SURIANO, BLITZ ENT.

Michael Clarke, Kyoshi 7th dan, Okinawan Goju-ryu, has trained in Karate since 1974. He has written over three hundred articles for international martial arts magazines and authored five books. A young 'street fighter' in England who became a disciplined student of budo in Okinawa, Clarke enthusiastically teaches traditional Goju-ryu Karate in his dojo near Launceston, Tasmania, Australia.

BOOKS FROM YMAA

6 HEALING MOVEMENTS
101 REFLECTIONS ON TAI CHI CHUAN
108 INSIGHTS INTO TAI CHI CHUAN
ADVANCING IN TAE KWON DO
ANALYSIS OF SHAOLIN CHIN NA 2ND ED
ANCIENT CHINESE WEAPONS
THE ART AND SCIENCE OF STAFF FIGHTING
ART OF HOJO UNDO
ARTHRITIS RELIEF, 3RD ED.
BACK PAIN RELIEF, 2ND ED.
BAGUAZHANG, 2ND ED.
CARDIO KICKBOXING ELITE
CHIN NA IN GROUND FIGHTING
CHINESE FAST WRESTLING
CHINESE FITNESS
CHINESE TUI NA MASSAGE
CHOJUN
COMPREHENSIVE APPLICATIONS OF SHAOLIN
    CHIN NA
CONFLICT COMMUNICATION
CROCODILE AND THE CRANE: A NOVEL
CUTTING SEASON: A XENON PEARL MARTIAL ARTS THRILLER
DEFENSIVE TACTICS
DESHI: A CONNOR BURKE MARTIAL ARTS THRILLER
DIRTY GROUND
DR. WU'S HEAD MASSAGE
DUKKHA HUNGRY GHOSTS
DUKKHA REVERB
DUKKHA, THE SUFFERING: AN EYE FOR AN EYE
DUKKHA UNLOADED
ENZAN: THE FAR MOUNTAIN, A CONNOR BURKE MARTIAL ARTS
    THRILLER
ESSENCE OF SHAOLIN WHITE CRANE
EXPLORING TAI CHI
FACING VIOLENCE
FIGHT BACK
FIGHT LIKE A PHYSICIST
THE FIGHTER'S BODY
FIGHTER'S FACT BOOK
FIGHTER'S FACT BOOK 2
FIGHTING THE PAIN RESISTANT ATTACKER
FIRST DEFENSE
FORCE DECISIONS: A CITIZENS GUIDE
FOX BORROWS THE TIGER'S AWE
INSIDE TAI CHI
KAGE: THE SHADOW, A CONNOR BURKE MARTIAL ARTS
    THRILLER
KATA AND THE TRANSMISSION OF KNOWLEDGE
KRAV MAGA PROFESSIONAL TACTICS
KRAV MAGA WEAPON DEFENSES
LITTLE BLACK BOOK OF VIOLENCE
LIUHEBAFA FIVE CHARACTER SECRETS
MARTIAL ARTS ATHLETE
MARTIAL ARTS INSTRUCTION
MARTIAL WAY AND ITS VIRTUES
MASK OF THE KING
MEDITATIONS ON VIOLENCE
MERIDIAN QIGONG
MIND/BODY FITNESS
THE MIND INSIDE TAI CHI
THE MIND INSIDE YANG STYLE TAI CHI CHUAN
MUGAI RYU
NATURAL HEALING WITH QIGONG
NORTHERN SHAOLIN SWORD, 2ND ED.
OKINAWA'S COMPLETE KARATE SYSTEM: ISSHIN RYU
POWER BODY

PRINCIPLES OF TRADITIONAL CHINESE MEDICINE
QIGONG FOR HEALTH & MARTIAL ARTS 2ND ED.
QIGONG FOR LIVING
QIGONG FOR TREATING COMMON AILMENTS
QIGONG MASSAGE
QIGONG MEDITATION: EMBRYONIC BREATHING
QIGONG MEDITATION: SMALL CIRCULATION
QIGONG, THE SECRET OF YOUTH: DA MO'S CLASSICS
QUIET TEACHER: A XENON PEARL MARTIAL ARTS THRILLER
RAVEN'S WARRIOR
REDEMPTION
ROOT OF CHINESE QIGONG, 2ND ED.
SCALING FORCE
SENSEI: A CONNOR BURKE MARTIAL ARTS THRILLER
SHIHAN TE: THE BUNKAI OF KATA
SHIN GI TAI: KARATE TRAINING FOR BODY, MIND, AND SPIRIT
SIMPLE CHINESE MEDICINE
SIMPLE QIGONG EXERCISES FOR HEALTH, 3RD ED.
SIMPLIFIED TAI CHI CHUAN, 2ND ED.
SIMPLIFIED TAI CHI FOR BEGINNERS
SOLO TRAINING
SOLO TRAINING 2
SUDDEN DAWN: THE EPIC JOURNEY OF BODHIDHARMA
SUMO FOR MIXED MARTIAL ARTS
SUNRISE TAI CHI
SUNSET TAI CHI
SURVIVING ARMED ASSAULTS
TAE KWON DO: THE KOREAN MARTIAL ART
TAEKWONDO BLACK BELT POOMSAE
TAEKWONDO: A PATH TO EXCELLENCE
TAEKWONDO: ANCIENT WISDOM FOR THE MODERN WARRIOR
TAEKWONDO: DEFENSES AGAINST WEAPONS
TAEKWONDO: SPIRIT AND PRACTICE
TAO OF BIOENERGETICS
TAI CHI BALL QIGONG: FOR HEALTH AND MARTIAL ARTS
TAI CHI BALL WORKOUT FOR BEGINNERS
TAI CHI BOOK
TAI CHI CHIN NA: THE SEIZING ART OF TAI CHI CHUAN, 2ND ED.
TAI CHI CHUAN CLASSICAL YANG STYLE, 2ND ED.
TAI CHI CHUAN MARTIAL APPLICATIONS
TAI CHI CHUAN MARTIAL POWER, 3RD ED.
TAI CHI CONNECTIONS
TAI CHI DYNAMICS
TAI CHI QIGONG, 3RD ED.
TAI CHI SECRETS OF THE ANCIENT MASTERS
TAI CHI SECRETS OF THE WU & LI STYLES
TAI CHI SECRETS OF THE WU STYLE
TAI CHI SECRETS OF THE YANG STYLE
TAI CHI SWORD: CLASSICAL YANG STYLE, 2ND ED.
TAI CHI SWORD FOR BEGINNERS
TAI CHI WALKING
TAIJIQUAN THEORY OF DR. YANG, JWING-MING
TENGU: THE MOUNTAIN GOBLIN, A CONNOR BURKE MARTIAL
    ARTS THRILLER
TIMING IN THE FIGHTING ARTS
TRADITIONAL CHINESE HEALTH SECRETS
TRADITIONAL TAEKWONDO
TRAINING FOR SUDDEN VIOLENCE
WAY OF KATA
WAY OF KENDO AND KENJITSU
WAY OF SANCHIN KATA
WAY TO BLACK BELT
WESTERN HERBS FOR MARTIAL ARTISTS
WILD GOOSE QIGONG
WOMAN'S QIGONG GUIDE
XINGYIQUAN

DVDS FROM YMAA

more products available from . . .
YMAA Publication Center, Inc. 楊氏東方文化出版中心
1-800-669-8892 • info@ymaa.com • www.ymaa.com